T0293667

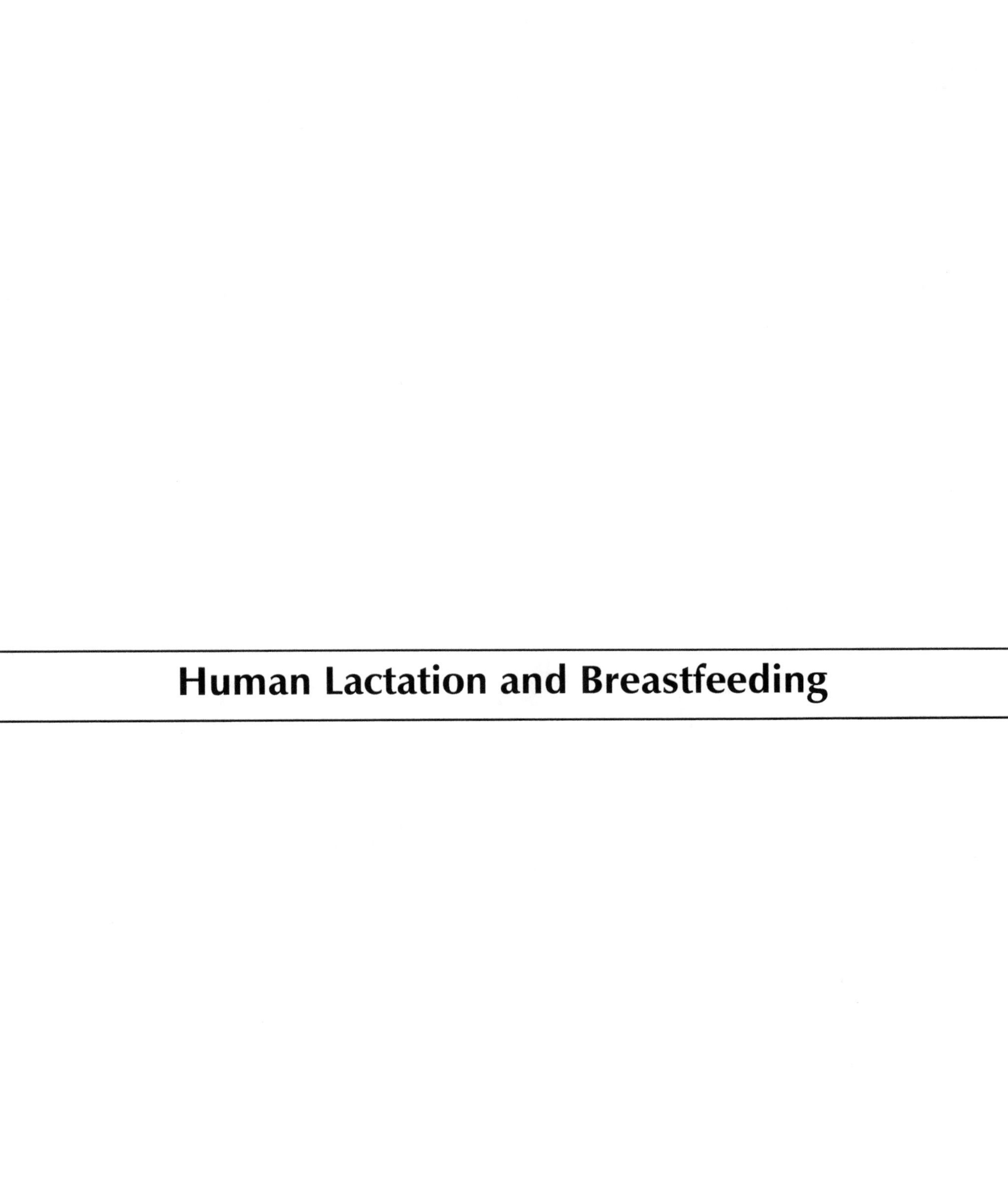

Human Lactation and Breastfeeding

Human Lactation and Breastfeeding

Editor: Emily Belcher

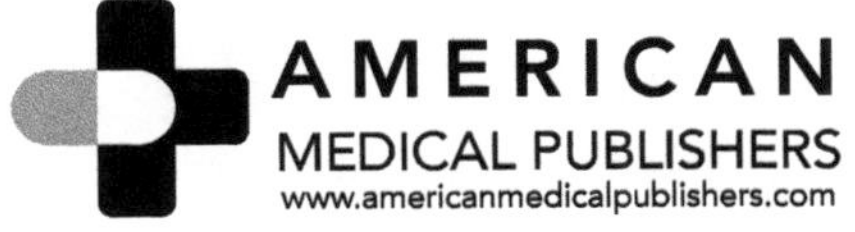

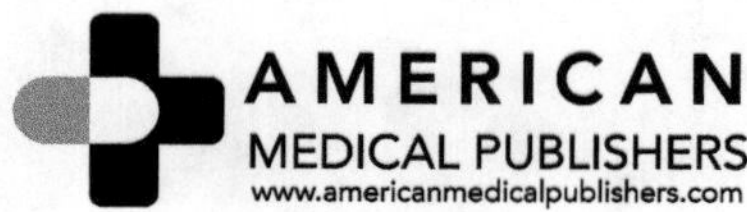

Cataloging-in-Publication Data

Human lactation and breastfeeding / edited by Emily Belcher.
p. cm.
Includes bibliographical references and index.
ISBN 978-1-63927-694-3
1. Breastfeeding. 2. Lactation. 3. Infants--Nutrition. 4. Lactation--Nutritional aspects.
5. Breastfeeding--Physiological aspects. I. Belcher, Emily.
RJ216 .H86 2023
649.33--dc23

American Medical Publishers,
41 Flatbush Avenue,
1st Floor, New York,
NY 11217, USA

ISBN 978-1-63927-694-3 (Hardback)

Contents

Preface

Every book is a source of knowledge and this one is no exception. The idea that led to the conceptualization of this book was the fact that the world is advancing rapidly; which makes it crucial to document the progress in every field. I am aware that a lot of data is already available, yet, there is a lot more to learn. Hence, I accepted the responsibility of editing this book and contributing my knowledge to the community.

Lactation is the secretion of milk from the mammary glands located in the breasts of sexually mature females. The mammary glands have various parts which work together in order to produce milk, which include alveoli, milk ducts, areola and nipple. Lactation is the biological response which takes place during and after pregnancy for feeding a newborn baby. The breastfeeding phase can continue till two or more years, and it has a significant role in the infant's development and lifelong health. Nutrition in the early life provides an opportunity for improving the health of an infant in the short and long term. This helps in the reduction of risk of various diseases, like sudden infant death syndrome (SIDS), respiratory tract infections, diarrhea and ear infections. Furthermore, breastfeeding can help in decreasing the risk of diabetes, food allergies, and asthma. This book provides comprehensive insights on lactation and breastfeeding. It is a resource guide for experts as well as students.

While editing this book, I had multiple visions for it. Then I finally narrowed down to make every chapter a sole standing text explaining a particular topic, so that they can be used independently. However, the umbrella subject sinews them into a common theme. This makes the book a unique platform of knowledge.

I would like to give the major credit of this book to the experts from every corner of the world, who took the time to share their expertise with us. Also, I owe the completion of this book to the never-ending support of my family, who supported me throughout the project.

Editor

1

Comprehensive Preterm Breast Milk Metabotype Associated with Optimal Infant Early Growth Pattern

Marie-Cécile Alexandre-Gouabau [1,*], Thomas Moyon [1], Agnès David-Sochard [1], François Fenaille [2], Sophie Cholet [2], Anne-Lise Royer [3], Yann Guitton [3], Hélène Billard [1], Dominique Darmaun [1,4], Jean-Christophe Rozé [1,4] and Clair-Yves Boquien [1,5]

1 INRA, UMR1280, Physiopathologie des Adaptations Nutritionnelles, Institut des maladies de l'appareil digestif (IMAD), Centre de Recherche en Nutrition Humaine Ouest (CRNH), Nantes F-44093, France; Thomas.Moyon@univ-nantes.fr (T.M.); agnes.david@univ-nantes.fr (A.D.-S.); helene.billard@univ-nantes.fr (H.B.); dominique.darmaun@chu-nantes.fr (D.D.); jeanchristophe.roze@chu-nantes.fr (J.-C.R.); clair-yves.boquien@univ-nantes.fr (C.-Y.B.)

2 Service de Pharmacologie et d'Immunoanalyse, Laboratoire d'Etude du Métabolisme des Médicaments, CEA, INRA, Université Paris Saclay, MetaboHUB, F-91191 Gif-sur-Yvette, France; francois.fenaille@cea.fr (F.F.); sophie.cholet@cea.fr (S.C.)

3 LUNAM Université, ON;IRIS, Laboratoire d'Etude des Résidus et Contaminants dans les Aliments (LABERCA), USC INRA 1329, Nantes F-44307, France; anne-lise.royer@oniris-nantes.fr (A.-L.R.); yann.guitton@oniris-nantes.fr (Y.G.)

4 CHU, Centre Hospitalo-Universitaire Hôtel-Dieu, Nantes F-44093, France

5 EMBA, European Milk Bank Association, Milano I-20126, Italy

* Correspondence: Marie-Cecile.Alexandre-Gouabau@univ-nantes.fr

Abstract: Early nutrition impacts preterm infant early growth rate and brain development but can have long lasting effects as well. Although human milk is the gold standard for feeding new born full-term and preterm infants, little is known about the effects of its bioactive compounds on breastfed preterm infants' growth outcomes. This study aims to determine whether breast milk metabolome, glycome, lipidome, and free-amino acids profiles analyzed by liquid chromatography-mass spectrometry had any impact on the early growth pattern of preterm infants. The study population consisted of the top tercile-Z score change in their weight between birth and hospital discharge ("faster grow", $n = 11$) and lowest tercile ("slower grow", $n = 15$) from a cohort of 138 premature infants (27–34 weeks gestation). This holistic approach combined with stringent clustering or classification statistical methods aims to discriminate groups of milks phenotype and identify specific metabolites associated with early growth of preterm infants. Their predictive reliability as biomarkers of infant growth was assessed using multiple linear regression and taking into account confounding clinical factors. Breast-milk associated with fast growth contained more branched-chain and insulino-trophic amino acid, lacto-N-fucopentaose, choline, and hydroxybutyrate, pointing to the critical role of energy utilization, protein synthesis, oxidative status, and gut epithelial cell maturity in prematurity.

Keywords: breast milk metabolome; glycome; lipidome; free amino acid; preterm infant; growth trajectory

---

1. Introduction

A growing body of evidence supports the impacts on lifelong health of exposure to multiple factors in early life [1]. Therefore, studying the influence of intrauterine environments and perinatal exposure are keys to understanding early growth and development and health throughout life. Indeed, putative benefits of breastfeeding in new born full-term infants are, at least in part, due to its complex composition in various macronutrients, micronutrients, and other bioactive compounds [2–4]. Maternal breast milk is the recommended nutrition for feeding pre-mature infants [5], due to its reported health benefits such as (i) a significant decrease in the risk of developing prematurity-related morbidities [6,7], including necrotizing enterocolitis [8] and infection [8,9]; (ii) a significant decrease in the feeding intolerance [8,10]; and (iii) an improvement in neurodevelopmental outcomes [8,11]. However, feeding unfortified human milk may lead to insufficient or inadequate postnatal nutritional intake for many preterm infants in the first few weeks of extra-uterine life, particularly the very preterm infants born with a low birth weight and before 28 weeks gestation. Additionally, it is often associated with extra-uterine growth restriction [11,12], which could have severe adverse consequences in term of developmental delay [13–15]. Fortification of human milk is therefore recommended by the European Society for Paediatric Gastroenterology Hepatology and Nutrition (EPSGHAN) [16]. Yet, even among preterm infants receiving protein-fortified human milk, a large range of variation is observed in the early postnatal growth patterns [17].

The host of low-molecular-weight metabolites present in breast milk fully justifies the application of metabolomics/lipidomics, a promising holistic approach in neonatology used, by our [18–20] and other laboratories [21–23]. Metabolomics have been shown to generate new insights when investigating human milk [20,24–26] during the first month of lactation [27] or pre-term and full-term human milk metabolomes over a full lactation period [28]. We also reported, for the first time, the association of early growth trajectory with a specific lipidomic signature in the human milk of mothers delivering preterm infants over the first month of lactation [20]. Human milk oligosaccharides (HMO) are other unique components known to affect the gut microbiota and may contribute to the reduced incidence of necrotizing enterocolitis [28–30], improved brain development [31], and growth patterns observed in breastfed infants [32,33]. Additionally, amino acid [34] and fatty acid [35] metabolism by mammary gland were suggested to affect milk production and infant growth, leading to a metabolic imprinting, which may persist into adulthood. To the best of our knowledge, this is the first study to explore in depth the relationships between the metabolome, lipidome, and glycome of human milk, and the early preterm infant growth during hospital stays in neonatal intensive care units. To fill this gap, we tested the potential of the liquid chromatography-mass spectrometry-based phenotypic approach to investigate the composition of human breast milk from mothers delivering a preterm newborn during the early course of lactation. More in detail, the current study aims at shedding light on the relationships between breast milk composition, characterized using targeted free amino acid pattern and non-targeted metabolomic, lipidomics and glycomic signatures, and the early growth of preterm infants nourished by their own mother's milk. As in our earlier reported pilot study [20], the present work was conducted within a larger prospective-monocentric-observational early birth LACTACOL cohort in which we selected two groups of preterm infants presenting very different growth trajectories during hospital stays. We previously reported in details [20] the breast milk lipidome in link with both infant growth groups, during the first month of lactation. The aims of the present work therefore are three-fold: (i) to assess metabolome, glycome and free amino acids pattern in the breast milk provided to preterms infants from week two to week four of lactation; (ii) to evaluate, initially and in week three-expressed breast milk samples, the interactions between human breast milk metabolome, lipidome and glycome and their association with the weight gain of infants between birth and time of discharge; and (iii) to identify a set of breast milk biomarkers with predictive ability on the postnatal weight growth trajectory of the preterm infants, taking into account confounding clinical factors. We hypothesized that our holistic approach, incorporating data from multiple breast milk compartments (i.e., metabolome, glycome, lipidome, and free amino acids), would considerably enhance our understanding of the molecular mechanisms linking breast milk composition to optimal early-growth of preterm infants.

2. Materials and Methods

2.1. Study Design and Population

The present pilot study was conducted within a larger prospective study of the previously published LACTACOL birth cohort of preterm infant mother dyads [20], whose primary objective was to explore the impact of breast milk protein content received by preterm infants during hospital stays, on neurodevelopmental outcomes at 2 years of age. A total of 118 mothers and 138 infants born between 27–34 weeks of gestational age with no severe congenital pathology and no major diseases, except prematurity and who received, for a minimum of 28 days, their own mother's breast milk only, were finally enrolled in the LACTACOL cohort (Figure 1). The current data were obtained on both sub-groups of infants selected among infants enrolled in the LACTACOL cohort and in the ancillary study, whose aim was to assess the relationship between breast milk composition (metabolome, lipidome, glycome, and amino acids) and preterm infant's growth pattern during the first month of life. These 26 selected infants presented no severe neonatal morbidity or necrotizing enterocolitis or retinopathy of prematurity.

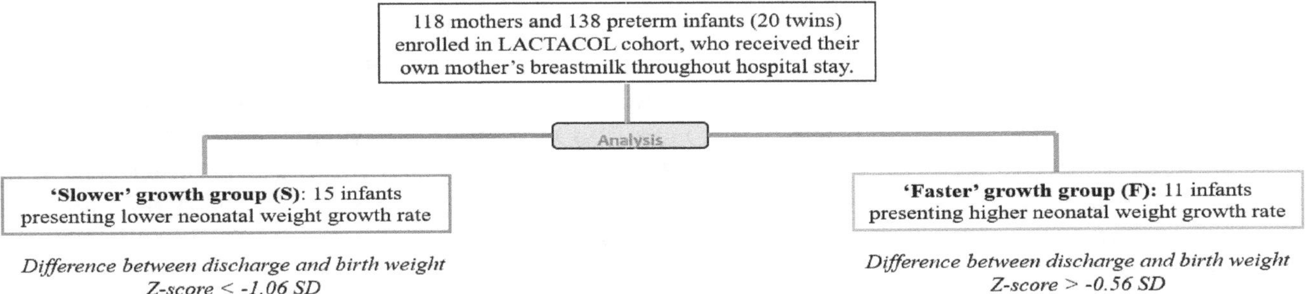

Figure 1. Study flowchart of infants enrolled in the ancillary study of the mono-centric prospective population-based LACTACOL (for global study flowchart of LACTACOL, see [20]). Among the 138 infants included in the LACTACOL cohort, no infant presented necrotizing enterocolitis (NEC), 4 infants had retinopathy of prematurity (ROP) of light severity, 3 presented intraventricular hemorrhage (IVH) of grade 2, 8 displayed bronchopulmonary dysplasia (BPD) at 28 days and 6 at 36 weeks' postmenstrual age. The 26 selected infants did not have NEC, ROP, or BPD.

Clinical characteristics were collected both on mothers and infants, including: maternal age, educational level, pre-gravid body mass index (BMI), adverse events during pregnancy and delivery, infants' gestational ages, birth weight, and head circumference, growth trajectory through hospital discharge, and events during hospital stays in neonatology. According to the EPSGHAN recommendations [16], preterm infants received parenteral nutrition and minimal enteral feeding with expressed breast milk predominantly provided by their own mother and fortified using Eoprotine® (Milupa, 1564 Domdidier, Suisse) and FortiPré® (Guigoz, 77186 Noisiel, France) for protein and carbohydrate intakes, and Liquigen® (Nutricia, 93406 Saint-Ouen, France) for lipid intakes, as previously detailed [20].

2.2. Ranking Infants according to Early Growth Trajectory

Infants enrolled in the LACTACOL cohort were ranked according to their change in weight Z-score (expressed in units of Standard Deviation (SD) and calculated as previously described [20] between birth and hospital discharge). For the first time, we chose to limit our longitudinal analysis of human breast milk composition to a small number of preterm mother infant dyads with no formal sample size calculation due to the exploratory nature of this pilot study. Then, the present study population consisted of the top tercile-Z score change in their weight between birth and hospital discharge ("faster grow", n = 11 infants) and lowest tercile ("slower grow", n = 15 infants), from our population of 138 enrolled preterm babies (born before 32 weeks gestation) (Figure 1).

2.3. Ethics

This research study was approved by the National Data Protection Authority (Commission Nationale de l'Informatique et des Libertés, N° 8911009) and the appropriate ethics Committee for the Protection of People Participating in Biomedical Research (CPP-Ouest I, reference CPP RCB-2011-AOO292-39). The current data were obtained in the ancillary study number three of the LACTACOL cohort registered at www:clinicaltrials.gov under #NCT01493063. The milk biobank was approved by the Committee for the Protection of Persons in medical research (CPP CB-2010-03). Parents received oral and written information in the maternity ward or neonatal unit and lactation support and training on proper sample collection from the study lactation consultant. A written consent was obtained from all parents at enrolment.

2.4. Human Milk Collection and Targeted Free Amino Acid (FAA) Analysis

Weekly representative 24-h breast milk expression was performed manually by mothers at home during all the lactation periods corresponding to their infant hospital stay, then processed, aliquoted, and frozen at −80 °C until analysis, as previously described [20]. FAA concentrations were determined in expressed breast milk samples collected from week two to week four of lactation using Ultra Performance Liquid Chromatography-High-Resolution-Mass Spectrometry (UPLC-HR-MS), as previously described [36]. Briefly, following a delipidation step by centrifugation and a deproteinization step by addition of sulfosalicylic acid and centrifugation, free amino acids (FAA) from supernatant were derivatized using AccQ®TagTM Ultra reagent (Waters Corporation, Milford, MA, USA)), separated on an Acquity H-Class® UPLC system (Waters Corporation, Milford, MA, USA), combined with a Xevo TQD® mass spectrometer (Waters Corporation, Milford, MA, USA), then identified and quantified, using the Waters TargetLinks™ software (Waters Corporation, Milford, MA, USA).

2.5. Breast Milk Liquid Chromatography-High-Resolution-Mass Spectrometry (LC-HRMS)–Based Glycomic Profiling

The extraction and reduction of oligosaccharides in human milk collected from week two to week four of lactation were performed as previously described [37]. Briefly, 10 μL of human milk were diluted by adding 450 μL of water and then delipidated by centrifugation. The lower phase was reduced with an NaBH4 solution and loaded onto a porous graphitized PGC cartridge (Hyperseb Hypercarb®, Thermo Scientific, San Jose, CA, USA). Milk reduced oligosaccharides were separated on a Hypercarb® column (2.1 mm i.d. × 100 mm, 3 μm particle size, Thermo Scientific, San Jose, CA, USA) on an Ultimate 3000 HPLC system (Thermo Scientific, San Jose, CA, USA). HMO chromatographic separation was performed at 30 °C with a flow rate of 300 μL/min using the gradient conditions with mobile phases A (water containing 0.1% formic acid) and B (acetonitrile containing 0.1% formic acid), as described by Oursel et al. [37]. Column effluent was directly introduced into the electrospray source of a hybrid quadruple time-of-flight (Q-TOF Impact HD) instrument (Bruker Daltonics, Bremen, Germany) operating in the positive ion mode. The source parameters were the following: 3700 V for the capillary voltage, 8.0 L/min for the dry gas, and 200 °C for the dry heater.

2.6. Breast Milk Liquid Chromatography-High-Resolution-Mass Spectrometry (LC-HRMS)–Based Lipidomic and Metabolomic Profiling

The organic and aqueous layers, following Bligh-Dyer extraction [38] of the same milk samples, were collected from week two to week four of lactation, dried separately, and subsequently reconstituted in acetonitrile-isopropanol-water (ACN: IPA: H_2O 65:30:5, $v/v/v$) and in water-acetonitrile (H_2O: ACN 95:5, v/v) for lipid and polar species, respectively. Then, lipidomic and metabolomic profilings were performed using separation on a 1200 infinity series® HPLC-system (Agilent Technologies, Santa Clara, CA, USA) coupled to an Exactive Orbitrap® MS (Thermo Fisher Scientific, Bremen, Germany) equipped with a heated electrospray (H-ESI II) source (operating in polarity switch mode), as previously described [20]. Concerning lipidomic profiling, a reverse phase

CSH® C_{18} (100 × 2.1 mm^2 i.d., 1.7 μm particle size) column (Waters Corporation, Milford, MA, USA) was used for lipid species separation using ACN:H_2O (60:40) and IPA:ACN:H_2O (88:10:2) as solvent A and B, respectively, with both containing 10 mM ammonium acetate and 0.1% acetic acid [39]. Concerning metabolomics fingerprinting, polar species separation was performed on the same LC-HRMS system on a reverse phase with a Hypersil GOLD C18 column (1.9 μm particle size, 100 × 2.1 mm) using a mobile phase of water (95%) and acetonitrile (5%), each containing 0.1% acetic acid according to Courant et al. [40]. The precision associated with sample preparation and LC-HRMS measurement was determined on the basis of a quality control (QC) consisting of a pool of 10 mothers' milk provided by the milk bank of Nantes Hospital Center.

2.7. Lipidomic, Metabolomic and Glycomic Data Treatment and Metabolites Annotation

Lipidomics and metabolomics raw data files were preprocessed and converted to the *.mzXML open file format using Xcalibur 2.2® (Thermo Fisher Scientific, San Jose, CA, USA) and MSConvert® (http://proteowizard.sourceforge.net/), respectively [41]. Then, lipidomics and metabolomics data were extracted using (i) pre-processing with the open-source XCMS® [42] within Workflow4Metabolomics® (W4M) (http://workflow4metabolomics.org) [43] for nonlinear retention time alignment and automatic integration for each detected features combined with CAMERA® [44] for annotation of isotopes and adducts, and (ii) normalization of intra- and inter-batch effects using Quality Control (QC) samples [45]. A manual curation, for the quality of integration and a filtration of the resulting XCMS (m/z; Retention Time (RT)) features by a 30% relative SD cutoff within the repeated pooled QC injections [46] were performed. Thereafter, accurate mass measurement of each putative metabolite was submitted to LIPID Metabolites and Pathways Strategy (LipidMaps®, www.lipidmaps.org), Human Metabolite Data base (HMDB®, www.hmdb.ca), Biofluid Metabolites Database (MetLin®, metlin.scripps.edu), and Milk Metabolome Database (MCDB®, www.mcdb.ca) annotation. Moreover, the lipids and metabolites of interest were identified with the use of the (pseudo) tandem mass spectrometry spectrum generated by all ion fragmentation [39] combined with the use of in-house reference databanks [47]. Metabolite's identification level was level one, for metabolites definitively annotated with our home data base (i.e., based upon characteristic physicochemical properties of a chemical reference standard (m/z, RT) and their M/MS spectra compared to those of breastmilk QC) or level two, for metabolites putatively annotated (i.e., without chemical reference standards, based upon physicochemical properties and MS/MS spectral similarity with public/commercial spectral libraries, e.g., LipidMaps®, MetLin®, and MCDB®). Monosaccharide compositions of HMOs were deduced from accurately measured masses (<5 ppm on average) and previously determined retention times were obtained through the use of some commercial HMO molecules [37]. Complementary MS/MS experiments were then performed to confirm putative structures. When it was not possible to clearly determine HMO structures, HMOs were named according to their monosaccharide compositions and denoted as hexose (Hex), N-acetylhexosamine (HexNAc), fucose (Fuc), and N-acetylneuraminic acid (NeuAc) numbers. In addition, isomeric forms were distinguished by a lower-case letter added after the monosaccharide composition (e.g., 4230a and 4230b). Overall, 89 (45 monosaccharide compositions) distinct HMOs were detected. Relative HMO abundances were calculated by dividing absolute HMO peak area by each sample's total HMO peak areas.

2.8. Statistical Analyses

In Tables 1–4, values were reported as medians and 25% and 75% percentiles. Statistical analyses were carried out using GraphPad Prism® software version 6.00 (La Joya, CA, USA), SIMCA P® version 14 (Umetrics AB, Sweden) and R version 3.4. (R Development Core Team, 2013; http://www.R-project.org). For all data analyses, the significance level (α) was set to 5%. Multivariate statistical models were applied separately on each glycomic, lipidomic, metabolomics, fatty acids and free amino acids data matrix considering the *a priori* structure into "faster" vs. "slower" infants' growth groups. We chose to take into account the higher (compared to glycomic data) variability in magnitude for lipidomic and metabolomic features; this is the reason why a Log Pareto scaling [48] was performed. Lipidomic or metabolomic data were submitted to the statistical workflow previously used with success on lipidomic profiling [20] in order to: (i) select the lipid/metabolic species providing a clear separation between the two infant postnatal growth subgroups from week two to week four of lactation, using the Analysis of Variance-PLS (AoV-PLS) combined with a Fisher's Linear Discriminant Analysis (LDA) procedure [49]; (ii) check the selected biomarkers predictive ability for infant weight growth, using Mann-Whitney *U*-test combined with multiple testing filtering (FDR); and (iii) confront them to the various confound clinical variables (mother's body mass index, birth weight, gestational age, complementary parenteral and enteral nutrition with the protein, lipid and energy intakes, duration of parenteral feeding and ventilation, and length of hospital-stay) and, in turn, test their reliability as biomarkers of infant's growth, by using multiple linear regression (MLR) combined to FDR on the remaining variables candidates as biomarkers, i.e., 80, 60, or 35 models for metabolomic, lipidomic or glycomic data, respectively. Moreover, we hypothesized that high-level data fusion, resulting in a meaningful synthesis, was expected to provide a holistic picture of the preterm breast milk composition. In order to integrate multiple–omics analytical sources and chemometrics for a comprehensive metabolic profiling of human preterm milk associated with an optimal infant weight growth, we used clustering or classification methods aiming at discriminating groups of milks using "omics" data. In order to simplify the model, we discarded the time lactation point factor of the present study and focused on "omics" data provided at week three of lactation, which had previously been shown to display the higher discriminating effect on preterm breast milk lipidome [20]. Additionally, as including an excessive amount of irrelevant variables would deteriorate the models, and in order to ovoid overfitting, all variables provided by AoV-PLS-DA scores with variables of importance in the projection (VIP)-index below 1.5 were removed in both metabolomic and lipidomic data and only the annotated representative metabolites and lipid species were kept. The input resulting metabolomic and lipidomic Log Pareto-scaled blocks were concatenated with mean and deviation standard-scaled blocks (i.e., glycomic profiling, fatty acid, and free amino acid patterns). Then, we tested on the super-matrix thus obtained an unsupervised unfold principal components analysis (UPCA-clustering method) [50] and supervised multi-block partial least squares analysis (MB-PLS- classification method) [51] strategies that searched for directions of similar sample distributions in the multidimensional spaces defined by each block of "omics" data, i.e., common components. Variables of interest for the discrimination of milk metabotype were selected according to their coordinates on the common components axes in the MB-PLS model.

3. Results

3.1. *Subject Characteristics*

The median difference between discharge and birth weight *Z*-score was −0.479 SD and −1.538 SD, for infants with "faster growth" and "slower growth", respectively. Two sets of twins belonged to the "slower" growth group, and two others sets of twins followed opposite trajectories regarding their weight *Z*-score difference between birth and hospital discharge, i.e., one twin belonged to the "faster" growth group, whereas the other twin belonged to the "slower" growth group. Table 1 displays the median maternal and infants' characteristics. Despite similar gestational age and hospital stay-lengths, the group of infants with 'faster' growth presented a 25% lower birth weight and a 69% greater gain in weight *Z*-score compared to the group of infants with "slower" growth. This negative correlation between birth weight and weight *Z*-score at time of discharge was previously reported in the large LIFT cohort of 2277 preterm infants by our team [52] and in another cohort [53].

Table 1. Maternal and preterm infants' characteristics.

Characteristics	"Faster" Growth Rate	"Slower" Growth Rate	p-Value
Maternal characteristics	11	11	
Age (years)	29.00 ± 4.52 (25.00; 35.00)	30.00 ± 4.12 (26.00; 33.00)	0.908
BMI before gestation (kg/m^2)	22.32 ± 5.26 (19.14; 28.91)	24.00 ± 5.11 (20.83; 30.80)	0.789
Infants characteristics at birth	11 (7 males and 4 females)	15 (10 males and 5 females)	
Neonatal Morbidity (number of events) *	0	0	
Gestational age (weeks)	31.00 ± 1.37 (30.0; 32.00)	30.00 ± 1.68 (29.00; 32.00)	0.288
Length of hospital stay (days)	51.50 ± 3.16 (37.25; 56.25)	49.50 ± 4.21 (36.75; 54.75)	0.849
Birth weight (kg)	1.200 ± 0.293 (1.020; 1.445)	1.605 ± 0.211 (1.465; 1.705)	**0.005**
Birth weight Z-score (SD)	−1.592 ± 0.958 (−2.079; −0.571)	0.564 ± 0.718 (−0.290; 0.842)	**0.000**
BMI at birth (kg/m^2)	7.694 ± 1.573 (7.139; 9.884)	9.455 ± 0.857 (8.843; 9.900)	0.161
Discharge weight (kg)	2.340 ± 0.320 (2.029; 2.520)	2.565 ± 0.270 (2.355; 2.720)	**0.041**
Discharge weight Z-score (SD)	−1.878 ± 0.857 (−2.264; −1.127)	−1.142 ± 0.682 (−1.552; −0.953)	0.146
BMI at Discharge (kg/m^2)	11.98 ± 0.485 (11.66; 12.28)	12.67 ± 0.955 (11.78; 13.36)	**0.047**
Difference between discharge and birth weight Z-score (SD)	−0.479 ± 0.189 (−0.668; −0.294)	−1.538 ± 0.417 (−1.953; −1.230)	**<0.001**

*: The development of comorbidities was clearly described in the same pilot study [20]. Values are medians and 25% and 75% percentiles. p values for comparison between "faster" and "slower" growth groups were derived using Mann-Whitney U test. Parameters in bold presented a significant p-value < 0.05.

Initially, time course breast milk compositional changes were detected, during the first month of lactation in our two sub-groups of 11 mothers delivering preterm newborns, who presented very different growth trajectories during their hospital stays using (i) targeted free amino-acids quantification combined with (ii) metabolomic (and lipidomic) and (iii) glycomic signatures. Then, multi- and univariate statistical models were applied to identify significant changes in metabolites that are associated with early postnatal infant growth. For second time, we focused (iv) our "omics" data fusion models on one representative time of lactation (week 3) to identify similar expression changes in various molecules and, in turn, highlight a few biological pathways of interest associated with optimal preterm infant growth.

3.2. Targeted Free Amino Acid Quantification

In the present pilot study, breast milk provided to the "faster" growth group presented a slightly higher essential amino acid content combined with a significantly higher content of branched-chain, insulinotrophic and gluconeogenic amino acids, as well as a decrease in sulfur amino acid content (with only taurine and methionine quantified). More specifically, breast milk arginine and tyrosine concentrations were significantly higher in the "faster" growth group than that in the "slower" growth group, whereas glycine and taurine levels were lower in the "faster" growth group with a trend toward lower glutamate and glutamine concentrations. Considering the predictive ability of free amino acid for infant weight growth during hospital stay, branched-chain and insulinotrophic amino acids were significant using multiple linear regression combined with multiple correction and taking into account maternal and infant clinical variables, whereas sulfur amino acids (taurine and methionine) presented only a trend (Table 2).

Table 2. Concentration levels of free amino acids in breast milk provided to preterm infants with "faster" or "slower" growth during the W2 to W4 lactation period.

Free Amino Acids (µM)	W2 to W4 Median (25% and 75% Percentile)		Mann-Whitney p-Value from W2 to W4	FDR Corrected MW q-Value from W2 to W4	MLR p-Value From W2 to W4	FDR Corrected MLR q-Value from W2 to W4
	"Slower" Growth (n = 38)	"Faster" Growth (n = 29)				
EAA	234.4 (216.9–278.5)	277.1 (221.4–343.5)	0.0675 ^{t}	0.18	0.06 #	0.08 #
Arginine	11.02 (7.56–21.84)	18.34 (11.45–28.13)	0.0079 **	0.05 *	0.10 #	0.08 #
Isoleucine	10.12 (7.56–14.51)	10.70 (8.12–18.01)	0.2224	0.29	0.08 #	0.44
Leucine	30.23 (19.93–35.46)	32.25 (24.00–39.02)	0.2407	0.29	0.05 #	0.40
Proline	30.21 (26.56–37.13)	30.32 (26.16–38.80)	0.9425	0.49	0.85	0.83
Methionine	5.29 (3.11–8.35)	6.27 (3.88–8.90)	0.6038	0.43	0.44	0.74
Phenylalanine	12.43 (8.81–15.47)	12.42 (7.25–16.43)	0.9277	0.48	0.48	0.77
Threonine	86.71 (74.34–115.7)	78.62 (66.76–107.5)	0.3197	0.31	0.39	0.71
Tryptophan	2.48 (1.89–4.23)	2.73 (1.97–4.22)	0.7676	0.45	0.59	0.21
Valine	51.13 (38.90–55.06)	52.09 (37.75–56.30)	0.8034	0.45	0.41	0.71
NEAA	2610 (2146–3280)	2512 (1753–3182)	0.2592	0.32	0.78	0.25
Alanine	206.7 (186.9–332.4)	201.0 (166.5–254.3)	0.5466	0.43	0.78	0.83
Aspartic acid & asparagine	66.93 (39.53–90.83)	57.39 (29.92–80.49)	0.3382	0.31	0.86	0.83
Glutamine	455.9 (211.4–902.3)	375.0 (134.4–572.0)	0.0838 ^{t}	0.17	0.14	0.52
Glutamic acid	1319 (898.5–1449)	1220 (906.3–1480)	0.6567	0.43	0.27	0.62
Glx	1838 (1381–2259)	1754 (1177–2098)	0.0613 ^{t}	0.14	0.52	0.21
Glycine	89.25 (68.99–105.2)	69.60 (54.38–103.09)	0.0126 *	0.05 *	0.18	0.56
Serine	86.01 (68.78–116.2)	86.01 (63.81–112.3)	0.8034	0.46	0.23	0.59
Tyrosine	11.64 (6.70–15.56)	14.49 (11.47–21.00)	0.0349 *	0.10	0.11	0.49
Taurine	313.9 (275.5–428.2)	270.0 (174.0–313.2)	0.0031 **	0.03 *	0.14	0.51
BCAA	85.15 (71.48–93.3)	101.1 (84.99–121.5)	0.0075 **	0.04 *	0.06 #	0.08 #
Insulino-trophic amino acid	182.0 (166.6–219.2)	224.9 (175.7–275.0)	0.0427 *	0.10 ^{t}	0.07 #	0.08 #
SAA	327.9 (297.0–430.7)	227.9 (168.6–355.1)	0.0019 **	0.03 *	0.13	0.09 #

Values are medians (25% and 75% percentiles) from amino acid concentrations from week 2 to week 4 of lactation period. EAA: essential amino acids; NEAA: non-essential amino acids; FAA: free amino acid; Glx: glutamine + glutamic acid; BCAA: branched chain amino-acids (valine + leucine + isoleucine); Insulinotrophic and glycemic amino acids = valine + leucine + isoleucine + threonine + arginine. Sulfur amino acids (SAA): taurine and methionine. Variables were considered as significantly modified between the two groups of infants' growth (Mann-Whitney U test) when their multiple comparisons adjusted P-values (i.e., False Discovery Rate (FDR) corrected-MW q-value) was < 0.05. *: MW p-value or FDR-corrected MW q-value < 0.05; **: MW p-value or FDR-corrected MW q-value < 0.01; t: MW p-value or FDR-corrected MW q-value < 0.1. Multiple linear regression (MLR) for infant weight Z-score (p-value) was also combined to FDR and predictive ability for infant weight growth was considered reliable when MLR q-value was < 0.1 (#).

3.3. *Lipidomics and Metabolomcs Profiling*

Lipidomic analysis of the human breast milk provided (from week two to week four of lactation) to the 26 infants selected in the present pilot study was previously reported [20]. The most discriminant features associated with infant growth during hospital stays corresponded to a cluster of 1256 VIP-based lipid species. Among the 50 AoV-PLS/LDA- and FDR-selected annotated lipid biomarkers, nine lipid species appeared of paramount interest due to their significant (10% threshold) MLR q-value for delta weight Z-score (data from Table 4, [20]). Similarly, metabolomic LC-HRMS (ESI^+/ESI^-) data obtained on preterm breast milk from week two to week four of lactation, were processed using AoV-PLS procedure [49] to assess the association between the metabolites and the *a priori* grouping structure ("faster" vs. "slower" infant growth). The score plots clearly highlighted the separation between breast milk metabotypes associated with 'faster' or 'slower' infant growth in both positive (Figure 2a) and negative (supplementary Figure S1) ionization modes with the breast milk metabolomic profiles, corresponding to the four sets of twins plotted between both clusters (depicted with blue symbols in Figure 2a and Figure S1a). Then, the selected appropriate components of AoV-PLS (for both ionization modes) were subjected to a Fisher's linear discriminant analysis (LDA) to test the significance of growth factor (Figure 2b and Figure S1b). Their cross-validation error rates of the LDA canonical variables for positive and negative mode were both equal to 7.14%. The most discriminant features associated with infant growth during hospital stay corresponded to a cluster of 125 (resp. 119) VIP-based metabolites species (VIP-index above 1.5) in the positive (resp. negative) ionization mode leading to 68 features that could be annotated (Table 3).

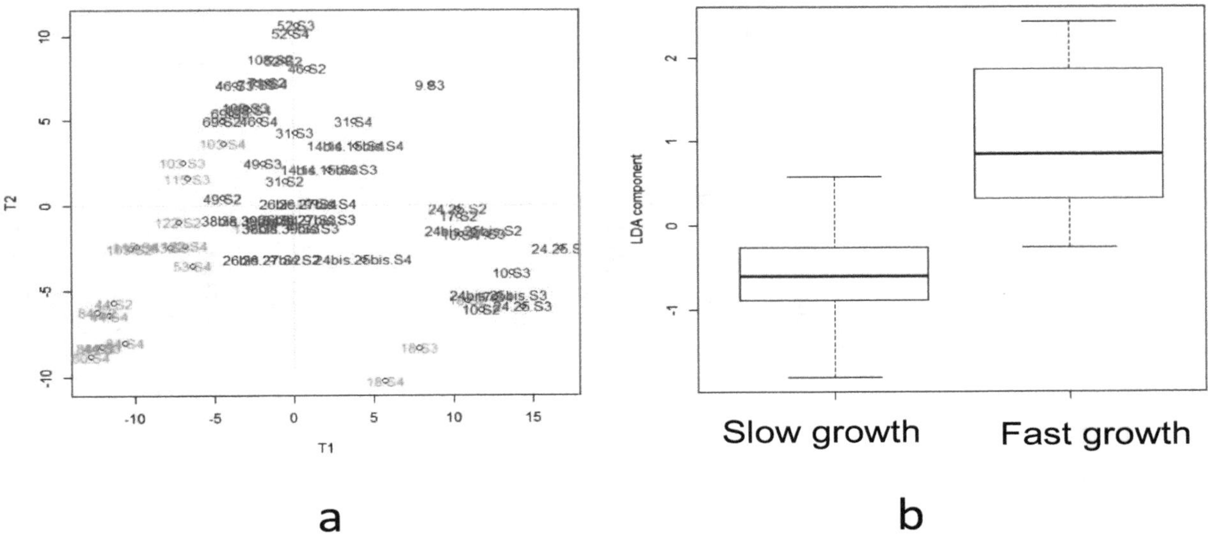

Figure 2. Analysis of Variance (AoV)-PLS and linear discriminant analysis (LDA) models based on the LC-ESI^+-HRMS metabolomics profiles of human preterm milk on the factor weight Z-score (discharge-birth): AoV-PLS score plot with 56% of variance (R2Y = 34%) on components 1–2 (**a**) and LDA (built on components of AoV-PLS) with a *p*-value = 0) (**b**). Breast milk provided to preterm infants who experienced "faster" (green) or "slower" (red) growth and to twin infants with discordant growth rate, one twin with high growth rate and the other one with low growth rate, (blue).

Table 3. Abundance (10^6) of annotated metabolites that discriminated metabotypes of breast milk provided to preterm infants with "faster" or "slower" growth during the W2 to W4 lactation period.

Metabolites (Annotation Level)	a, b, c	mz	Abundance of Metabolites (10^6)			
			Median (25% and 75% Percentile), W2 to W4			
			"Slower" Growth (n = 38)	"Faster" Growth (n = 29)	Mann-Whitney p-Value (FDR-Corrected MW q-Value in Exposant)	MLR p-Value (FDR-Corrected MLR q-Value in Exposant)
Amino acid						
Hippuric acid [1]	a	180.0654 $(M+H)^+$	1.36 (0.79–1.81)	1.36 (0.88–2.20)	0.86	0.33
2-hydroxyhippuric acid [2]	a, b, c	194.0459 $(M-H)^-$	0.07 (0.05–0.126)	0.08 (0.05–0.15)	0.25	0.04
Valine [1]	a	118.0865 $(M+H)^+$	2.81 (1.72–3.23)	2.67 (0.91–3.17)	0.79	0.17
Leucine [1]	a, c	130.0872 $(M-H)^-$	1.92 (1.45–2.87)	2.99 (1.61–4.66)	0.02 **	0.92
N-Carbamoylsarcosine [2]	a, c	133.0609 $(M+H)^+$	0.96 (0.66–1.45)	1.69 (1.18–2.38)	0.0003 **	0.96
Tryptophan metabolism						
Tryptophan [1]	a, c	205.0970 $(M+H)^+$	4.20 (3.59–4.77)	4.76 (3.51–7.95)	0.18	0.79
Kynurenine [1]	a, c	192.0653 $(M\text{-}NH3+H)^+$	0.97 (0.64–1.55)	0.72 (0.59–0.93)	*0.06* [t]	0.80
1H-Indole-3-carboxaldehyde [2]	a, b	146.0599 $(M+H)^+$	2.18 (1.55–2.81)	2.26 (1.66–3.63)	0.27	0.98
Indole-3-ethanol [2]	a	184.0732 $(M+Na)^+$	9.66 (6.11–13.01)	9.59 (6.62–12.06)	0.82	0.14
3-Methylindole [2]	a	132.0806 $(M+H)^+$	0.43 (0.35–0.55)	0.47 (0.39–0.63)	0.10	0.70
Tyrosine metabolism						
hydroxyphenylacetic acid [1]	a, c	151.0399 $(M-H)^-$	0.32 (0.25–0.37)	0.30 (0.21–0.37)	0.61	0.08
p-Cresol (4-methylphenol) [2]	a, b, c	107.0501 $(M-H)^-$	1.84 (1.16–2.85)	1.37 (0.09–2.21)	0.04 *	0.20
p-Cresol sulfate [2]	a	187.0070 $(M-H)^-$	5.28 (4.14–9.27)	4.89 (2.67–6.79)	0.13 [t]	0.17
Sulphur metabolism						
Cystathionine [2]	a	240.1015 $(M+NH_4)^+$	0.67 (0.51–0.80)	0.87 (0.66–1.35)	0.02 *	0.90
Methionin [1]	a, c	150.0580 $(M+H)^+$	1.82 (1.49–2.19)	1.81 (1.63–2.69)	0.36	0.89
Se-Adenosylselenohomocysteine [2]	a	228.0314 $(M+H+Na)^+$	0.22 (0.17–0.25)	0.19 (0.13–0.24)	0.15 [t]	*0.09*
S-Adenosylhomocysteine [2]	a	365.1048 $(M-H_2O\text{-}H)^+$	6.53 (5.02–7.63)	4.48 (3.92–6.84)	0.007 *	0.20
Hydrogen sulfite [2]	a, b, c	79.9573 $(M-H)^-$	0.52 (0.38–0.85)	0.44 (0.31–0.67)	*0.07* [t]	0.23
Thiocyanic acid [2]	a, c	150.0018 $(M-H)^-$	0.75 (0.64–0.83)	0.57 (0.51–0.76)	0.02 *	0.69
Aromatic compound						
Benzoic acid [1]	a	121.0294 $(M-H)^-$	3.14 (2.27–4.18)	2.49 (2.09–2.95)	0.01 *	0.16
Hydroxyphenyllactic acid [2]	a	241.0730 $(M+Hac\text{-}H)^-$	0.14 (0.11–0.16)	0.11 (0.08–0.18)	0.17	0.96
Pyridines and Derivatives/Nucleosides						
Niacinamide [1]	a	123.0554 $(M+H)^+$	6.45 (5.27–10.82)	11.00 (6.17–13.84)	0.029 *	0.16

Table 3. *Cont.*

Metabolites (Annotation Level)	a, b, c	mz	Abundance Des Ions (10^6)			
			Median (25% and 75% Percentile), W2 to W4			
			"Slower" Growth (n = 38)	"Faster" Growth (n = 29)	Mann-Whitney p-Value (FDR-Corrected MW q-Value in Exposant)	MLR p-Value (FDR-Corrected MLR q-Value in Exposant)
Energy metabolism						
Hydroxyhexanoylcarnitine [2]	a	276.1803 $(M + H)^+$	0.11 (0.04–0.22)	0.08 (0.05–0.21)	0.84	0.52
Oxoicosanoyl-CoA [2]	a, b	547.2129 $(M + H+ NH4)^+$	0.66 (0.53–0.89)	0.81 (0.63–1.20)	0.04 *	0.87
3-Hydroxypimelyl-CoA [2]	a	943.2103 $(M + NH4)^+$	1.77 (1.66–2.02)	1.79 (1.61–2.04)	0.98	0.91
Hexanoylglycine [2]	a, b	174.1123 $(M + H)^+$	0.20 (0.12–0.26)	0.13 (0.08–0.19)	0.02 *	0.15
Heptanoylglycine [2]	a	229.1544 $(M + H)^+$	0.64 (0.50–0.97)	0.65 (0.49–0.81)	0.58	0.69
Gamma-Butyrolactone/	a	85.0293 $(M - H)^-$	42.9 (25.08–58.13)	48.37 (34.67–65.61)	0.32	0.68
But-2-enoic/Isocrotonic acid [2]	a, b	631.3089 $(M - H)^-$	0.01 (0.00–0.03)	0.02 (0.01–0.06)	0.01 *	0.63
butyl 2-dodecanoic acid/ 5-Tetra dodecanoic acid [2]	a	225.1859 $(M - H)^-$	0.09 (0.04–0.19)	0.06 (0.01–0.10)	*0.05* [t]	0.81
caproic acid [1]	a	115.0763 $(M - H)^-$	0.13 (0.11–0.15)	0.14 (0.11–0.18)	0.46	0.26
3-hydroxycapric acid [2]	a, b, c	187.1339 $(M - H)^-$	0.43 (0.26–0.81)	0.62 (0.50–1.11)	0.01 *	0.97
Geranic acid [2]		167.1077 $(M - H)^-$	0.09 (0.07–0.22)	0.08 (0.06–0.16)	0.13	0.03
Sebacic acid [1]	a, c	261.1345 $(M\text{-}CH3COO)^-$	0.10 (0.07–0.18)	0.13 (0.08–0.19)	0.18 [t]	0.72
3-Hydroxysebacic acid [2]	a, c	217.1081 $(M - H)^-$	0.04 (0.03–0.06)	0.06 (0.03–0.07)	*0.07* [t]	0.68
3,4-Methylenesebacic acid [2]	a	225.1132 $(M - H)^-$	0.04 (0.03–0.06)	0.03 (0.02–0.04)	0.12 [t]	0.82
2-Hydroxybutyric acid [1]	a, b, c	103.0399 $(M - H)^-$	2.93 (2.35–3.72)	3.85 (3.05–4.81)	0.005 *	0.77
2-hydroxy-3-methylbutyric acid [1]	a, b, c	117.0555 $(M - H)^-$	0.99 (0.81–1.82)	1.52 (1.07–2.07)	0.01 *	*0.06*
pyridosine [2]	a, c	253.1195 $(M - H)^-$	0.20 (0.09–0.28)	0.11 (0.07–0.22)	*0.06* [t]	0.17
Glycerophosphorylcholine [2]	a, c	292.0724 $(M - H)^-$	0.68 (0.49–0.96)	0.58 (0.41–0.71)	*0.07* [t]	0.40
N-Heptanoylglycine [2]	a, b	186.1135 $(M - H)^-$	0.93 (0.47–1.83)	0.61 (0.40–1.16)	*0.07* [t]	0.14
Butyryl glycine/Saccharopine [2]	a	335.1455 * $(M + Fa - H)^-$	0.22 (0.11–0.53)	0.28 (0.08–0.51)	0.58	0.62
2-Phenylglycine [2]	a, c	150.0559 $(M - H)^-$	0.14 (0.09–0.22)	0.17 (0.10–0.29)	0.11 [t]	*0.08*
Cis-aconitic acid [1]	a	154.9983 $(M\text{-}H_2O - H)^-$	1.33 (0.58–2.27)	1.73 (1.28–2.49)	*0.09* [t]	0.85
Pyruvic acid [1]	a, b, c	147.0297 $(M\text{-}CH3COO)^-$	2.15 (1.27–3.49)	3.55 (1.94–6.10)	0.03 *	0.95
Citraconic [1]	a, b, c	129.0192 $(M - H)^-$	13.82 (9.49–26.19)	21.43 (13.82–29.91)	0.02 *	0.95
2-Keto-glutaramic acid [2]	a, c	144.0302 $(M - H)^-$	0.38 (0.30–0.44)	0.37 (0.31–0.58)	0.21	0.44
Panthothenic acid [1]	a, c	200.0929 $(M\text{-}H_2O - H)^-$	0.09 (0.06–0.11)	0.10 (0.08–0.11)	0.51	0.007
4-Heptenal [2]	a, b	111.0814 $(M - H)^-$	0.43 (0.33–0.50)	0.35 (0.26–0.45)	0.04 *	0.55
2-Methylpentanal [2]	a	99.0814 $(M - H)^-$	0.12 (0.09–0.13)	0.10 (0.09–0.12)	*0.06* [t]	0.98
Undecenal [2]	a, b, c	167.1440 $(M - H)^-$	0.08 (0.06–0.12)	0.06 (0.04–0.13)	0.006 *	0.02
Methyl 2-octynoate [2]	a	153.0919 $(M - H)^-$	0.10 (0.07–0.13)	0.07 (0.06–0.11)	*0.09* [t]	0.06

Table 3. *Cont.*

Metabolites (Annotation Level)	a, b, c	mz	Abundance Des Ions (10^6)			
			Median (25% and 75% Percentile), W2 to W4			
			"Slower" Growth ($n = 38$)	"Faster" Growth ($n = 29$)	Mann-Whitney p-Value (FDR-Corrected MW q-Value in Exposant)	MLR p-Value (FDR-Corrected MLR q-Value in Exposant)
4-Methylphenyl-acetaldehyde [2]	a	133.0658 $(M-H)^-$	0.07 (0.05–0.11)	0.06 (0.05–0.09)	0.04 *	0.14
4-Hydroxynonenal [2]	a, c	155.1077 $(M-H)^-$	0.06 (0.04–0.09)	0.07 (0.05–0.10)	0.13 ^{t}	0.79
cis-4-Decenedioic acid [2]	a, b, c	199.0973 $(M-H)^-$	0.07 (0.05–0.11)	0.10 (0.07–0.16)	0.01 *	0.94
Tetradecanedioic acid [1]	a, c	257.1761 $(M-H)^-$	0.08 (0.05–0.12)	0.12 (0.08–0.19)	*0.07* ^{t}	0.62
Dodecanedioic acid [2]	a, c	229.1445 $(M-H)^-$	0.41 (0.30–0.56)	0.35 (0.30–0.54)	0.42	0.01
Heptanoic acid [2]	a, c	129.0920 $(M-H)^-$	0.17 (0.14–0.21)	0.14 (0.10–0.19)	*0.06* ^{t}	0.74
2-benzyloctanoic acid [2]	a, b, c	233.1544 $(M-H)^-$	1.45 (0.78–2.31)	0.87 (0.61–1.45)	0.007 *	0.81
N-methylethanolaminium phosphate [2]	a, b, c	136.0165 $(M-H_2O-H)^-$	0.36 (0.27–0.51)	0.26 (0.19–0.30)	<0.0001 **	0.81
Phosphorylcholine [1]	a,	206.0551 $(M+Na)^+$	5.78 (4.26–6.63)	4.03 (0.68–5.67)	0.001 *	0.21
Glycerophosphocholin [2]	a	280.0917 $(M+Na)^+$	18.88 (9.66–30.18)	16.98 (3.54–24.57)	0.12 ^{t}	0.57
Choline [1]	a,	105.11080 $(M+H)^+$	2.67 (2.25–3.66)	3.30 (2.74–4.65)	0.008 *	0.02
Glucuronide/oligosides						
Dihydrocaffeic acid 3-O-glucuronide [2]	a, b, c	383.0763 $(M+Na)^+$	1.15 (0.87–1.29)	1.05 (0.86–1.23)	0.49	0.51
2-Fucosyllactose [2]	a, c	511.1629 $(M+H)^+$	106.6 (82.1–152.5)	122.6 (98.5–148.7)	0.34	0.79
N-acetyl-D-glucosamine [2]	a	244.0788 $(M+Na)^+$	2.94 (2.71–3.51)	3.20 (2.55–3.81)	0.74	0.68
Lacto-N-fucopentaose-2 [2]	a, b	876.2936 $(M+Na)^+$	9.29 (7.62–12.68)	10.56 (8.07–15.04)	0.15 ^{t}	0.72
Saccharopine [2]	a, c	335.1455 $(M\text{-}CH3COO)^-$	0.22 (0.11–0.53)	0.28 (0.08–0.51)	0.58	0.62

Values are medians (25% and 75% percentiles) from metabolites abundances from week 2 to week 4 of lactation period. Metabolites' annotation level in brackets: 1: identification level, definitively annotated with our home data base (i.e., based upon characteristic physicochemical properties of chemical reference standards (m/z, RT) and their MS/MS spectra compared to those of breastmilk QC); 2: putatively annotated compounds (i.e., without chemical reference standards, based upon physicochemical properties and MS/MS spectral similarity with public/commercial spectral libraries). (**a**) VIP in AoV-PLS/LDA ESI^+ or ESI^- model, (**b**) loadings in MB-PLS model, (**c**) loadings in ACC model; when the letters (a, b or c) are in italic, that means that the significance of metabolites, as VIP or loadings in statistical models, is just a trend. Variables were considered as significantly modified between the two groups of infants' growth (Mann-Whitney U test) when their multiple comparisons adjusted P-values (i.e., FDR corrected-MW q-value) was < 0.05. FDR-corrected MW q-value was labelled in exposant: *: FDR-corrected q-value < 0.05; **: FDR-corrected MW q-value < 0.01; t: FDR-corrected MW q-value < 0.1. Predictive ability of metabolites for infant weight growth was considered reliable when FDR-corrected MLR q-value was < 0.1 (and labelled in exposant as #).

We identified (Table 3) the association between our two groups of preterm infant's growth and breast milk metabolites (VIP in AoV-PLS models) that manually map to pathways such as the arginine-creatinine pathway, aromatic amino acid metabolism (including intermediate products of tryptophan, tyrosine, and/or phenylalanine catabolism), nicotinamide adenine dinucleotide precursors (such as nicotinamide and tryptophan), sulfur metabolism, oligosaccharides (e.g., 2′-Fucosyllactose and Lacto-N-FucoPentaose), mitochondrial fatty acid beta-oxidation, (including metabolites such as acylglycine and several analytes of the tricarboxylic acid cycle), pyruvic, citraconic, and aconitic acids, and choline metabolism. Many metabolites were significantly different between both groups of infants' growth when their multiple comparisons adjusted P-values (i.e., q-value after false discovery rate (FDR)) was <0.1, such as higher levels in orotic acid, nicotinamide, hydroxybutyric acid, pyruvic and citraconic acids, and choline in the "faster" group besides lower abundance in cresol and benzoic acid, for example. Among these metabolites, only a few metabolites predicted early infant growth (significant MLR p-value but unsuccessful for multiple correction testing, FDR-corrected MLR q-value), including: hydroxy-3-methylbutyric acid, undecenal, dodecanedioic acid and choline.

3.4. Glycomics Profiling

Milk samples were analyzed for changes in their HMO profiles from W2 to W4 of lactation in association with postnatal weight growth trajectory during hospital stay. On the PLS-DA score plot of PLS components (PCs 1 and 2) (Figure 3a), as expected, there was a clear difference in milk HMO profiles depending on secretor status in preterm milk samples, as the milk samples were separated into secretor (21 mothers) or non-secretor (five mothers) groups. The overal percentage of non-secretor mothers in our sub-cohort of LACTACOL was consistent with the proportions in most human populations, i.e., approximately 20% [28], but was significantly higher for mothers of infants ranked in the "slower" growth group (36%, i.e., 4 non-secretor mothers) versus those ranked in the "faster" growth group (10%, i.e., only one non-secretor mother). In this study, secretor or non-secretor status (i.e., mothers expressing or not the 1,2-fucosyl-transferase 2) was essentially defined by either high or low 2′Fucosyllactose (2′FL) levels, respectively, as measured by LC-MS [28,54]. Milk from mothers that was classified as non-secretors showed very low or even no detectable levels of 2′-FL, whereas milk from mothers classified as secretors contained high amounts of 2′-FL. Interestingly, exclusion of the five HMO profiles from non-secretor mothers in the statistical PLS-DA model improved the separation between the milks of the "faster" and "slower" infant growth groups (Figure 3b). As shown in Table 4, relative abundances of several measured HMOs differed significantly between breast milks provided to preterm infants with "faster" or "slower" growth during the W2 to W4 lactation period with higher overall levels of HMOs in milk given to fast-growing infants. In detail, and regardless of the maternal secretor status, breast milk provided to infants with optimal growth contained more total fucosylated HMOs (essentially due to the mono-fucosylayed, Lacto-N-FucoPentaose I (LNFPI percentage), both di-fucosylated HMOs, an isomer of Lacto-N-difucosyl-hexaose (LNDFH with the following monosaccharides structure: 3210, i.e., 3 Hex//1 HexNac/2 Fuc/0 NeuAc) 4210d, and neutral HMOs such as pLNH (lacto-N-hexaose), but contained less neutral HMO 3000 and di-fucosylated HMO 4210b. Many of these HMOs were found to be variables of interest for breast milk glycome discrimination (VIP-PLS-DA index above 1.0, as reported in Table 4). Of note, breast milk presented no between-group differences in any sialylated HMOs. As reported in Table 4, many HMOs were significantly predictive of infant weight Z-score, as they successfully passed the multiple linear regression test (MLR p-value), following adjustment for maternal and infant confounding factors and after multiple correction testing (FDR-corrected MLR q-value significant, i.e., <0.1). Indeed, the fucosylated LNFP I, an isomer of LNDFH 3′FL (3′-fucosyllactose) and the neutral pLNH were predictive of infant weight Z-score for secretor mothers only, whereas, the four minor di-fucosylated HMOs (4230c, 4230b, 4240b, and 4210d) remained predictive of infant weight Z-score regardless of the secretor or non-secretor status of mothers.

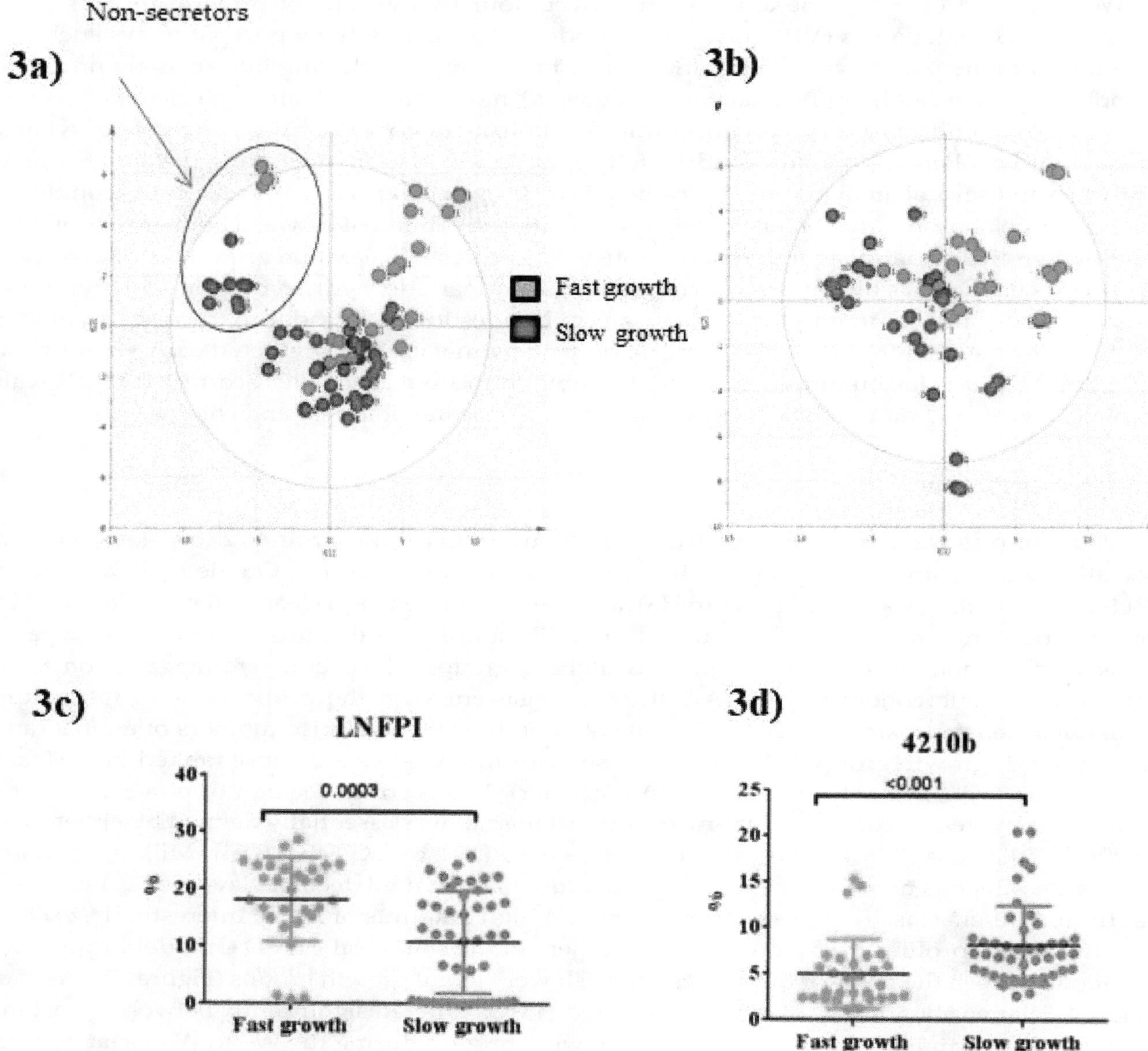

Figure 3. PLS-DA score plot based on the LC- HRMS glycomics profiles of human preterm milk of all mothers (**a**) (with non-secretor mothers circled on the basis of on the concentration of 2′-FL in their milks) or only of secretor mothers (**b**), on the factor weight *Z*-score (discharge-birth) with 45–39% of variance (R2Y = 37–45%), respectively, on components 1–2. Scatter plot (median) from W2 to W4 of lactation period (with secretor and non-secretor mothers) for two representative HMOs selected among VIP of interest: LNFPI (**c**) and 4210b (**d**), respectively. *P* values for comparison between "faster" and "slower" growth groups were derived using Mann-Whitney *U* test.

Table 4. Major HMOs detected in breast milk glycome and provided to preterm infants with "faster" or "slower" growth during the W2 to W4 lactation period.

HMOs	Composition						Median (25% and 75% Percentile) from W2 to W4 (Secretors and Non Secretors Mothers)		Mann-Whitney p-Value (FDR-Corrected MW q-Value in Exposant)		VIP –PLS-DA (C1–C2)		MLR-p-Value (FDR-Corrected MLR q-Value in Exposant)	
	mz	RT	Hex	HexNac	Fuc	NeuAc	"Slower" Growth (n = 38)	"Faster" Growth (n = 29)	Secretors and Non Secretors	Secretors Only	Secretors and Non Secretors	Secretors Only	Secretors and Non Secretors	Secretors Only
Fucosylated							61.46 (50.28–65.13)	62.82 (60.20–65.19)	0.1847 ^{t}	0.1370				0.73
Sialylated							8.47 (6.97–9.40)	7.45 (6.70–9.11)	0.2545	0.2773				0.37
Fucosylated./Sialylated							1.95 (1.50-2.32)	1.63 (1.33–2.30)	*0.0973* ^{t}	0.1422				0.35
Neutral							28.30 (26.78–38.23)	26.87 (25.92–29.57)	0.0352 *	0.6966				0.95
Mono Fucosylated							28.49 (19.06–34.74)	36.95 (31.83–39.21)	0.0020	0.0669				0.19
Di Fucosylated							26.64 (23.83–28.53)	23.12 (19.14–26.77)	0.0026	0.0054 *				0.10
Tri Fucosylated							3.52 (2.96–4.00)	2.85 (2.63–3.26)	0.0061	*0.0883*				0.43
Tetra Fucosylated							3.20 (2.54–4.07)	2.94 (1.77–3.83)	0.1520	0.0243 *				0.004 *
LNFPI≠	856.3280	10.2	3	1	1	0	11.99 (0.36-18.65)	19.86 (15.00–23.69)	0.0003 **	0.0045 *	1.22	1.26	0.63	0.03 *
pLNH≠	1075.4023	18	4	2	0	0	0.26 (0.14–0.35)	0.38 (0.26–0.54)	0.0014 **	0.0013 *	1.44	1.75	0.50	0.10 *
2′-FL≠	491.1958	8.5	2	0	1	0	11.22 (0.10–13.87)	12.58 (10.29–15.09)	*0.0882* ^{t}	0.9433	1.10	1.08	0.63	0.22 *
6′-SL	636.2333	9.6	2	0	0	1	2.50 (2.30–3.06)	2.47 (1.81–3.05]	0.3219	0.9433	0.65	0.29	0.26	0.31 *
LNnH≠	1075.4023	15.1	4	2	0	0	0.82 (0.32–1.44)	0.95 (0.58–2.31)	*0.0689* ^{t}	0.8116	1.25	1.22	0.67	0.52 ^{t}
LNT/LNnT≠	710.2701	10.9	3	1	0	0	22.52 (20.29–35.65)	22.46 (20.04–25.21)	0.1991 ^{t}	0.2591	1.00	0.81	0.48	0.62 ^{t}
LSTc/b	1001.3655	18.4	3	1	0	1	2.59 (2.00–3.57)	2.63 (2.25–3.41)	0.7012	0.1422	0.89	0.87	0.78	0.65 ^{t}
LNDFH I	1002.3859	5.7	3	1	2	0	4.26 (0.44–6.25)	5.10 (0.51–6.96)	0.3986	0.8903	0.55	0.74	0.22	0.50 ^{t}
3′ FL	491.1958	1.8	2	0	1	0	0.03 (0.00–0.08)	0.00 (0.00–0.03)	0.0133 *	0.1697	0.94	0.70	0.12	0.09 *
3′SL	636.2333	18.9	2	0	0	1	0.15 (0.13–0.21)	0.14 (0.11–0.18)	0.1555 ^{t}	0.9433	0.46	0.48	0.26	0.16 *
LNDFH ≠	1002.3859	9.6	3	1	2	0	0.26 (0.14-0.36)	0.36 (0.27-0.45)	0.0020 **	0.1050	1.12	1.05	0.43	0.04 *
LNDFHx	1002.3859	6.8	3	1	2	0	0.26 (0.11–1.11)	0.14 (0.07–0.24)	0.0293 *	*0.0726* ^{t}	0.97	1.04	0.15	0.06 *
4230c≠	1513.5760	13.5	4	2	3	0	0.11 (0.00–0.18)	0.07 (0.04–0.14)	0.5405	0.0002 **	1.90	1.55	0.0062 *	0.07 *
4210d≠	1221.4602	17.4	4	2	1	0	0.18 (0.00–0.39)	0.47 (0.27–1.31)	0.0005 **	0.0142 *	1.69	1.66	0.10	0.04 *
4220e≠	1367.5181	13	4	2	2	0	1.59 (0.37–2.43)	1.75 (1.35–2.77)	0.1799 ^{t}	0.6128	1.28	1.76	0.86	0.78 ^{t}
4230b≠	1513.576	8.2	4	2	3	0	0.65 (0.00–1.49)	0.61 (0.06–1.20)	0.7967	*0.0893* ^{t}	1.38	1.33	0.0095 *	0.09 *
3000≠	507.1907	6.4	3	0	0	0	0.26 (0.19–0.31)	0.16 (0.12–0.23)	<0.0001 ***	0.0022 *	2.06	0.90	0.53	0.22 *
5300 (2+)	720.7709	18.1	5	3	0	0	0.15 (0.10–0.23)	0.16 (0.14–0.32)	0.0771 ^{t}	0.6305	1.41	1.39	0.72	0.37 *
6420c (2+)≠	1049.3949	18.1	6	4	2	0	0.44 (0.09–0.64)	0.50 (0.32–0.72)	0.1893 ^{t}	0.5220	1.11	0.67	0.30	0.76 ^{t}
6430d (2+)≠	1122.4238	16.8	6	4	3	0	0.14 (0.00–0.26)	0.15 (0.10–0.24)	0.2102 ^{t}	0.2663	1.18	1.00	0.34	0.87 ^{t}
5310c	1586.5924	18	5	3	1	0	0.29 (0.22–0.38)	0.38 (0.25–0.46)	0.0428 *	0.4094	0.90	1.02	0.95	0.16 *
2110a	694.2752	3.6	2	1	1	0	0.01 (0.00–0.27)	0.24 (0.00–0.51)	0.0811 ^{t}	0.6772	0.90	1.49	0.48	0.60 ^{t}
4240b≠	1659.6339	13.9	4	2	4	0	0.04 (0.00–0.11)	0.04 (0.00–0.08)	0.9654	0.0457 *	1.29	0.68	0.0007 **	0.05 *
2020a≠	637.2537	11.1	2	0	2	0	0.49 (0.04–0.61)	0.55 (0.45–0.66)	0.0840 ^{t}	0.9700	1.10	1.23	0.72	0.20 *
5310b	1586.5924	17	5	3	1	0	0.24 (0.13–0.31)	0.16 (0.09–0.27)	0.1091 ^{t}	0.0420 *	0.93	0.97	0.84	0.40 *

Table 4. *Cont.*

HMOs	Composition						Median (25% and 75% Percentile) from W2 to W4 (Secretors and Non Secretors Mothers)		Mann-Whitney *p*-Value (FDR-Corrected MW *q*-Value in Exposant)		VIP –PLS-DA (C1–C2)		MLR-*p*-Value (FDR-Corrected MLR *q*-Value in Exposant)	
	mz	RT	Hex	HexNAc	Fuc	NeuAc	"Slower" Growth ($n = 38$)	"Faster" Growth ($n = 29$)	Secretors and Non Secretors	Secretors Only	Secretors and Non Secretors	Secretors Only	Secretors and Non Secretors	Secretors Only
4220a	684.2627	7.7	4	2	2	0	0.20 (0.14–0.29)	0.11 (0.07–0.25)	0.0216 *	*0.0911* ^{t}	0.49	0.52	0.10	0.82 ^{t}
4220b≠	1367.5181	8.8	4	2	2	0	0.31 (0.09–1.78)	0.23 (0.07–0.33)	0.0895 ^{t}	0.3352	1.02	0.99	0.15	0.14 *
4210b≠	1221.4602	12.6	4	2	1	0	7.19 (5.03–8.90)	3.75 (2.37–6.33)	<0.0001 ***	0.0003 **	1.05	1.84	0.30	0.07 *
5330b	1878.7082	13.9	5	3	3	0	0.23 (0.00–0.39)	0.29 (0.00–0.38)	0.3749	0.4106	0.96	1.10	0.05	0.26 *
5320a	1732.6503	12.9	5	3	2	0	0.27 (0.13–0.70)	0.13 (0.05–0.22)	0.0004 **	0.0045 *	1.06	1.37	0.47	0.16 *

Relative HMO abundances (%) were calculated by dividing absolute HMO peak area by each sample's total HMO peak areas. Values are medians (25% and 75% percentiles) from relative HMOs abundances from week 2 to week 4 of lactation period. P values for comparison between "faster" and "slower" growth groups were derived using Mann-Whitney *U* test. Variables were considered as significantly modified between the two groups of infants' growth when their multiple comparisons adjusted *P*-values (e.g., q-value after false discovery rate) was < 0.05. *: FDR-corrected MW *q*-value < 0.05; **: FDR-corrected MW *q*-value < 0.01; ***: FDR-corrected MW *q*-value < 0.001; *t*: FDR-corrected MW *q*-value < 0.1. Multiple Linear Regression (MLR) for infant weight Z-score (p-value) was also combined with FDR, and predictive ability for infant weight growth was considered reliable when MLR *q*-value was < 0.05. *: FDR-corrected MLR *q*-value < 0.05; *t*: FDR-corrected MLR *q*-value < 0.1. ≠: variables of importance for PLS-DA model (VIP > 1.0). LNDFH, Lacto-N-difucosyl-hexaose; LNT, lacto-N-tetraose; pLNH, p-Lacto-N-Hexaose; LNFP, lacto-N-fucopentaose; LNnT, lacto-N-neotetraose; LNT, lactoN-tetraose; LST, sialyl-lacto-N-tetraose; 2′-FL, 2′-fucosyllactose; 3-FL, 3-fucosyllactose; 3′-SL, 3′-sialyllactose; Hex, hexose; HexNac, N-acetylhexosamine; Fuc, fucose and NeuAc, N-acetylneuraminic acid. Fucosylation was further investigated to determine the differences in the abundance of mono, di, tri, and tetrafucosylation (based on the number of fucose residues).

3.5. Integration of Multi-Omics Data sets

The aim of the current pilot study was to determine whether multi-block modeling could be applied for relating MS-based metabolomic, lipidomic, glycomic, fatty acids, and free amino acids data with regard to the predictive component that is the infant growth trajectory. Due to the complexity of longitudinal study by extracting the relevant information from multiple "omics" data sources, we chose to focus on "omics" data obtained on one representative time of lactation (week three of lactation). More specifically, the horizontal concatenation of annotated VIP provided by the AoV-PLS-DA model applied on MS-based metabolomic (i.e., 68 metabolites), lipidomic (i.e., 143 lipid species previously selected in [20]), and glycomic (79 HMOs) data with all metabolites–species issues from free amino acid and total fatty acid quantification was a straightforward solution to providing an extended analytical coverage of the biochemical diversity characterizing the breast milk samples. Concerning the glycomics data set, we had to overcome the problem due to the breast milk clustering based on maternal secretor or non-secretor status. As the relatively substantial variation in HMOs between the high and low 2′FL levels clusters were recently reported not to impact term infant growth of either sex up to four months [54], we chose to perform, on glycomic data, a mean-centered scaling of HMOs abundances on maternal secretor or non-secretor status before the "omics" data fusion. Then, on the super-matrix thus obtained, we tested UPCA or MBPLS multi-block strategies. Following the fusion of 340 selected annotated variables resulting from the combination of five data sources (blocks), the unsupervised UPCA score plot (Figure 4a) showed—on the principal components PC 3–4 that reported 21.4% variance—a clustering of breast milk samples and indicated a specific metabotype in the milk provided to preterm infants with "faster" growth versus that fed to infants with "slower" growth. The supervised MB-PLS score plot (Figure 4b) clearly highlighted on components 1–2 (18.5% of variance for the five blocks data), two breast milk metabotypes associated with 'faster' or 'slower' infant growth. The breast milk profiles, corresponding to the four sets of twins and depicted with blue symbols in Figure 4 were plotted between both "faster" and "slower" clusters. The most discriminant features associated with infant growth during hospital stay corresponded to a cluster of 87 metabolites species selected according to their loadings on the first MB-PLS components PC1 and PC2, and including: (i) many HMOs, such as LNFPI and 4210d, positively correlated with PC1 (i.e., associated with "faster" growth) or 4230b and 4230c, negatively correlated with PC1 (i.e., associated with "slower" growth), (ii) a few free amino acids (such as valine and glycine associated with "slower" growth), (iii) several lipidomic-species that were associated with "faster" growth, such as medium-chain saturated fatty acids (MCSAT, e.g., pentadecanoic and myristic acid), triglycerides (TG(46:0) and TG(50:2)), phospholipids (PS(38:4) and PE(38:3)), or that were associated with "slower" growth, such as oleic acid, plasmalogen-derivatives (PC(P-34:2) and PE(P-36:0)), lyso-phosphatidylethanolamine-containing arachidonic acid (LysoPE(20:4)), ceramide (Cer(18:1/22:0)), and very long-chain TG (TG(54:4) and TG(58:7)) and finally, (iv) few metabolomic-species positively (3-hydroxycapric acid, dihydrocaffeic acid 3-O-glucuronide, LNFPII) or negatively (9-undecenal, heptanoyl- and hexanoyl-glycine, 3-hydroxy-adipic acid, valerenic acid) correlated to PC1. Among these metabolites, MCSAT and oleic acid were previously shown to be predictive of optimal early growth [20].

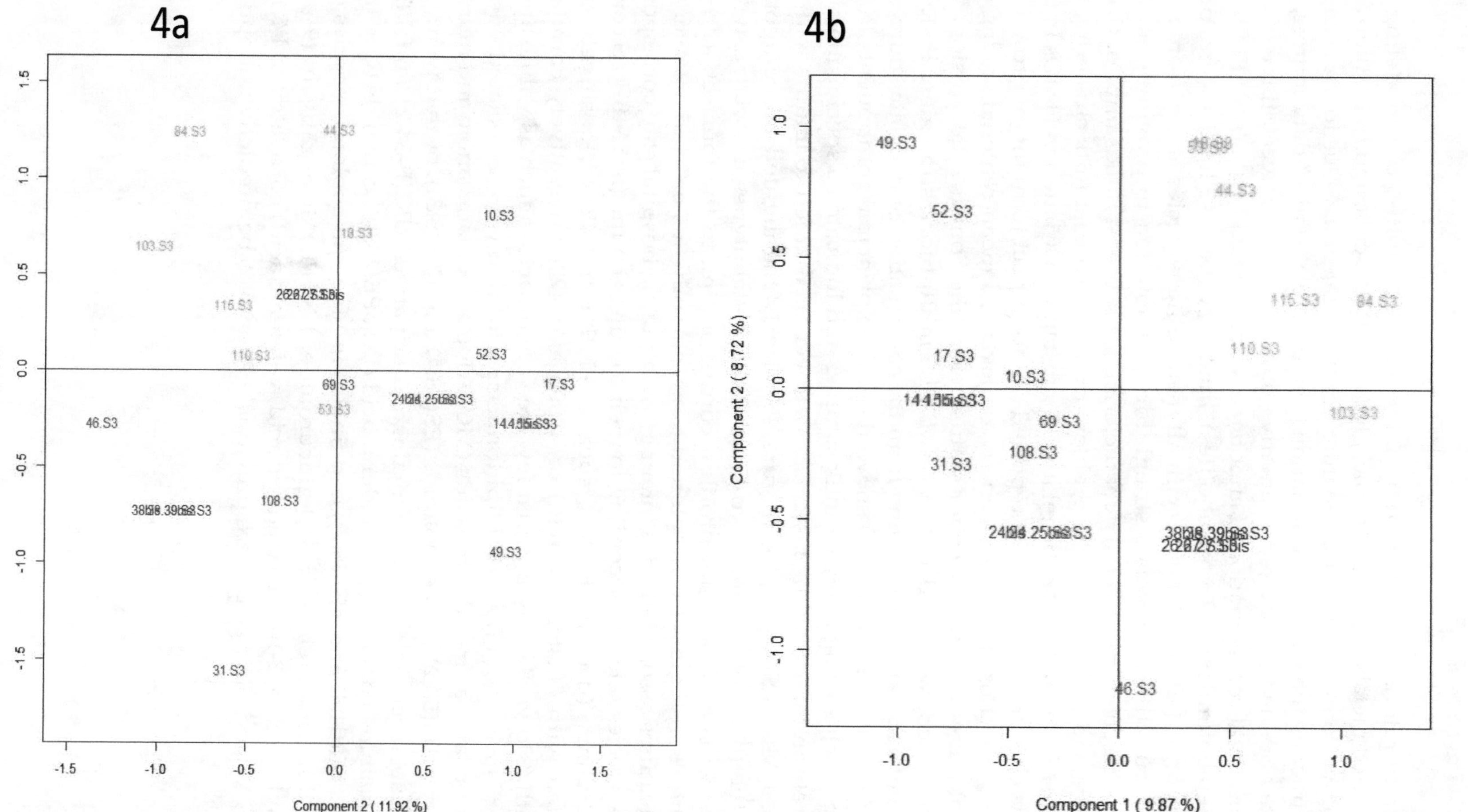

Figure 4. Score plot generated from UPCA (**a**) (with 21.4% of variance on components 3–4) and MB-PLS-DA (**b**) (with 18.5% of variance on components 1–2) based on the lipidomics/metabolomics/glycomics/FA/FAA profiles of human preterm milk at week 3 of lactation on the factor weight Z-score (discharge minus birth). Breast milk provided to preterm infants who experienced "faster" (green) or "slower" (red) growth and to twin infants with discordant growth rate, one twin with high growth rate and the other one with low growth rate (blue).

4. Discussion

To date, only a few metabolomics studies have been reported on preterm human milk in the first few weeks of lactation [27,28]. To the best of our knowledge, the current pilot study is the first to comprehensively characterize and compare the preterm human milk lipidome (previously reported in [20]), metabolome, glycome, total fatty acid, and free amino acid profiles in relation to the growth velocity of preterm infant early in life in a group of 26 breastfeeding mother infant dyads. Our findings strongly suggest that molecular species other than "classic" macronutrients in human breast milk might affect infant growth early in life.

4.1. Higher Breast Milk Content in Branched-Chain and Insulino-Trophic Amino Acid and in Tyrosine Associated to Optimal Infant Growth

The higher levels of total branched-chain amino acids (BCAA) in breast milk provided to infants who experienced a "faster" early growth was consistent with the muscle protein anabolic effects of BCAA reported in adult humans [55]. In a previous study conducted on obese mothers of full-term infants, we found a 20% higher BCAA content in the breast milk obtained from obese mothers compared with control, lean mothers [56]. Several authors argued that the higher BCAA content of most formulas compared to human milk may contribute to the higher early weight gain observed in bottle-fed (compared to breastfed) full-term infants [57,58]. However, whether a high milk BCAA content directly impacts the growth of the breast-fed child remains to be explored. Among the insulino-trophic amino acid, arginine, the sole endogenous source of nitric oxide (NO), and a precursor of polyamines and creatine may regulate angiogenesis, mammary gland development, enhance protein synthesis, and decrease protein degradation in mammary epithelial cells [59], thereby improving lactation performance [60,61]. In our study, the optimal early infant growth associated with higher breast milk contents of arginine and carbamoylsarcosine, an intermediate in the creatine-arginine pathway, might reflect the positive effects of arginine and polyamine on muscle protein synthesis and on immune response [61], its beneficial effects on the intestinal mucosa itself, the prevention of necrotizing enterocolitis [62–64] and its protective effect for the nervous system [61]. Higher availability of creatine may serve as a source for phosphorylation in muscle tissue and fat metabolism. The higher amounts of tyrosine combined with lower abundances of tyrosine catabolism products (hydroxyphenylacetic acid and cresol) [23] observed in the "faster" breast milk are consistent with the key role of tyrosine in infant growth as a precursor of thyroxine, a hormone involved in energy metabolism, and of dopamine, a neurotransmitter.

4.2. Enhanced Milk Fat Availability by Infants with an Early "Faster" Growth Velocity

Our data highlighted lower concentrations of two free amino acids involved in bile acid conjugation, glycine and taurine, in the "faster" growth group. These data were observed along with an enhanced total lipid content previously reported in "faster" milk [20]. We speculate that the lower milk content in glycin and taurine, under their free form, along with the higher fat content could be explained by enhanced bile acid conjugation in "faster" breast milk, which could, consequently, facilitate the solubilization of lipids, sterols, and fat-soluble vitamins by forming mixed micelles, and, in turn, the uptake of these nutrients into enterocytes despite gastrointestinal immaturity. This also is in agreement with higher coefficients of fat absorption reported in breast-fed vs. formula-fed new borns, and related to the bile salt-dependent lipase (BSL) present in human milk [65]. The "faster" breast milk also presented decreased glycine derivatives, including hexanoyl- and heptanoylglycine, which are products of the mitochondrial fatty acid beta-oxidation [66]. These findings suggest low rates of fatty acids utilization in mammary gland and/or breast milk, which could enhance fat availability for breast-fed preterm infants. Moreover, the "faster" breast milk contained higher amounts in beta-hydroxybutyrate, a ketone body involved in the mammary gland synthesis of triglycerides, leading to the formation of milk fat globules [34]. Apart from its pivotal role as an energy fuel for extrahepatic tissues like brain, heart, or skeletal muscle in newborns, hydroxybutyrate is reported to play a role as a signaling mediator, a driver of protein post-translational modification, and a modulator of inflammation and oxidative stress [67]; such mechanisms could explain the link between beta-hydroxybutyrate availability and optimal early growth in a context of prematurity. Moreover, preterm breast milk metabolome showed decreased levels of few odd medium unbranched- (heptanoic and undecenal) or branched-chain (BCFAs, as 2-benzyloctanoic acid and methyl-2-octynoic acids) fatty acids but enhanced levels in one specific BCFA, the citraconic acid (known as methylmaleate, an odd and methyl-branched short chain unsaturated dicarboxylic fatty acid) in the "faster" group. Interestingly, mother's milk BCFAs [68] have been reported to reduce the occurrence of necrotizing enterocolitis in a mouse model due to their active roles in reducing inflammation and altering microbiota in the gut [69]. However, the potential effects of BCFAs on the infant health and development remain to be examined [68], as Wongtangtintharn et al. [70] suggested that BCFA lowers fatty acid synthesis [71]. Indeed, the higher lipid content we previously reported in the "faster" breast milk lipidome [20] seems to be consitent with the lower levels of many BCFA observed in the present study. Additionally, the fact that odd chain saturated fatty acid are reported to pass into the milk of lactating cows [72] suggests that these fatty acids may also cross the blood-brain barrier and act on early postnatal brain development. Finally, the higher availability of niacinamide in "faster" milk suggests niacinamide could act, through its role as a precursor of co-enzymes NAD and NADP, and impact fatty acid utilization since NAD^+ is used as a coenzyme in energy production (glycolysis, mitochondrial respiration) and improves gastrointestinal tract repair after damage as well as immune response [73].

Taken together, our findings suggest that the "faster" milk supplied (i) a higher content in energy, with calories supplied under a more digestible form of the preterm newborns, to overcome the immaturity of their digestive tractus, (ii) larger amounts or amino acids that promoted protein anabolism, and (iii) bioactive molecule, that played critical roles in energy homeostasis and gastrointestinal function, contributing to an optimal early-growth in infants born preterm. These findings also suggest that the higher lipid content in breast milk metabotype associated with preterm infants with optimal weight growth during hospitalization is used for enhanced fat oxidation rather than fat deposition, promoting tissue growth and likely a preferential fat-free mass deposition, which might in turn contribute to the recovery of the body composition and optimization of neurodevelopmental outcomes [74]. Moreover, the high BCAA and arginine intakes in breast milk provided to infants who belong to the "faster" group are also in agreement with this putative fat-free mass accretion in preterm infants, which could explain an optimal weight gain.

Additionally, the higher content in phosphatidylcholine and sphingomyelin previously reported in the "faster" milk of the same pilot study [20] is consistent with the higher amounts of choline observed in breast milk metabolome provided to infants with optimal early-growth trajectory. Choline plays a key role as a precursor for acetylcholine (a neuromediator) and betaine (a source of labile methyl groups), which could increase the availability of methionine and choline and also enhance liver glycogenesis [75]. Indeed, this higher choline content may have a profound benefic impact upon the homestatic mechanisms and upon the physiological function in preterm infants, leading to an optimal growth during their hospitalization.

4.3. *Di-Fucosylated HMOs Associated to Early Preterm Infant Growth*

We found similar proportions of fucosylated and sialylated HMOs in preterm milk in good agreement with an earlier study from another team [31] but with slight differences in HMO-fucosylation level (according to the number of fucose residues carried) in both growth groups, such as a higher abundance of mono-(LNFPI) and a lower abundance of di- and tri-fucosylated oligosaccharides in breast milk provided to infants with "faster" growth. Given the small number of non-secretor mothers in this pilot study (five among 26 mothers) and because only one preterm milk sample was collected from a non-secretor mother who delivered a preterm infant with a "faster" growth, meaningful conclusions regarding differences in "faster" and "slower" growth milk on the basis of maternal secretor status cannot be drawn. There are scarce data to clarify the putative relationship between the maternal milk fucosyl-transferase 2 (FUT2)-dependent oligosaccharide status and infant anthropometry [32,54]. Recently, a specific FUT2-dependent HMO, LNFP I, but not 2'FL, was reported to be associated with the weight of full term infants at six months of age [32], but that association was not observed on growth curves over the first four months of life in groups of healthy, full term infants [54]. In our cohort, we observed consistent effects of the minor di-fucosylated HMOs (4230c, 4230b, 4240b, and 4210d) but not 2'FL and of the mono-fucosylated LNFP I (considering only secretors mother infant dyads) concentrations in breast milk on preterm infant growth up to 4 weeks of lactation. After multiple linear regression combined with multiple corrections and adjustment for confounding maternal and infant factors, the ability of the latter HMOs to predict early weight gain persisted. These di-fucosylated HMOs were also selected as discriminant metabolites in our MB-PLS model built on the five blocks of milk components. However, given the small sample size included in this exploratory study, future work would be needed in larger samples with longer follow-up to identify the exact contribution of specific HMOs to preterm infant growth. The impact of HMOS may involve effects on intestinal epithelium and gut microbiome, as fucosylated HMOs (and particularly LNFPI) support increased *bifidobacteria*, which dominate the microbiota of breastfed infants [76] but also on immune development and/or protection from infection through systemic effects [32], thereby likely affecting infant growth and body composition.

5. Conclusions

Previous studies have shown breastfeeeding is associated with many health benefits in pre-term infants. However, whether such benefits are due to mother's milk constituents, *per se*, remains unclear. Breastmilk may not always be adequate for pre-term infants with high nutrition density requirements, which may lead to insufficient weight gain. We believe this to be the first study to document the changes in the metabolomics/lipidomics/glycomics/amino acids profiles of pre-term human milk during the first month of lactation, related to preterm infant growth during hospital stays. We showed that specific differences in milk metabolites exist between breast milk provided to preterm infants with optimal or non-optimal early growth, and a set of few milk metabolites were identified as predictive of infant growth parameters in the present pilot study, pointing to the critical role of energy utilization, protein synthesis, oxidative status, gut epithelial cell maturity, or more indirectly, gut microbiome in the context of prematurity. In particular, our findings highlighted robust biomarkers, i.e., arginine, tyrosine, hydroxybutyrate, niacinamide, choline, and lacto-N-fucopentaose I, that displayed a good ability to predict weight gain during hospital stays. Moreover, this preterm milk metabolomic signature suggests that the optimal early growth trajectory during hospital stays of preterm infants could be combined with preferential fat utilization and fat-free mass accretion. A clear limitation of our pilot study is its small population sample size and slight differences in birth weight between the groups. Although it has long been known that infants born with a lower birth weight grow faster [36,37], matching groups for birth weight would have been nearly impossible. We therefore have to admit that it cannot be ascertained whether the difference in breastmilk composition is programmed by infant antenatal growth or, alternatively, is one among the many determinant factors of postnatal growth trajectory. This study is also limited by the statistical method we applied because the Mann-Whitney *U* test has a lower power than the parametric method. Before the metabolites identified here can be considered valid biomarkers, they need to be quantified in the entire preterm newborn LACTACOL cohort and, ideally, validated in other longitudinal birth cohorts. Nevertheless, this pioneer integrative analysis for human breast milk might open the way to novel strategies using human milk as a tool to improve the outcome of a frail population of newborn infants. Indeed, providing optimal individual nutrition remains a daunting challenge and the subject of heated debate between neonatalogists on the issue of "individualized" fortification of human milk to improve growth and long term outcomes for all preterm infants.

Author Contributions: M.-C.A.-G., C.-Y.B., J.-C.R.: had full access to all of the data in the study and took responsibility for the integrity of the data and the accuracy of the data analysis designed research; C.-Y.B., J.-C.R.: conceived the LACTACOL study and design; H.B. and C.-Y.B.: managed the LACTACOL cohort; M.-C.A.-G.: conceived and supervised the present metabolomics study conducted on a subset of infants of LACTACOL cohort; T.M.: conceived the appropriate statistical tools and/or performed the statistical analysis; A.D.-S., A.-L.R., Y.G., F.F., S.C.: conducted metabolomics analysis and/or metabolites identification using MS; M.-C.A.-G.: drafted the manuscript; T.M., F.F., C.-Y.B. and D.D.: critically revised the manuscript for important intellectual content; and all authors: acquired, analyzed, or interpreted the data, and read and approved the final manuscript.

Acknowledgments: This work was part of the LACTACOL project. The LACTACOL projet was funded by Région Pays-de-la-Loire (2011–2012) and by the 'Fonds Européen de Développement Economique et Régional » (FEDER, Grant 38395, Project 6226, 2013–2015). We thank lactating mothers for having accepted donation of breast milk for the LACTACOL protocol, andCécile Boscher, Laure Simon, and Evelyne Gauvard for caring mothers and their infants as well as guarantying the collection of maternal milk. We also thank the Biological Resource Centre for biobanking (CHU Nantes, Hôtel Dieu, Centre de Ressources Biologiques (CRB), Nantes, F-44093, France (BRIF: BB-0033-00040)) for storing human milk samples in the milk biobank (DC-2009-982). Metabolomics LC-HRMS experiments, bioinformatics tool development and data treatment were performed on the LABERCA, a technical plateau from CORSAIRE Metabolomics platform (Biogenouest network) with the collaborative portal dedicated to metabolomic data processing, analysis and annotation 'Workflow4Metabolomics'. Glycomics LC-HRMS experiments were performed on the CEA-Saclay plateau (MetaboHUB, France). The authors would like to acknowledge Lauriane Rambaud (LABERCA, Nantes, France) for her technical assistance in breast milk metabobolome annotation.

Abbreviations

AoV-PLS	analysis of variance combined to partial least squares regression
BCFA	branched-chain fatty acids
ESI	electrospray ionization
FDR	false discovery rate
GA	gestational age
HMO	human milk oligosaccharides
LC-HR-MS	Liquid-Chromatography-High-Resolution-Mass-Spectrometry
MG PLS-DA	multi-group partial least squares discriminant analysis
MLR	multiple linear regression
MCSAT	medium-chain saturated fatty acid
U-PCA	unfold principal component analysis
SD	standard deviation
W4M	Workflow4Metabolomics®

References

1. Victora, C.G.; Bahl, R.; Barros, A.J.; França, G.V.; Horton, S.; Krasevec, J.; Murch, S.; Sankar, M.J.; Walker, N.; Rollins, N.C.; et al. Breastfeeding in the 21st century: Epidemiology, mechanisms, and lifelong effect. *Lancet* **2016**, *387*, 475–490. [CrossRef]
2. Mills, S.; Ross, R.P.; Hill, C.; Fitzgerald, G.F.; Stanton, C. Milk intelligence: Mining milk for bioactive substances associated with human health. *Int. Dairy J.* **2011**, *21*, 377–401. [CrossRef]
3. Andreas, N.J.; Kampmann, B.; Le-Doare, K.M. Human breast milk: A review on its composition and bioactivity. *Early Hum. Dev.* **2015**, *91*, 629–635. [CrossRef] [PubMed]
4. Mosca, F.; Giannì, M.L. Human milk: Composition and health benefits. *La Pediatria Medica e Chirurgica* **2017**, *39*. [CrossRef] [PubMed]
5. Boquien, C.Y. Human milk: An ideal food for nutrition of preterm newborn. *Front. Pediatr.* **2018**, *6*. [CrossRef] [PubMed]

6. Johnson, T.J.; Patel, A.L.; Bigger, H.R.; Engstrom, J.L.; Meier, P.P. Economic benefits and costs of human milk feedings: A strategy to reduce the risk of prematurity-related morbidities in very-low-birth-weight infants. *Adv. Nutr. Int. Rev. J.* **2014**, *5*, 207–212. [CrossRef] [PubMed]
7. Sankar, M.J.; Sinha, B.; Chowdhury, R.; Bhandari, N.; Taneja, S.; Martines, J.; Bahl, R. Optimal breastfeeding practices and infant and child mortality: A systematic review and meta-analysis. *Acta Paediatr.* **2015**, *104*, 3–13. [CrossRef] [PubMed]
8. Quigley, M.; McGuire, W. Formula versus donor breast milk for feeding preterm or low birth weight infants. *Cochrane Database Syst. Rev.* **2014**. [CrossRef] [PubMed]
9. Corpeleijn, W.E.; de Waard, M.; Christmann, V.; van Goudoever, J.B.; Jansen-van der Weide, M.C.; Kooi, E.M.; Koper, J.F.; Kouwenhoven, S.M.; Lafeber, H.N.; Mank, E.; et al. Effect of donor milk on severe infections and mortality in very low-birth-weight infants: The early nutrition study randomized clinical trial. *JAMA Pediatr.* **2016**, *170*, 654–661. [CrossRef] [PubMed]
10. Boyd, C.A.Q.; Quigley, M.A.; Brocklehurst, P. Donor breast milk versus infant formula for preterm infants: Systematic review and meta-analysis. *Arch. Dis. Child. Fetal Neonatal Ed.* **2007**, *92*, F169–F175. [CrossRef] [PubMed]
11. Rozé, J.C.; Darmaun, D.; Boquien, C.Y.; Flamant, C.; Picaud, J.C.; Savagner, C.; Claris, O.; Lapillonne, A.; Mitanchez, D.; Branger, B.; et al. The apparent breastfeeding paradox in very preterm infants: Relationship between breast feeding; early weight gain and neurodevelopment based on results from two cohorts; EPIPAGE and LIFT. *BMJ Open* **2012**, *2*, e000834. [CrossRef] [PubMed]
12. Curtis, M.; Rigo, J. Extrauterine growth restriction in very-low-birthweight infants. *Acta Paediatr.* **2004**, *93*, 1563–1568. [CrossRef] [PubMed]
13. Ehrenkranz, R.A.; Dusick, A.M.; Vohr, B.R.; Wright, L.L.; Wrage, L.A.; Poole, W.K. Growth in the neonatal intensive care unit influences neurodevelopmental and growth outcomes of extremely low birth weight infants. *Pediatrics* **2006**, *117*, 1253–1261. [CrossRef] [PubMed]
14. Larroque, B.; Ancel, P.Y.; Marret, S.; Marchand, L.; André, M.; Arnaud, C.; Pierrat, V.; Rozé, J.C.; Messer, J.; Thiriez, G.; et al. Neurodevelopmental disabilities and special care of 5-year-old children born before 33 weeks of gestation (the EPIPAGE study): A longitudinal cohort study. *Lancet* **2008**, *371*, 813–820. [CrossRef]
15. Frondas-Chauty, A.; Simon, L.; Branger, B.; Gascoin, G.; Flamant, C.; Ancel, P.Y.; Darmaun, D.; Rozé, J.C. Early growth and neurodevelopmental outcome in very preterm infants: Impact of gender. *Arch. Dis. Child. Fetal Neonatal Ed.* **2014**, *99*, F366–F372. [CrossRef] [PubMed]
16. Agostoni, C.; Buonocore, G.; Carnielli, V.P.; De Curtis, M.; Darmaun, D.; Decsi, T.; Domellöf, M.; Embleton, N.D.; Fusch, C.; Genzel-Boroviczeny, O.; et al. Enteral nutrient supply for preterm infants: Commentary from the European Society of Paediatric Gastroenterology; Hepatology and Nutrition Committee on Nutrition. *J. Pediatr. Gastr. Nutr.* **2010**, *50*, 85–91. [CrossRef] [PubMed]
17. Henriksen, C.; Westerberg, A.C.; Rønnestad, A.; Nakstad, B.; Veierød, M.B.; Drevon, C.A.; Iversen, P.O. Growth and nutrient intake among very-low-birth-weight infants fed fortified human milk during hospitalisation. *Brit. J. Nutr.* **2009**, *102*, 1179–1186. [CrossRef] [PubMed]
18. Alexandre-Gouabau, M.C.; Courant, F.; Le Gall, G.; Moyon, T.; Darmaun, D.; Parnet, P.; Coupé, B.; Antignac, J.P. Offspring metabolomic response to maternal protein restriction in a rat model of intrauterine growth restriction (IUGR). *J. Proteome Res.* **2011**, *10*, 3292–3302. [CrossRef] [PubMed]
19. Alexandre-Gouabau, M.C.; Courant, F.; Moyon, T.; Küster, A.; Le Gall, G.; Tea, I.; Antignac, J.P.; Darmaun, D. Maternal and cord blood LC-HRMS metabolomics reveal alterations in energy and polyamine metabolism, and oxidative stress in very-low birth weight infants. *J. Proteome Res.* **2013**, *12*, 2764–2778. [CrossRef] [PubMed]
20. Alexandre-Gouabau, M.-C.; Moyon, T.; Cariou, V.; Antignac, J.-P.; Qannari, E.M.; Croyal, M.; Soumah, M.; Guitton, Y.; Billard, H.; Legrand, A.; et al. Breast milk lipidome is associated with early growth trajectory in preterm infants. *Nutrients* **2018**, *10*, 164. [CrossRef] [PubMed]
21. Fanos, V.; Atzori, L.; Makarenko, K.; Melis, G.B.; Ferrazzi, E. Metabolomics application in maternal-fetal medicine. *BioMed Res. Int.* **2013**, *9*. [CrossRef] [PubMed]
22. Demmelmair, H.; Koletzko, B. Variation of metabolite and hormone contents in human milk. *Clin. Perinatol.* **2017**, *44*, 151–164. [CrossRef] [PubMed]

23. Carraro, S.; Baraldi, E.; Giordano, G.; Pirillo, P.; Stocchero, M.; Houben, M.; Bont, L. Metabolomic Profile of Amniotic Fluid and Wheezing in the First Year of Life—A Healthy Birth Cohort Study. *J. Pediatr.* **2018**, *196*, 264–269. [CrossRef] [PubMed]
24. Marincola, F.C.; Noto, A.; Caboni, P.; Reali, A.; Barberini, L.; Lussu, M.; Murgia, F.; Santoru, M.L.; Atzori, L.; Fanos, V.J. A metabolomic study of preterm human and formula milk by high resolution NMR and GC/MS analysis: Preliminary results. *Matern. Fetal Neonatal Med.* **2012**, *25*, 62–67. [CrossRef] [PubMed]
25. Wu, J.; Domellöf, M.; Zivkovic, A.M.; Larsson, G.; Öhman, A.; Nording, M.L. NMR-based metabolite profiling of human milk: A pilot study of methods for investigating compositional changes during lactation. *Biochem. Biophys. Res. Comm.* **2016**, *469*, 626–632. [CrossRef] [PubMed]
26. George, A.; Gay, M.; Trengove, R.; Geddes, D. Human Milk Lipidomics: Current Techniques and Methodologies. *Nutrients* **2018**, *10*, 1169. [CrossRef] [PubMed]
27. Spevacek, A.R.; Smilowitz, J.T.; Chin, E.L.; Underwood, M.A.; German, J.B.; Slupsky, C.M. Infant Maturity at Birth Reveals Minor Differences in the Maternal Milk Metabolome in the First Month of Lactation. *J. Nutr.* **2015**, *45*, 1698–1708. [CrossRef] [PubMed]
28. Sundekilde, U.K.; Downey, E.; O'Mahony, J.A.; O'Shea, C.A.; Ryan, C.A.; Kelly, A.L.; Bertram, H.C. The effect of gestational and lactational age on the human milk metabolome. *Nutrients* **2016**, *8*, 304. [CrossRef] [PubMed]
29. Maffei, D.; Schanler, R.J. Human milk is the feeding strategy to prevent necrotizing enterocolitis! *Semin. Perinatol.* **2017**, *41*, 36–40. [CrossRef] [PubMed]
30. Bode, L. Human Milk Oligosaccharides in the Prevention of Necrotizing Enterocolitis: A journey from in vitro and in vivo models to mother-infant cohort studies. *Front Pediatr.* **2018**, *6*, 385. [CrossRef] [PubMed]
31. De Leoz, M.L.A.; Gaerlan, S.C.; Strum, J.S.; Dimapasoc, L.M.; Mirmiran, M.; Tancredi, D.J.; Smilowitz, J.T.; Kalanetra, K.M.; Mills, D.A.; German, J.B.; et al. Lacto-N-tetraose; fucosylation; and secretor status are highly variable in human milk oligosaccharides from women delivering preterm. *J. Proteome Res.* **2012**, *11*, 4662–4672. [CrossRef] [PubMed]
32. Alderete, T.L.; Autran, C.; Brekke, B.E.; Knight, R.; Bode, L.; Goran, M.I.; Fields, D.A. Associations between human milk oligosaccharides and infant body composition in the first 6 mo of life. *Am. J. Clin. Nutr.* **2015**, *102*, 1381–1388. [CrossRef] [PubMed]
33. Charbonneau, M.R.; O'Donnell, D.; Blanton, L.V.; Totten, S.M.; Davis, J.C.; Barratt, M.J.; Cheng, J.; Guruge, J.; Talcott, M.; Bain, J.R.; et al. Sialylated milk oligosaccharides promote microbiota-dependent growth in models of infant undernutrition. *Cell* **2016**, *164*, 859–871. [CrossRef] [PubMed]
34. Rezaei, R.; Wu, Z.; Hou, Y.; Bazer, F.W.; Wu, G. Amino acids and mammary gland development: Nutritional implications for milk production and neonatal growth. *J. Anim. Sci. Biotechnol.* **2016**, *7*, 20. [CrossRef] [PubMed]
35. Metrustry, S.J.; Karhunen, V.; Edwards, M.H.; Menni, C.; Geisendorfer, T.; Huber, A.; Reichel, C.; Dennison, E.M.; Cooper, C.; Spector, T.; et al. Metabolomic signatures of low birthweight: Pathways to insulin resistance and oxidative stress. *PLoS ONE* **2018**, *13*, e0194316. [CrossRef] [PubMed]
36. Ferchaud-Roucher, V.; Desnots, E.; Naël, C.; Martin Agnoux, A.; Alexandre-Gouabau, M.C.; Darmaun, D.; Boquien, C.Y. Use of UPLC-ESI-MS/MS to quantitate free amino acid concentrations in micro-samples of mammalian milk. *SpringerPlus* **2013**, *2*, 622. [CrossRef] [PubMed]
37. Oursel, S.; Junot, C.; Fenaille, F. Comparative analysis of native and permethylated human milk oligosaccharides by liquid chromatography coupled to high resolution mass spectrometry. *J. Chromatogr. B* **2017**, *1071*, 49–57. [CrossRef] [PubMed]
38. Bligh, E.G.; Dyer, W.J. A rapid method of total lipid extraction and purification. *Can. J. Biochem. Physiol.* **1959**, *37*, 911–917. [CrossRef] [PubMed]
39. Gallart-Ayala, H.; Courant, F.; Severe, S.; Antignac, J.P.; Morio, F.; Abadie, J.; Le Bizec, B. Versatile lipid profiling by liquid chromatography-high resolution mass spectrometry using all ion fragmentation and polarity switching. Preliminary application for serum samples phenotyping related to canine mammary cancer. *Anal. Chim. Acta* **2013**, *796*, 75–83. [CrossRef] [PubMed]
40. Courant, F.; Royer, A.L.; Chéreau, S.; Morvan, M.L.; Monteau, F.; Antignac, J.P.; Le Bizec, B. Implementation of a semi-automated strategy for the annotation of metabolomic fingerprints generated by liquid chromatography-high resolution mass spectrometry from biological samples. *Analyst* **2012**, *137*, 4958–4967. [CrossRef] [PubMed]

41. Kessner, D.; Chambers, M.; Burke, R.; Agus, D.; Mallick, P. ProteoWizard: Open source software for rapid proteomics tools development. *Bioinformatics* **2008**, *24*, 2534–2536. [CrossRef] [PubMed]
42. Smith, C.A.; Want, E.J.; O'Maille, G.; Abagyan, R.; Siuzdak, G. XCMS: Processing mass spectrometry data for metabolite profiling using nonlinear peak alignment, matching, and identification. *Anal. Chem.* **2006**, *78*, 779–787. [CrossRef] [PubMed]
43. Giacomoni, F.; Le Corguillé, G.; Monsoor, M.; Landi, M.; Pericard, P.; Pétéra, M.; Duperier, C.; Tremblay-Franco, M.; Martin, J.F.; Jacob, D.; et al. Workflow4Metabolomics: A collaborative research infrastructure for computational metabolomics. *Bioinformatics* **2014**, *31*, 1493–1495. [CrossRef] [PubMed]
44. Kuhl, C.; Tautenhahn, R.; Bottcher, C.; Larson, T.R.; Neumann, S. CAMERA: An integrated strategy for compound spectra extraction and annotation of liquid chromatography/mass spectrometry data sets. *Anal. Chem.* **2011**, *84*, 283–289. [CrossRef] [PubMed]
45. Van Der Kloet, F.M.; Bobeldijk, I.; Verheij, E.R.; Jellema, R.H. Analytical error reduction using single point calibration for accurate and precise metabolomic phenotyping. *J. Prot. Res.* **2009**, *8*, 5132–5141. [CrossRef] [PubMed]
46. Dunn, W.B.; Broadhurst, D.; Begley, P.; Zelena, E.; Francis-McIntyre, S.; Anderson, N.; Brown, M.; Knowles, J.D.; Halsall, A.; Haselden, J.N.; et al. Procedures for large-scale metabolic profiling of serum and plasma using gas chromatography and liquid chromatography coupled to mass spectrometry. *Nat. Protoc.* **2011**, *6*, 1060. [CrossRef] [PubMed]
47. Ferchaud-Roucher, V.; Croyal, M.; Krempf, M.; Ouguerram, K. Plasma lipidome characterization using UHPLC-HRMS and ion mobility of hypertriglyceridemic patients on nicotinic acid. *Atherosclerosis* **2015**, *241*, e123–e124. [CrossRef]
48. Van den Berg, R.A.; Hoefsloot, H.C.; Westerhuis, J.A.; Smilde, A.K.; van der Werf, M.J. Centering, scaling, and transformations: Improving the biological information content of metabolomics data. *BMC Genom.* **2006**, *7*, 142. [CrossRef] [PubMed]
49. El Ghaziri, A.; Qannari El, M.; Moyon, T.; Alexandre-Gouabau, M.-C. ANOVA-PLS: A new method for the analysis of multivariate data depending on several factors. *Electron. J. Appl. Stat. Anal.* **2015**, *8*, 214–235. [CrossRef]
50. Henrion, R. N-way principal component analysis theory; algorithms and applications. *Chemometr. Intell. Lab.* **1994**, *25*, 1–23. [CrossRef]
51. Westerhuis, J.A.; Kourti, T.; MacGregor, J.F. Analysis of multiblock and hierarchical PCA and PLS models. *J. Chemometr.* **1998**, *12*, 301–321. [CrossRef]
52. Simon, L.; Frondas-Chauty, A.; Senterre, T.; Flamant, C.; Darmaun, D.; Rozé, J.C. Determinants of body composition in preterm infants at the time of hospital discharge. *Am. J. Clin. Nutr.* **2014**, *100*, 98–104. [CrossRef] [PubMed]
53. Steward, D.K.; Pridham, K.F. Growth patterns of extremely low-birth-weight hospitalized preterm infants. *J. Obstet. Gynaecol. Neonat. Nurs.* **2002**, *31*, 57–65. [CrossRef]
54. Sprenger, N.; De Castro, C.A.; Steenhout, P.; Thakkar, S.K. Longitudinal change of selected human milk oligosaccharides and association to infants' growth, an observatory, single center, longitudinal cohort study. *PLoS ONE* **2017**, *12*, e0171814. [CrossRef] [PubMed]
55. Lynch, C.J.; Adams, S.H. Branched-chain amino acids in metabolic signalling and insulin resistance. *Nat. Rev. Endocrinol.* **2014**, *10*, 723. [CrossRef] [PubMed]
56. De Luca, A.; Hankard, R.; Alexandre-Gouabau, M.C.; Ferchaud-Roucher, V.; Darmaun, D.; Boquien, C.Y. Higher concentrations of branched-chain amino acids in breast milk of obese mothers. *Nutr. J.* **2016**, *32*, 1295–1298. [CrossRef] [PubMed]
57. McCormack, S.E.; Shaham, O.; McCarthy, M.A.; Deik, A.A.; Wang, T.J.; Gerszten, R.E.; Clish, C.B.; Mootha, V.K.; Grinspoon, S.K.; Fleischman, A. Circulating branched-chain amino acid concentrations are associated with obesity and future insulin resistance in children and adolescents. *Pediatr. Obes.* **2013**, *8*, 52–61. [CrossRef] [PubMed]
58. Kirchberg, F.F.; Harder, U.; Weber, M.; Grote, V.; Demmelmair, H.; Peissner, W.; Rzehak, P.; Xhonneux, A.; Carlier, C.; Ferre, N.; et al. Dietary protein intake affects amino acid and acylcarnitine metabolism in infants aged 6 months. *J. Clin. Endocr. Metab.* **2015**, *100*, 149–158. [CrossRef] [PubMed]
59. Ma, Q.; Hu, S.; Bannai, M.; Wu, G. L-Arginine regulates protein turnover in porcine mammary epithelial cells to enhance milk protein synthesis. *Amino Acids* **2018**, *50*, 621–628. [CrossRef] [PubMed]

60. Kim, S.W.; Wu, G. Regulatory role for amino acids in mammary gland growth and milk synthesis. *Amino Acids* **2009**, *37*, 89–95. [CrossRef] [PubMed]
61. Tan, C.; Zhai, Z.; Ni, X.; Wang, H.; Ji, Y.; Tang, T.; Ren, W.; Long, H.; Deng, B.; Deng, J.; et al. Metabolomic profiles reveal potential factors that correlate with lactation performance in sow milk. *Sci. Rep. UK* **2018**, *8*. [CrossRef] [PubMed]
62. Bode, L. Recent advances on structure; metabolism; and function of human milk oligosaccharides. *J. Nutr.* **2006**, *136*, 2127–2130. [CrossRef] [PubMed]
63. Plaza-Zamora, J.; Sabater-Molina, M.M.; Rodríguez-Palmero, M.; Rivero, M.; Bosch, V.; Nadal, J.M.; Zamora, S.; Larqué, E. Polyamines in human breast milk for preterm and term infants. *Br. J. Nutr.* **2013**, *3*, 1–5. [CrossRef] [PubMed]
64. Shah, P.S.; Shah, V.S.; Kelly, L.E. Arginine supplementation for prevention of necrotising enterocolitis in preterm infants. *Cochrane Database Syst. Rev.* **2017**. [CrossRef] [PubMed]
65. Blazquez, A.M.; Cives-Losada, C.; Iglesia, A.; Marin, J.J.; Monte, M.J. Lactation during cholestasis: Role of ABC proteins in bile acid traffic across the mammary gland. *Sci. Rep. UK* **2017**, *7*, 7475. [CrossRef] [PubMed]
66. Luan, H.; Liu, L.F.; Tang, Z.; Zhang, M.; Chua, K.K.; Song, J.X.; Mok, V.C.; Li, M.; Cai, Z. Comprehensive urinary metabolomic profiling and identification of potential noninvasive marker for idiopathic Parkinson's disease. *Sci. Rep. UK* **2015**, *5*. [CrossRef] [PubMed]
67. Puchalska, P.; Crawford, P.A. Multi-dimensional roles of ketone bodies in fuel metabolism; signaling; and therapeutics. *Cell Metab.* **2017**, *25*, 262–284. [CrossRef] [PubMed]
68. Dingess, K.A.; Valentine, C.J.; Ollberding, N.J.; Davidson, B.S.; Woo, J.G.; Summer, S.; Peng, Y.M.; Guerrero, M.L.; Ruiz-Palacios, G.M.; Ran-Ressler, R.R.; et al. Branched-chain fatty acid composition of human milk and the impact of maternal diet: The Global Exploration of Human Milk (GEHM) Study. *Am. J. Clin. Nutr.* **2016**, *105*, 177–184. [CrossRef] [PubMed]
69. Ran-Ressler, R.R.; Khailova, L.; Arganbright, K.M.; Adkins-Rieck, C.K.; Jouni, Z.E.; Koren, O.; Ley, R.E.; Brenna, J.T.; Dvorak, B. Branched chain fatty acids reduce the incidence of necrotizing enterocolitis and alter gastrointestinal microbial ecology in a neonatal rat model. *PLoS ONE* **2011**, *6*. [CrossRef] [PubMed]
70. Wongtangtintharn, S.; Oku, H.; Iwasaki, H.; TODA, T. Effect of branched-chain fatty acids on fatty acid biosynthesis of human breast cancer cells. *J. Nutr. Sci. Vitaminol.* **2004**, *50*, 137–143. [CrossRef]
71. Vlaeminck, B.; Fievez, V.; Cabrita, A.R.J.; Fonseca, A.J.M.; Dewhurst, R.J. Factors affecting odd-and branched-chain fatty acids in milk: A review. *Anim. Feed Sci. Tech.* **2006**, *131*, 389–417. [CrossRef]
72. Jenkins, B.; West, J.; Koulman, A. A review of odd-chain fatty acid metabolism and the role of pentadecanoic acid (C15: 0) and heptadecanoic acid (C17: 0) in health and disease. *Molecules* **2015**, *20*, 2425–2444. [CrossRef] [PubMed]
73. Gill, B.D.; Indyk, H.E. Development and application of a liquid chromatographic method for analysis of nucleotides and nucleosides in milk and infant formulas. *Int. Dairy J.* **2007**, *17*, 596–605. [CrossRef]
74. Gianni, M.L.; Roggero, P.; Mosca, F. Human milk protein vs. formula protein and their use in preterm infants. *Cur. Opin. Clin. Nutr.* **2019**, *22*. [CrossRef] [PubMed]
75. Zeisel, S.H. Choline: Critical role during fetal development and dietary requirements in adults. *Annu. Rev. Nutr.* **2006**, *26*, 229–250. [CrossRef] [PubMed]
76. Newburg, D.S.; Morelli, L. Human milk and infant intestinal mucosal glycans guide succession of the neonatal intestinal microbiota. *Pediatr. Res.* **2015**, *77*, 115–120. [CrossRef] [PubMed]

2

Fat Loss in Continuous Enteral Feeding of the Preterm Infant: How Much, What and When is it Lost?

Carlos Zozaya [1,*], Alba García-Serrano [2], Javier Fontecha [2], Lidia Redondo-Bravo [3], Victoria Sánchez-González [1], María Teresa Montes [1] and Miguel Saenz de Pipaón [1,4]

1 Neonatology Department, La Paz University Hospital, Autonomous University of Madrid, 28046 Madrid, Spain; vickysg85@hotmail.com (V.S.-G.); maitemontesb@gmail.com (M.T.M.); miguel.saenz@salud.madrid.org (M.S.d.P.)

2 Bioactivity and Food Analysis Department, Institute of Food Science Research (CIAL, CSIC-UAM), Autonomous University of Madrid, 28049 Madrid, Spain; albamaria.garcia.serrano@csic.es (A.G.-S.) j.fontecha@csic.es (J.F.)

3 Preventive Medicine and Public Health Department, La Paz University Hospital, Autonomous University of Madrid, 28046 Madrid, Spain; lidiaredondobravo@gmail.com

4 Carlos III Health Institute, Maternal and Child Health and Development Research Network, 48903 Barakaldo, Bizkaia, Spain

* Correspondence: czozayan@gmail.com

Abstract: Human milk fat is a concentrated source of energy and provides essential and long chain polyunsaturated fatty acids. According to previous experiments, human milk fat is partially lost during continuous enteral nutrition. However, these experiments were done over relatively short infusion times, and a complete profile of the lost fatty acids was never measured. Whether this loss happens considering longer infusion times or if some fatty acids are lost more than others remain unknown. Pooled breast milk was infused through a feeding tube by a peristaltic pump over a period of 30 min and 4, 12 and 24 h at 2 mL/h. Adsorbed fat was extracted from the tubes, and the fatty acid composition was analyzed by gas chromatography-mass spectrometry. Total fat loss (average fatty acid loss) after 24 h was $0.6 \pm 0.1\%$. Total fat loss after 24 h infusion was $0.6 \pm 0.1\%$ of the total fat infused, although the highest losses occur in the first 30 min of infusion ($13.0 \pm 1.6\%$). Short-medium chain (0.7%, $p = 0.15$), long chain (0.6%, $p = 0.56$), saturated (0.7%, $p = 0.4$), monounsaturated (0.5%, $p = 0.15$), polyunsaturated fatty (0.7%, $p = 0.15$), linoleic (0.7%, $p = 0.25$), and docosahexaenoic acids (0.6%, $p = 0.56$) were not selectively adsorbed to the tube. However, very long chain fatty (0.9%, $p = 0.04$), alpha-linolenic (1.6%, $p = 0.02$) and arachidonic acids (1%, $p = 0.02$) were selectively adsorbed and, therefore, lost in a greater proportion than other fatty acids. In all cases, the magnitude of the loss was clinically low.

Keywords: preterm infant; enteral nutrition; lipids; omega-3 fatty acids; omega-6 fatty acids; Docosahexaenoic acid; Arachidonic acid; long-chain polyunsaturated fatty acids

---

1. Introduction

Fat is an important nutrient for preterm infants [1]. Lipids provide infants most of their energy needs. Lipids also offer specific supplies critical for growth and development like long and very long chain polyunsaturated fatty acids (LCPUFA) including essential fatty acids (Alpha-linolenic and Linoleic acids) and their main derivatives: Docosahexaenoic acid (DHA) and Arachidonic acid (ARA). DHA and ARA seem to be semi-essential for the preterm infant [2]. Both are major components of the brain, and retinal cell membranes and might be related to neurodevelopment and visual function. In case of an early deficit of these fatty acids, there is an increased risk of prevalent preterm morbidities, like sepsis and bronchopulmonary dysplasia [3]. Unfortunately, this early deficit might be common, as current nutritional practices (early parenteral nutrition, with lipid emulsions not designed specifically for the preterm infant) do not deliver the same amount of LCPUFA than a fetus of the same gestational ages would receive in-utero [4].

Human milk (HM) is the recommended diet for all infants, including very low birth weight (VLBW) infants. For the latter, HM is usually delivered via an enteral feeding tube until the preterm infant can be fed orally. Continuous enteral feeding is used in the neonatal intensive care unit as an alternative to bolus/gavage feeding in some clinical scenarios (e.g., enteral intolerance or persistent hypoglycemia) [5]. In 1978, Brooke and Barley reported for the first time that human milk fat delivery was reduced when milk was continuously infused [6]. During the 80's and 90's different authors had similar results, reporting total fat losses up to 90% after 8 h of infusion of freshly collected human milk [7]. To limit fat loss, several strategies have been tested (higher infusion flow rates, syringe angulation, milk refrigeration, use of eccentric nozzle syringes, use of peristaltic syringe pumps, previous and frequent milk homogenization, etc.). These interventions proved to be useful to a certain degree [7–13]. However, concern about fat loss during continuous enteral nutrition is a recurrent issue that still appears to be a problem. Recent research studies have reported total fat losses between 4 and 25% [13–16]. Whether fat loss is important enough to be clinically relevant in real conditions remains to be clarified. It is important to note that the infusion time of all these studies has been shorter than 8 h, whereas feeding tubes are usually used for longer times in real conditions. Previous reports suggested that lipid losses were not constant over time, but timing of the greater losses (at the beginning of the infusion or later on) is still a controversial issue [6,15,17,18]. Moreover, there are other aspects related to fat loss during continuous enteral nutrition that have not yet been investigated. To date, most reports have focused on total fat losses or have only described what happens to lipid fractions (i.e., triglycerides), but we have no data on possible different losses of individual fatty acids depending on fatty acid characteristics (i.e., chain length or degree of unsaturation). Not all fatty acids have the same biological functions, and some of them are essential in humans or semi-essential for the preterm infant.

We conducted an in vitro experiment, which mirrors in vivo current clinical practice, over a 24-h period. Our objectives were: (1) to determine whether fat losses are constant over the infusion time and, if not, when they are more pronounced over the 24-h period; and (2) to test whether there is a selective loss of individual or groups of fatty acids depending on chain length and degree of unsaturation.

2. Materials and Methods

Pooled donor, non-pasteurized HM (1100 mL) was used in this experiment. The HM used in this experiment was progressively collected and was kept frozen for a mean period of 2.5 months (range 1.9–4.7) at −20 °C. It was defrosted before the experiment keeping the sample in refrigeration conditions (5 °C) over 24 h.

The experiment reproduced our standard clinical practices. HM was infused through a 4-French diameter and 40-cm polyvinyl chloride (PVC) di-(2-ethylhexyl) phthalate (DEHP)-free feeding tube (Nutrisafe 2, Vygon, Écouen, France) attached to a PVC system 150 cm in length and 1.5 × 2.5 mm in diameter (Nutrisafe 2, Vygon) by a peristaltic pump (Alaris Enteral, CareFusion, San Diego, CA, USA). The feeding tube and part of the attached system were inside an incubator (Incubator 8000 SC Dräger, Lübeck, Germany). The incubator was set at 33 °C and 60% humidity. The syringe, pump and the rest of the connecting systems were outside the incubator. Average room temperature was 23.8 °C (range 22.7–24.7 °C), and the humidity was 36.9% (range 35–39%). The entire experiment was done within the same 24 h. HM was loaded into 20-mL syringes for enteral nutrition. Then the syringe was hand shaken to homogenize the milk and placed in the pump, with the syringe maintained in a vertical position (tip upwards). Infusions then were programmed at 2 mL/h. When infusion finished, feeding tubes and systems were washed with a distilled water bolus (5 mL) to remove the remaining milk. Then, the feeding tubes and connecting systems were collected and immediately stored at −20 °C.

This whole procedure was repeated infusing milk over 30 min, 4, 12 and 24 h, in quadruplicate for each infusion time. To reproduce a real 12 and 24-h infusion, both the HM and the syringes were changed every 4 h. The pooled HM was kept refrigerated (5 °C) during the experiment day. Aliquots (20 mL) were extracted and then left at room temperature for 30 min before filling the syringes, to warm the HM, according to our standard practice. Pre-infusion HM samples were collected at time zero, and at 12 and 24 h from the beginning of the experiment. Following collection, the milk samples were stored at −20 °C.

2.1. Total Fat Extraction and GC-MS Analysis

The milk fat adsorbed inside the tubes was extracted using high-performance liquid chromatography-grade hexane as a solvent. More commonly used extraction solutions, such as chloroform 2/methanol 1 (Folch) and hexane/isopropanol (Hara and Radin), were initially used, but they extracted silicones from the tube's inner surfaces, contaminating the sample and raising concerns about chromatogram reliability. We subsequently verified that hexane allows extraction of the total fat, given no compounds of dairy fatty acids were detected at the retention times when the tubes were ultimately washed according to the Folch [19] or the Hara and Radin method [20]. Blank control tubes ($n = 3$) were washed with the same solvent but without having passed any milk.

The lipid extracts obtained were concentrated by removing the organic solvent under a gentle stream of nitrogen. Then, the lipid extracts were weighed and analyzed as fatty acid methyl esters (FAMEs) obtained by direct derivatization of samples, as described by Castro-Gómez et al. [21]. Briefly, lipid extracts were transferred to borosilicate glass tubes with an acid/heat resistant cap containing 100 µL of tritridecanoin in hexane as internal standard (1.3 mg/mL). Then, 1 mL of 3 M H_2SO_4 in methanol was added to each tube and heated for 30 min at 98 °C. After incubation, the samples were cooled in ice for 5 min, and 1 mL of hexane was added. The samples were vortexed for 30 s, and the reaction was then stopped with 7.5 mL of 6% solution of sodium hydrogen carbonate and centrifuged at 1000× *g*, at 4 °C, for 5 min. The upper organic layer containing the FAME was collected and transferred to amber vials for GC–MS injection and 1 µL (at 1:10 split ratio) was injected into a 6890 Agilent gas chromatograph (Palo Alto, CA, USA) fitted with a mass spectrometry (MS) (Agilent 5973 N) detector in a 100-m CPSil-88 capillary column (100 m × 0.25 mm inner diameter × 0.2 µm film thickness (Chrompack, Middelburg, The Netherlands). The GC-MS temperature program and conditions were those previously reported by Rodriguez-Alcala and Fontecha [22]. Briefly, the column was maintained at 100 °C for 1 min after injection and temperature-programmed at 7 °C/min to 170 °C, maintained there for 55 min, and then raised 10 °C/min to 230 °C and maintained there for 33 min. The injector temperature was set at 250 °C. Helium was used as carrier gas with a column inlet pressure of 30 psi. MS detector conditions were a transfer line temperature of 250 °C, a source temperature of 230 °C, a quad temperature of 150 °C and electron impact ionization at 70 eV. For peak identification, mass spectra obtained in our analysis were compared with those in the National Institute of Standards and Technology Library (Gaithersburg, MD, USA). For the qualitative and quantitative analyses, response factors were calculated using anhydrous milk fat (reference material BCR-164) and Supelco 37 FAME mix (Sigma, St. Louis, MO, USA). Tritridecanoin as internal standard (200 µL; 1.3 mg/mL) was also used. Assays were performed in triplicate.

Losses of total fat and fatty acids at each time point were expressed as percentages of the total infused amount recovered from the tube. Percentages were calculated according to the formula:

$$\% \text{ Loss} = R \times 100/(C \times V), \tag{1}$$

where "R" stands for the raw amount of fatty acid / total fat (mg) recovered from the tube, "C" means milk's fatty acid concentration (mg/mL) and "V" is the volume infused through the tube over the set time (1 mL over 30 min, 8, 24 and 48 mL over 4, 12 and 24 h, respectively).

A fatty acid was classified as very-long-chain fatty acid (VLCFA) if it had >18 carbon atoms, long-chain fatty acid (LCFA) when it had 16 or 18 carbon atoms and short-medium chain fatty acid (SMCFA) if it had between 6 and 14 carbon atoms.

2.2. Statistical Analysis

The statistical analysis was performed using SPSS 20 statistical software (IBM Corporation, Armonk, NY, USA). Descriptive data are presented as mean (± standard deviation) and frequency (%) as appropriate. The Mann–Whitney U test was used to calculate median differences between total fat (which is equivalent to mean fatty acid loss) and individual/families of fatty acid rate losses at 24 h. The Kruskal–Wallis rank test was performed to compare median losses among more than two groups according to the fatty acid composition in various time periods (30 min, 4, 12 and 24 h). A selected one-to-one post hoc analysis was performed correcting significance according to the Dunn-Bonferroni method. Losses of total fat (average fatty acid loss) and individual selected fatty acids over time were analyzed with a curvilinear regression model. For these models, we selected the most abundant fatty acids in the HM or those which seem to be more clinically relevant (essential fatty acids and LCPUFA).

2.3. Ethical Issues

The La Paz University Hospital research ethics committee approved the study, and our donors provided informed consent to use their milk for research purposes.

3. Results

The fatty acid composition of the pooled HM used in this study is described in Table 1. Samples were analyzed at time zero, 12 and 24 h on the experiment day to rule out oxidative changes affecting the relative fatty acid composition of the HM before it was infused. There were no statistically significant differences regarding saturated fatty acids (SFA), monounsaturated fatty acids (MUFA) and polyunsaturated fatty acids (PUFA) nor regarding chain length (short-medium, long and very long fatty acids) relative composition. Furthermore, individual LCPUFA: alpha-linolenic acid (ALA), linoleic acid (LNA), DHA and ARA concentrations (mg/100 mg of fat) remained stable throughout the study period of 24 h (differences were not statistically significant).

Table 1. The fatty acid composition of the pooled human milk used in this experiment.

Fatty Acids	mg/100 mg of Fat
6:0	0.2 ± 0.10
8:0	0.3 ± 0.10
10:0	1.4 ± 0.20
12:0	5 ± 0.30
14:0	5.2 ± 0.10
15:0	0.2 ± 0.02
16:0	21.5 ± 0.20
17ai	0.1 ± 0.01
16:1t	0.3 ± 0.03
16:1 n7	1.3 ± 0.10
17:0	0.2 ± 0.02
18:0	8.3 ± 0.20
18:1 n9	40.6 ± 0.30
18:1 n11	1.7 ± 0.10
18:2 n6 (LNA)	11.6 ± 0.20
20:0	0.1 ± 0.02
18:3 n3 (ALA)	0.3 ± 0.05

Table 1. *Cont.*

Fatty Acids	mg/100 mg of Fat
20:1 n9	0.3 ± 0.10
20:3 n6	0.15 ± 0.10
20:4 n6 (ARA)	0.2 ± 0.03
22:6 n3 (DHA)	0.25 ± 0.02
Traces (<0.2%)	0.85 ± 0.20
∑SFA	42.6 ± 0.60
∑MUFA	44.8 ± 0.30
∑PUFA	12.5 ± 0.30
∑SMCFA	12.4 ± 0.70
∑LCFA	86.4 ± 0.50
∑VLCFA	1.2 ± 0.20

ALA: α-linolenic acid; LNA: linoleic acid; AA: arachidonic acid; DHA: docosahexaenoic acid; SFA: saturated fatty acid; MUFA: monounsaturated fatty acid; PUFA: polyunsaturated fatty acid; SMCFA: short-medium chain fatty acids; LCFA: long-chain fatty acid, and VLCFA: Very long chain fatty acid.

Over 24 h, the mean total fat loss was 0.6 ± 0.1% of the total fat infused. However, fat loss was not constant. The highest fat losses occur in the first 30 min of infusion (13.0 ± 1.6%) and then fat loss progressively decreased at 4 and 12 h to 2% ± 0.4% and 0.87% ± 0.04%, respectively ($R^2 = 0.98$; $p < 0.0001$) (Figure 1).

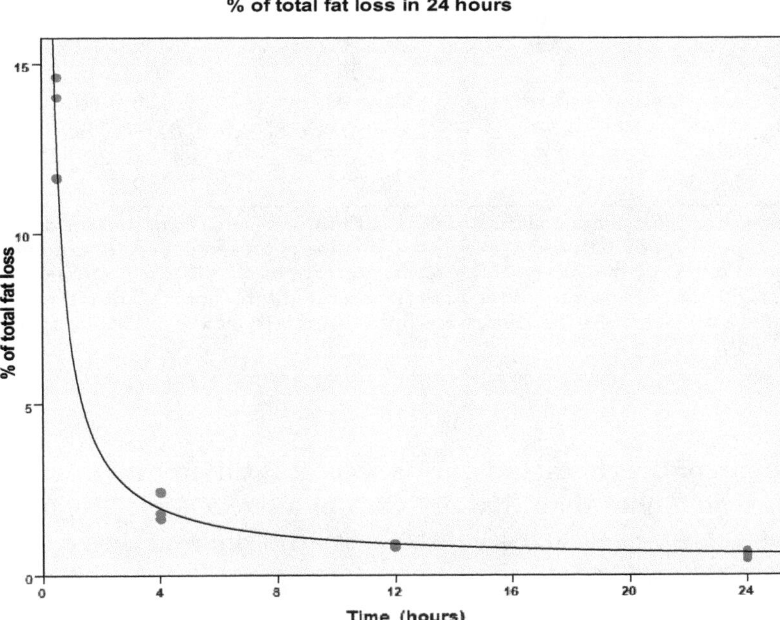

Figure 1. Amount of the total fat loss as % of the fat adsorbed in the tube in relation with the total fat infused during 24 h.

Fatty acids were lost in different percentages, at different time points, according to the degree of unsaturation of the fatty acid chain (Table 2). Saturated fatty acids were lost in a higher proportion than monounsaturated fatty acids at 30 min (30.6% vs. 5.8%, $p = 0.01$) and 12 h of infusion (1.1% vs. 0.6%, $p = 0.02$), whereas we found no differences when comparing saturated or monounsaturated with polyunsaturated fatty acids. At 24 h, there were no significant differences among the three groups.

Table 2. Percentage of fatty acid loss (% of the total amount of FA initially infused that was recovered from the tube after the infusion time).

Fatty Acid	30 min	4 h	12 h	24 h
6:0	80.4 ± 13.2	8.3 ± 2.90	2.0 ± 0.30	1.2 ± 0.20
8:0	26.4 ± 0.60	4.5 ± 0.80	1.7 ± 0.10	1.1 ± 0.30
10:0	23.8 ± 8.20	5.5 ± 1.10	2.4 ± 0.40	1.5 ± 0.40
12:0	9.5 ± 1.80	2.4 ± 0.60	1.1 ± 0.10	0.8 ± 0.10
14:0	9.0 ± 0.01	1.3 ± 0.40	0.5 ± 0.10	0.4 ± 0.10
15:0	13.6 ± 3.80	2.0 ± 0.50	0.6 ± 0.20	0.4 ± 0.10
16:0	24.0 ± 1.60	2.9 ± 0.40	1.0 ± 0.10	0.6 ± 0.10
16:1 n7	8.0 ± 2.00	2.1 ± 0.80	1.1 ± 0.10	0.8 ± 0.20
17:0	23.4 ± 2.00	2.8 ± 0.50	1 ± 0.10	0.6 ± 0.10
18:0	31.4 ± 2.10	3.5 ± 0.60	1.2 ± 0.10	0.7 ± 0.10
18:1 n9	5.6 ± 1.80	1.3 ± 0.50	0.6 ± 0.10	0.5 ± 0.10
18:1 n11	4.7 ± 2.00	1.1 ± 0.50	0.5 ± 0.10	0.4 ± 0.10
18:2 n6 (LNA)	7 ± 2.10	1.8 ± 0.70	0.9 ± 0.10	0.7 ± 0.10
18:3 n3 (ALA)	10.5 ± 2.60	3.8 ± 1.80	2.2 ± 0.30	1.6 ± 0.30
20:0	64.4 ± 5.20	10.2 ± 2.10	3.4 ± 0.50	2.1 ± 0.60
20:3 n6	9.5 ± 4.20	2.5 ± 1.00	1.3 ± 0.20	0.9 ± 0.10
20:4 n6 (ARA)	11.6 ± 3.60	3.0 ± 1.00	1.5 ± 0.20	1.0 ± 0.20
22:6 n3 (DHA)	8.4 ± 2.10	1.6 ± 0.80	0.8 ± 0.20	0.6 ± 0.10
ΣSFA	30.6 ± 2.60a	2.9 ± 0.40	1.1 ± 0.10b	0.7 ± 0.10
ΣMUFA	5.8 ± 1.30a	1.3 ± 0.50	0.6 ± 0.10b	0.5 ± 0.10
ΣPUFA	7.5 ± 2.00	1.9 ± 0.70	1.0 ± 0.10	0.7 ± 0.10
p-value *	0.015	0.06	0.02	0.08
ΣSMCFA	13.8 ± 6.10	2.4 ± 0.50	1.0 ± 0.10	0.7 ± 0.10
ΣLCFA	14 ± 4.50	2.0 ± 0.40c	0.8 ± 0.01d	0.6 ± 0.10e
ΣVLCFA	23.5 ± 2.50	3.7 ± 0.50c	1.4 ± 0.20d	0.9 ± 0.20e
p-value *	0.09	0.02	0.007	0.04

Results are expressed as mean % ± standard deviation. Distributions were compared for degree of unsaturation and length chain at every time point by Kruskal-Wallis test (* *p*-value is presented). A, b, c, d and e, indicate significant differences in the one to one post-hoc analysis (Dunn-Bonferroni test). ALA: α-linolenic acid; LNA: linoleic acid; AA: arachidonic acid; DHA: docosahexaenoic acid; SFA: saturated fatty acid; MUFA: monounsaturated fatty acid; PUFA: polyunsaturated fatty acid; SMCFA: short-medium chain fatty acids; LCFA: long-chain fatty acid; VLCFA: Very long chain fatty acid.

Regarding the length of the chain, fatty acids were lost differently from 4 h of infusion onwards (Table 2). VLCFA loss was higher than that of LCFA at 4 h (3.7% vs. 2%, $p = 0.02$), at 12 h (1.4% vs. 0.8%, $p = 0.005$) and, at 24 h (0.9% vs. 0.6%, $p = 0.03$). We did not find differences between VLCFA and SMCFA or between SMCFA and LCFA at any time.

We also studied the loss of some individual fatty acids. The most abundant fatty acids in the HM (16:0 and 18:1n-9) or those which are especially relevant for the preterm infant (essential fatty acids—LNA and ALA—and their derivatives DHA and ARA) were selected. Total fat loss after 24 h was considered as a reference. Some fatty acids were not lost in a higher proportion than total fat, as in the cases of 18:1n-9 (0.5% ± 0.1%, $p = 0.15$), LNA (0.7% ± 0.1%, $p = 0.25$) and DHA (0.6% ± 0.1%, $p = 0.56$). However, in other cases, losses of some fatty acids were significantly greater than total fat loss, as with ALA (1.6% ± 0.3%, $p = 0.02$) and ARA (1% ± 0.2%, $p = 0.02$). In all cases, the magnitude of the loss was small after 24 h (Table 2). In Table 3 we presented curvilinear regression models predicting losses after 24 h of these selected fatty acids.

Table 3. Curvilinear regression models to predict loss of some selected fatty acids after 24 h of HM infusion. ALA: α-linolenic acid; LNA: linoleic acid; AA: arachidonic acid; DHA: docosahexaenoic acid.

Fatty Acids	Coefficient of Determination (R^2)	Curvilinear Model Equation	*p*-Value
16:0	0.99	$y = -0.007 + 11.98/x$	<0.0001
18:1 n9	0.86	$y = 0.477 + 2.562/x$	<0.0001
18:2 n6 (LNA)	0.87	$y = 0.732 + 3.143/x$	<0.0001
18:3 n3 (ALA)	0.85	$y = 1.969 + 4.285/x$	<0.0001
20:4 n6 (ARA)	0.87	$y = 1.177 + 5.257/x$	<0.0001
22:6 n3 (DHA)	0.92	$y = 0.494 + 3.985/x$	<0.0001

4. Discussion

How much HM fat is lost during continuous enteral feeding, and when this loss occurs during the infusion, is controversial. In addition, there are no data in the literature about what is exactly lost, in terms of individual fatty acid losses. To answer these questions, we have introduced three different elements in our experimental design, compared to previous studies:

4.1. Our Total Experiment Time Was Longer (up to 24 h of Infusion), Although We Still Included Intermediate Times

Our first objective was to determine whether the previously reported fat losses percentages could be related, at least to a certain degree, with the duration of the experiments. Some authors have suggested losses were higher only after 4 h [17] or even after 8 h of infusion [18]. However, another recent article suggested that losses appear to be higher at the beginning of the infusion [15], although the experiments in that particular study did not last more than 60 min. Our results are consistent with this last report and show that the duration of the feeding affects overall fat delivery efficiency. Significant fat loss in the first 30 min of infusion suggests that binding sites in the tubes become saturated at the beginning of the infusion. Later, percentage of fat loss is smaller maybe because there are not as many available binding sites. Thus, after some time of infusion, fat delivery efficiency increases, even though infusion flow velocity remains the same. Experiment duration has varied in previous studies but, to our knowledge, it has never been longer than 8 h. However, feeding tubes are changed every 48–72 h in real practice [23]. Thus, we designed a study over a 24-h period to mimic longer infusion times, which is closer to actual practices. We did not prolong to 48–72 h to avoid potential fatty acid oxidation of the breast milk during the experiment. As we used the same pooled milk during the whole experiment, fatty acid oxidation could have limited our conclusions, because the pre-infusion milk would have become somewhat "different" during the experiment. We can assure that in our case this change in the milk fatty acid composition did not occur because the milk fatty acid profile remained unchanged at time zero, mid and end of the study day. The velocity of milk flow is another important factor associated with fat loss. The lower the velocity, the higher the losses [24]. We chose a very slow flow (2 mL/h) to reproduce a worse-case-possible real scenario (less than 2 mL/h would represent trophic feeds for many preterm infants). However, we adhered to the best standard of care, and we also implemented some proven preventive measures: an upward tip position and gentle homogenization of the milk before infusion, to minimize the loss as we would do in our patients [8,13].

4.2. Direct Measurement of Adhered Fat to Nasogastric Tubes Instead of a Pre- and Post-Infused Milk Analysis

We recovered the fat remaining in the tube after the HM infusion and then, we determined the fatty acid composition on these samples. On the other hand, in previous studies, the milk coming out of the tubes was collected and then, the percentage of fat lost was calculated knowing the composition of the milk going in. We believe direct determination is more accurate than calculation. Moreover, we have proved this method is feasible. So far, no clinical studies involving real patients have been done. Therefore, the ultimate clinical relevance of fat loss during continuous enteral nutrition has never been reported. Our method could be used in future clinical studies, to measure fat loss affecting real patients, collecting feeding tubes after having been used in real patients, instead of recreating clinical practices in experimental conditions. Doing so, we could eventually relate fat losses with clinical outcomes.

4.3. Outcome Variables (not only Total Fat but also Individual Fatty Acids)

To our knowledge, this is the first report of the fatty acid composition of HM fat loss during continuous enteral nutrition. We speculate that the more fluid a fatty acid, the more easily it flows through the tube. Saturated and longer chain fatty acids were the more retained fatty acids over short infusion times (which would be the beginning of the continuous infusion in a real patient). This finding could be related to the fatty acid structure, which determines its fluidity [25]. Unsaturated fatty acids have lower melting points than saturated fatty acids of the same length. In other words, saturated fatty acids are less fluid. Also, the longer a fatty acid is, the less its fluidity.

This study has some limitations. We only measured fat adhered to the feeding and connecting tubes but not to the syringes. Nevertheless, the capacity of the syringe is greater, and contact between the milk and binding sites of its surface is less likely, so we think its effect would be neglectable. Only one flow rate (2 mL/h) was tested. We cannot extrapolate our results directly to other flow speeds. However, we assumed that at higher velocities losses would be less based on previous studies. Finally, we did not run milk for more than 24 h, although feeding tubes are used for longer times before being replaced in real patients. We do not know what the actual fat delivery would be after 48–72 h using the same feeding tube. However, our regression model suggests that as of 12 h of infusion the losses remain somewhat constant and low.

According to our results, the clinical significance of HM fat loss after 24 h of continuous infusion seems to be trivial, both quantitatively and qualitatively. When fat is oxidized, every gram of it produces 9 kcal. Considering our results, if an infant is fed 120–150 mL/kg/day in continuous enteral infusion, fat loss would mean 0.2–0.3 kcal/kg/day. This represents around 0.2–0.25% of the total caloric intake recommended for a preterm infant on enteral nutrition. Regarding quality does not seem to be clinically significant either. As stated previously, LCPUFA delivery to the preterm infant is insufficient following current nutritional recommendations [26]; but this problem does not appear to be worsened significantly by additional fat losses during continuous enteral nutrition. Mean HM fat content is 3.2 g–3.6 g/100 mL [27]. Worldwide, DHA and ARA fatty acids represent 0.32% $\pm$ 0.22% and 0.47% $\pm$ 0.13% of HM fat, respectively [28]. Fetal accretion rates are 95 mg of ARA and 42 mg of DHA per day during the last five weeks of gestation [29]. Thus, losses in continuous enteral feeding over 24-h infusion in a 1.5 kg infant would lead to a daily loss of 0.1–0.15 mg of DHA and 0.3–0.4 mg of ARA.

5. Conclusions

We conclude that continuous enteral feeding over 24 h resulted in no substantial loss of human milk fat. Therefore, feeding over a 24-h period does not appear to be a barrier to the delivery of fatty acids, including DHA and ARA fatty acids.

Author Contributions: C.Z., J.F. and M.S.d.P. conceptualized the study; C.Z., V.S.-G. and M.T.M. performed the experiment and collected the samples; A.G.-S. and J.F. did the laboratory determinations; L.R.-B. work on the statistical analysis; C.Z. drafted the manuscript, which was critically reviewed by the rest of the authors.

Acknowledgments: We thank the technician Javier Megino and all Hospital La Paz NICU nurses and auxiliary nurses for their valuable assistance. We also thank the mothers who donate the milk to conduct this research.

References

1. Agostoni, C.; Buonocore, G.; Carnielli, V.P.; De Curtis, M.; Darmaun, D.; Decsi, T.; Domellöf, M.; Embleton, N.D.; Fusch, C.; Genzel-Boroviczeny, O.; et al. Enteral nutrient supply for preterm infants: Commentary from the European Society of Paediatric Gastroenterology, Hepatology and Nutrition Committee on Nutrition. *J. Pediatr. Gastroenterol. Nutr.* **2010**, *50*, 85–91. [CrossRef] [PubMed]
2. Martin, C.R. Fatty acid requirements in preterm infants and their role in health and disease. *Clin. Perinatol.* **2014**, *41*, 363–382. [CrossRef] [PubMed]
3. Martin, C.R.; Dasilva, D.A.; Cluette-Brown, J.E.; Dimonda, C.; Hamill, A.; Bhutta, A.Q.; Coronel, E.; Wilschanski, M.; Stephens, A.J.; Driscoll, D.F.; et al. Decreased postnatal docosahexaenoic and arachidonic acid blood levels in premature infants are associated with neonatal morbidities. *J. Pediatr.* **2011**, *159*, 743–749. [CrossRef] [PubMed]
4. Lapillonne, A.; Eleni Dit Trolli, S.; Kermorvant-Duchemin, E. Postnatal docosahexaenoic acid deficiency is an inevitable consequence of current recommendations and practice in preterm infants. *Neonatology* **2010**, *98*, 397–403. [CrossRef] [PubMed]
5. Klingenberg, C.; Embleton, N.D.; Jacobs, S.E.; O'Connell, L.A.F.; Kuschel, C.A. Enteral feeding practices in very preterm infants: An international survey. *Arch. Dis. Child.* **2012**, *97*, F56–F61. [CrossRef] [PubMed]
6. Brooke, O.; Barley, J. Loss of energy during continuous infusions of breast milk. *Arch. Dis. Child.* **1978**, *53*, 344–345. [CrossRef] [PubMed]
7. Lavine, M.; Clark, R.M. The effect of short-term refrigeration of milk and addition of breast milk fortifier on the delivery of lipids during tube feeding. *J. Pediatr. Gastroenterol. Nutr.* **1989**, *8*, 496–499. [CrossRef] [PubMed]
8. Spencer, S.A.; Hull, D. Fat content of expressed breast milk: A case for quality control. *Br. Med. J.* **1981**, *282*, 99–100. [CrossRef]
9. Narayanan, I.; Singh, B.; Harvey, D. Fat loss during feeding of human milk. *Arch. Dis. Child.* **1984**, *59*, 475–477. [CrossRef] [PubMed]
10. Greer, F.R.; McCormick, A.; Loker, J. Changes in fat concentration of human milk during delivery by intermittent bolus and continuous mechanical pump infusion. *J. Pediatr.* **1984**, *105*, 745–749. [CrossRef]
11. Martinez, F.E.; Desai, I.D.; Davidson, A.G.; Nakai, S.R.A. Ultrasonic homogenization of expressed human milk to prevent fat loss during tube feeding. *J. Pediatr. Gastroenterol. Nutr.* **1987**, *6*, 593–597. [CrossRef] [PubMed]
12. Rayol, M.R.S.; Martinez, F.E.; Jorge, S.M.; Goncalves, A.L.; Desai, I.D. Feeding premature infants banked human milk homogenized by ultrasonic treatment. *J. Pediatr.* **1993**, *123*, 985–988. [CrossRef]
13. García-Lara, N.R.; Escuder-Vieco, D.; Alonso Díaz, C.; Vázquez Román, S.; De la Cruz-Bértolo, J.; Pallás-Alonso, C.R. Type of Homogenization and Fat Loss during Continuous Infusion of Human Milk. *J. Hum. Lact.* **2014**, *30*, 436–441. [CrossRef] [PubMed]
14. Igawa, M.; Murase, M.; Mizuno, K.; Itabashi, K. Is fat content of human milk decreased by infusion? *Pediatr. Int.* **2014**, *56*, 230–233. [CrossRef] [PubMed]
15. Tabata, M.; Abdelrahman, K.; Hair, A.; Hawthorne, K.; Chen, Z.; Abrams, S. Fortifier and Cream Improve Fat Delivery in Continuous Enteral Infant Feeding of Breast Milk. *Nutrients* **2015**, *7*, 1174–1183. [CrossRef] [PubMed]
16. Jarjour, J.; Juarez, A.; Kocak, D.; Liu, N.J.; Tabata, M.M.; Hawthorne, K.M.; Ramos, R.F.; Abrams, S.A. A Novel Approach to Improving Fat Delivery in Neonatal Enteral Feeding. *Nutrients* **2015**, *7*, 5051–5064. [CrossRef] [PubMed]
17. Chan, M.M.; Nohara, M.; Chan, B.R.; Curtis, J.; Chan, G.M. Lecithin decreases human milk fat loss during enteral pumping. *J. Pediatr. Gastroenterol. Nutr.* **2003**, *36*, 613–615. [CrossRef] [PubMed]
18. Lemons, P.M.; Miller, K.; Eitzen, H.; Strodtbeck, F.; Lemons, J.A. Bacterial growth in human milk during continuous feeding. *Am. J. Perinatol.* **1983**, *1*, 76–80. [CrossRef] [PubMed]
19. Folch, J.M.; Lees, S.; Loane, S. A simple method for the isolation and purification of total lipides from animal tissues. *J. Biol. Chem.* **1957**, *226*, 497–509. [PubMed]
20. Hara, A.; Radin, N.S. Lipid extraction of tissues with a low-toxicity solvent. *Anal. Biochem.* **1978**, *90*, 420–426. [CrossRef]

21. Castro-Gómez, P.; Fontecha, J.; Rodríguez-Alcalá, L.M. A high-performance direct transmethylation method for total fatty acids assessment in biological and foodstuff samples. *Talanta* **2014**, *128*, 518–523. [CrossRef] [PubMed]
22. Rodríguez-Alcalá, L.M.; Fontecha, J. Hot topic: Fatty acid and conjugated linoleic acid (CLA) isomer composition of commercial CLA-fortified dairy products: Evaluation after processing and storage. *J. Dairy Sci.* **2007**, *90*, 2083–2090. [CrossRef] [PubMed]
23. Hurrell, E.; Kucerova, E.; Loughlin, M.; Caubilla-Barron, J.; Hilton, A.; Armstrong, R.; Smith, C.; Grant, J.; Shoo, S.; Forsythe, S. Neonatal enteral feeding tubes as loci for colonisation by members of the *Enterobacteriaceae*. *BMC Infect. Dis.* **2009**, *9*, 146. [CrossRef] [PubMed]
24. Mehta, N.R.; Hamosh, M.; Bitman, J.; Wood, D.L. Adherence of medium-chain fatty acids to feeding tubes during gavage feeding of human milk fortified with medium-chain triglycerides. *J. Pediatr.* **1988**, *112*, 474–476. [CrossRef]
25. Mostofsky, D.I.; Yehuda, S.; Salem, N. *Fatty Acids: Physiological and Behavioral Functions*; Humana Press: New York, NY, USA, 2001.
26. Lapillonne, A.; Groh-Wargo, S.; Lozano Gonzalez, C.H.; Uauy, R. Lipid needs of preterm infants: Updated recommendations. *J. Pediatr.* **2013**, *162*, S37–S47. [CrossRef] [PubMed]
27. Ballard, O.; Morrow, A.L. Human Milk Composition. *Pediatr. Clin. N. Am.* **2013**, *60*, 49–74. [CrossRef] [PubMed]
28. Brenna, J.T.; Varamini, B.; Jensen, R.G.; Diersen-Schade, D.A.; Boettcher, J.A.; Arterburn, L.M. Docosahexaenoic and arachidonic acid concentrations in human breast milk worldwide. *Am. J. Clin. Nutr.* **2007**, *85*, 1457–1464. [CrossRef] [PubMed]
29. Kuipers, R.S.; Luxwolda, M.F.; Offringa, P.J.; Rudi Boersma, E.; Dijck-Brouwer, D.A.; Muskiet, F.A. Fetal intrauterine whole body linoleic, arachidonic and docosahexaenoic acid contents and accretion rates. *Prostaglandins Leukot. Essent. Fat. Acids* **2012**, *86*, 13–20. [CrossRef] [PubMed]

3

Factors Associated with Increased Alpha-Tocopherol Content in Milk in Response to Maternal Supplementation with 800 IU of Vitamin E

Amanda de Sousa Rebouças [1], Ana Gabriella Costa Lemos da Silva [2], Amanda Freitas de Oliveira [2], Lorena Thalia Pereira da Silva [2], Vanessa de Freitas Felgueiras [2], Marina Sampaio Cruz [3], Vivian Nogueira Silbiger [3], Karla Danielly da Silva Ribeiro [2,*] and Roberto Dimenstein [1]

1 Department of Biochemistry, Federal University of Rio Grande do Norte, 59078-970 Natal-RN, Brazil; amandasousar2@hotmail.com (A.d.S.R.); rdimenstein@gmail.com (R.D.)
2 Department of Nutrition, Federal University of Rio Grande do Norte, 59078-970 Natal-RN, Brazil; gabriella_lemos_06@yahoo.com.br (A.G.C.L.d.S.); amandda_freitas@outlook.com (A.F.d.O.); lorenathaliaps@gmail.com (L.T.P.d.S.); vanessadffelgueiras@gmail.com (V.d.F.F.)
3 Department of Pharmacy, Federal University of Rio Grande do Norte, 59012-570 Natal-RN, Brazil; marinasmcruz@gmail.com (M.S.C.); viviansilbiger@hotmail.com (V.N.S.)
* Correspondence: karladaniellysr@yahoo.com.br

Abstract: Background: Vitamin E supplementation might represent an efficient strategy to increase the vitamin E content in milk. The present study aimed to evaluate the impact of supplementation with 800 IU RRR-alpha-tocopherol on the alpha-tocopherol content of milk and the factors associated with the increase in vitamin E. Methods: Randomized clinical trial with 79 lactating women from Brazil, who were assigned to the control group, or to the supplemented group (800 IU of RRR-alpha-tocopherol). Milk and serum were collected between 30 and 90 days after delivery (collection 1), and on the next day (collection 2). Alpha-tocopherol was analyzed using high-performance liquid chromatography. Results: In the supplemented group, the alpha-tocopherol content in serum and milk increased after supplementation ($p < 0.001$). In the multivariate analysis, only alpha-tocopherol in milk (collection 1) was associated with the level of this vitamin in milk after supplementation ($\beta = 0.927$, $p < 0.001$), and binary logistic regression showed that the dietary intake was the only determinant for the greater effect of supplementation in milk. Conclusion: The pre-existing vitamin level in milk and diet are determinants for the efficacy of supplementation in milk, suggesting that in populations with vitamin E deficiency, high-dose supplementation can be used to restore its level in milk.

Keywords: clinical trial; lactation; infants; breastfeeding; lactating women

---

1. Introduction

Breast milk contains all the essential nutrients and factors for the growth and development of the infant's gastrointestinal, cerebral and immune system [1,2]. Thus, exclusive breastfeeding is recommended during the first six months of life [3]. Among the vitamins present in milk, vitamin E, is an antioxidant responsible for protecting the lipoproteins and polyunsaturated fatty acids present in the cellular membranes against peroxidation [4]. Vitamin E deficiency in children and newborns, including preterm infants (birth <37 gestational weeks), can lead to intracranial hemorrhage, chronic pulmonary diseases, hemolytic anemia, retinopathy and childhood cognitive deficits [4]. The prevalence of vitamin E deficiency (SVD) in newborns can be up to 77% [5–7] and in Brazil, a study found low vitamin levels (<500 µg/dL) in 90% of newborns [8]. The transfer of vitamin E to breast milk depends on circulating lipoproteins, and this mechanism can be influenced by maternal factors, both intrinsic and extrinsic [2,9,10]. In colostrum milk, the actions of pregnancy hormones, such as estrogen, contributes to the increase in circulating lipoproteins, ensuring a greater transfer of vitamin E into milk [2,11]. However, in mature milk the vitamin E content decreases because of changes in fat globules, and other characteristics, such as maternal age, gestational age of delivery, and the fatty acid profile might that influence the vitamin E content in milk [8,9,12,13].

Studies analyzing this micronutrient in mature milk observed that even in lactating women with vitamin E deficiency, its concentration in milk was maintained, which suggested a possible mobilization of alpha-tocopherol from the adipose tissue, which is considered the largest extrahepatic vitamin E reserve [2,8,14,15].

One strategy to increase the concentrations of vitamin E in milk is maternal supplementation [9,10]. Garcia et al. [16] found that at 24 h after supplementation, alpha-tocopherol levels in the colostrum increased. Other studies [17,18] found that vitamin E supplementation in its naturally occurring form (RRR-alpha-tocopherol) is more efficient to increase its content in milk compared with supplementation with the synthetic form or with a blend of natural and synthetic forms. In the natural form, the lateral chain has the RRR conformation, whereas the synthetic form can present isomers with 2R- (RRR-, RSR-, RSS- and RRS-) and 2S- (SRR-, SRS-, SSR-, SSS-) conformations. This structural difference results in increased bioavailability of the RRR form because of its higher affinity for the liver alpha-tocopherol transfer protein (alpha-TPP) [18,19].

Single-dose supplementation with 400 IU RRR-alpha-tocopherol in the immediate postpartum period caused an increase in the vitamin in the transitional milk (between 7 and 15 days after delivery), but not in the mature milk [20,21]. The authors suggested that a higher dose of vitamin E could influence the duration of the response. This identified the need to investigate the effect of higher doses, because the studies only used 400 IU of alpha-tocopherol, and suggested that this supplementation should be provided in the mature milk phase, which comprises a period of greater stability in milk nutritional composition.

Interestingly, different responses to supplementation have been noted, where the same treatment caused a greater increase of the vitamin in the milk in some studies [20–22] and a smaller effect in others [17], however, these studies lacked an analysis of the factors that influenced this response. These observations should be considered, because maternal milk with a low alpha-tocopherol content has been found, which could expose infants to vitamin E deficiency (VED) [20,21,23–25]. By contrast, studies of vitamin E supplementation in a single dose and in greater quantity could reveal the previously unknown mechanism of vitamin transfer to the mammary gland.

Thus, given that maternal supplementation with vitamin E is an effective measure to increase this vitamin content in milk [21,22], the mother-child binomial should be protected from the adverse effects of VED, and that there are differences in the response to this supplementation, but no understanding of which characteristics contribute to this response. The objective of the present study was to evaluate the impact of supplementation with 800 IU RRR-alpha-tocopherol on the alpha-tocopherol level in mature milk and the factors associated with the increase, with the aim of improving our understanding of the mechanism the transfer of vitamin E in the lactation period.

2. Materials and Methods

2.1. Participants and Intervention

The study was a randomized, parallel-group trial. Participants were recruited at the Pediatric Ambulatory Care of the Onofre Lopes University Hospital (HUOL), Natal-RN, Brazil, and data collection took place between October 2017 and July 2018.

The present study was approved by the Ethics Committee of the Federal University of Rio Grande do Norte (UFRN), under the protocol number 2.327.614, CAAE 76779217.1.0000.5537, and was also registered in the Brazilian Registry of Clinical Trials—ReBec, under the code RBR-38nfg2, available at http://www.ensaiosclinicos.gov.br/rg/RBR-38nfg2/.

The sample calculation was performed using GPower software, Version 3.1.9 [26] considering two independent groups tested using one way analysis of variance (ANOVA) for repeated measures among factors, with alpha parameters equal to 5%, expected power at 80%, and the effect measure value equal to 0.25 [27]. The analysis showed that each group should have at least 33 individuals, totaling 66 participants.

The eligibility criteria included women between 30 and 90 days after delivery; who were breastfeeding their children, either exclusively or partially; who were residents of Natal, RN and its metropolitan regions; who were not diagnosed with a diseases (hypertension, diabetes, neoplasms, heart disease, diseases of the gastrointestinal and hepatic tract, syphilis or were HIV-positive); who were non-smokers; no multiple births and whose infants were not malformed. Exclusion criteria were women who did not have sufficient milk or blood for analysis of vitamin levels, users of illicit drugs, and those who made daily use of vitamin supplements containing vitamin E during lactation.

The eligible participants were informed of the study's objectives and those who agreed to participate signed the consent form. At recruitment, they were allocated in one of the study groups, depending on the day of the week: Monday and Thursday for the supplemented group and Tuesday and Wednesday for the control group, where only the supplemented group ingested two capsules containing 400 IU of RRR-alpha-tocopherol consecutively, totaling 800 IU (588 mg of alpha-tocopherol). The capsule contained 98% RRR-alpha-tocopherol acetate, as assessed according to the method of Lira (2017) [21]. The study complied with the Consolidated Standards of Reporting Trials—CONSORT (Figure 1).

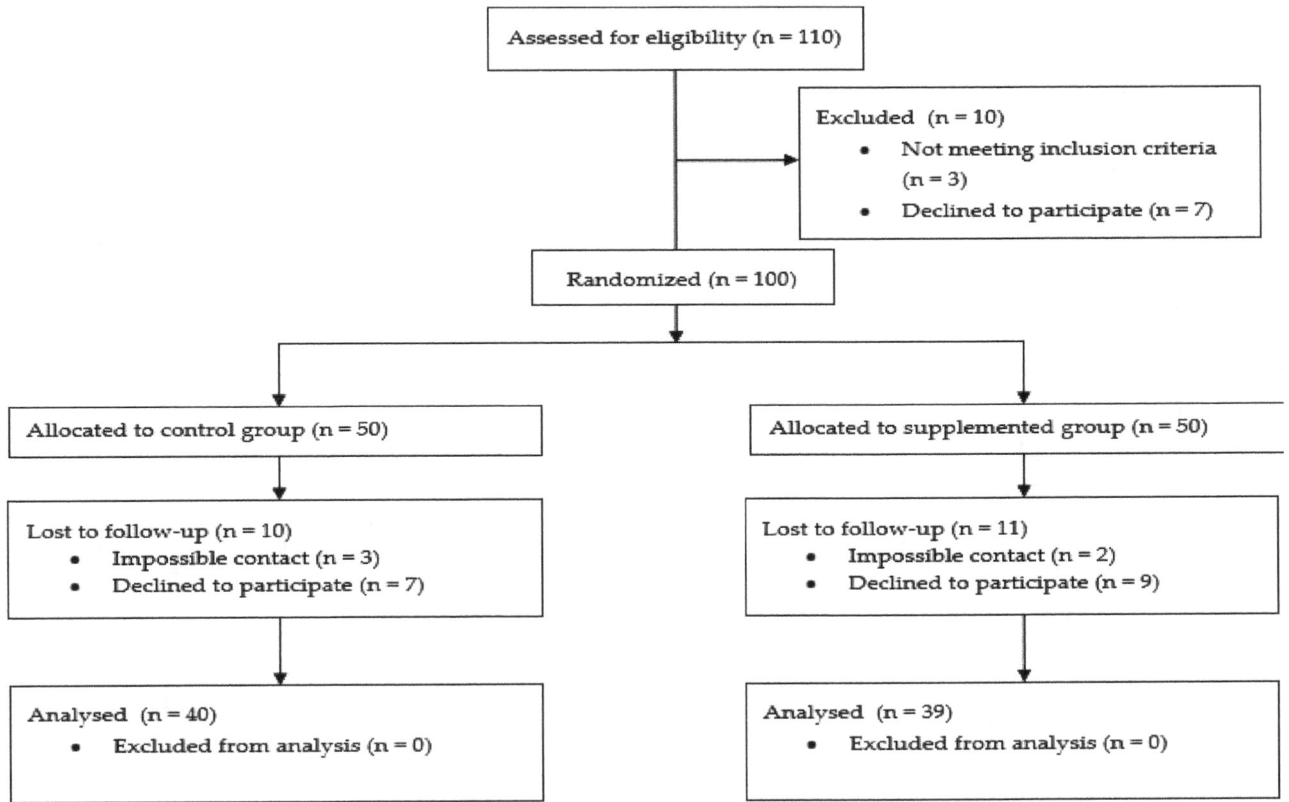

Figure 1. Consolidated Standards of Reporting Trials flow diagram (CONSORT).

2.2. Data Collection

A semi-structured questionnaire was used to collect data on socioeconomic aspects, such as family income, schooling and maternal age, as well as information on gestational age and type of delivery. Maternal height and current weight were also assessed and used to calculate the body mass index (BMI).

Milk and serum were collected from the participants at two time points. Collection 1 was performed at the hospital and collection 2 was performed at the participant's home the day after collection 1. In the supplemented group, supplementation with 800 IU of RRR-alpha-tocopherol was performed immediately after collection 1 of milk and serum.

A 2 mL sample of breast milk was collected by manual expression from a single breast that had not breastfed recently, and 5 mL of blood were collected by venipuncture. All the biological samples were collected after a 4 to 6 h fast, stored in polypropylene tubes packed in aluminum foil, and transported in refrigerated units. The breast milk was stored at −20 °C until the time of analysis. Before storage, the blood samples were centrifuged for 10 min (at 4000 rpm), to separate the serum for analysis of vitamin E and lipoproteins.

The dietary intake of vitamin E was evaluated by means of the 24 h dietary recall (24HR) applied at the two collection time points. Participants were asked about all foods, supplements and beverages consumed the day before the interview.

2.3. Determination of Alpha-Tocopherol and Lipid Profile in Biological Samples

The extraction of alpha-tocopherol from milk and serum was performed according to the method adapted by Lira et al. (2013) [28]. Ethanol (95%) was used to precipitate proteins (Vetec, Rio de Janeiro, Brazil), and hexane PA (Vetec, Rio de Janeiro, Brazil) was used as an extraction reagent. After evaporation in nitrogen, serum and milk residues were dissolved, respectively, in 250 μL of absolute ethanol (Vetec, Rio de Janeiro, Brazil) and 250 mL of dichloromethane (Vetec, Rio de Janeiro, Brazil): methanol (Sigma-Aldrich, St. Louis, Missouri, EUA) (2:1; *v*/*v*). The aliquots were then analyzed using high-performance liquid chromatography (HPLC).

HPLC consisted of an LC-20AT (Shimadzu, Kyoto, Japan) pump coupled to a CBM 20A communicator and an SPD-10A UV-VIS detector (Shimadzu, Kyoto, Japan). AC18 reversed phase column (LiChroCART 250-4, Merck, Darmstadt, Germany) was used for chromatographic separation. The mobile phase was 100% methanol in an isocratic system, with a flow rate of 1 mL/min and a wavelength of 292 nm was used to detect alpha-tocopherol. The identification and quantification of the vitamin in the samples were established by comparing the area of the peak obtained in the chromatogram with the area of the alpha-tocopherol standard (Sigma-Aldrich, São Paulo, Brazil). The concentration of the standard was confirmed by the specific extinction coefficient for alpha-tocopherol (e1%, alpha-tocopherol, 1 cm = 75.8 to 292 nm) in absolute ethanol (Vetec, Rio de Janeiro, Brazil) [29]. Women with serum alpha-tocopherol values less than 12 μmol/L were considered as deficient in vitamin E [30].

The transport of vitamin E from serum to breast milk involves lipoproteins; therefore, serum cholesterol and high-density lipoprotein (HDL) levels were analyzed with using a commercial kit (Labtest) and enzymatic colorimetric methods, by using an automatic biochemistry analyzer (Labmax plenno). Low-density lipoprotein (LDL) was quantified using the equation proposed by Martin et al. (2013) [31].

2.4. Dietary Intake of Vitamin E

Vitamin E intake was obtained using two 24 h dietary recall (24HR), applied using face-to-face interviews at the two data collection times in both groups. During this interview, the participants were asked about the food (and its preparation), supplements and beverages consumed in the last 24 h before the interview, in which the home measures described were converted to grams or milliliters [32,33] and the amount of vitamin E consumed was analyzed using the software Virtual Nutri Plus [34], from the database constructed by Rodrigues (2016) [8]. The dietary intake of vitamin E was corrected for total energy intake. The resulting values were obtained using SPSS, version 21.0 for Windows (SPSS Inc., Chicago, IL, USA) employing the residual method.

2.5. Statistical Analysis

Statistical analysis was performed using the statistical software IBM SPSS version 21.0 for Windows (SPSS Inc., Chicago, IL, USA). The Kolmogorov–Smirnov normality test was applied. Numerical data were expressed as the mean (standard deviation, SD), and categorical results were reported as absolute and relative frequencies. Student's t-test for dependent samples was used to verify intragroup differences, and the t-test for independent samples was used to analyze the differences between the groups. To evaluate the relationship between serum, breast milk and dietary vitamin E intake, the Pearson correlation coefficient was calculated. Linear multiple regression analysis was used to verify the ratio between alpha-tocopherol in milk after vitamin supplementation and in serum, the lipid profile, vitamin E intake and other maternal factors. The factors associated with the effect of supplementation on milk were also investigated. For this, the lactating women in the supplemented group were divided into quartiles according to the percentage increase in the milk alpha-tocopherol content between collection 1 and collection 2, being classified into a smaller effect (quartile 1) and greater effect (quartiles 2–4). The quartile categorization was used to identify the participants who presented lower effect and greater effects, because all participants should present higher alpha-tocopherol in milk values after supplementation. In addition to providing an analysis of the possible determinants for the milk supplementation response. The association of maternal variables with the effect of supplementation was evaluated according to binary multiple regression. All differences were considered significant when $p \leq 0.05$.

3. Results

3.1. General Characteristics of the Population

The socioeconomic characteristics of the lactating women are presented in Table 1. The mean age of the participants was 27 years, and the majority had completed high school. About 40% of the women were overweight according to their BMI values, and exclusive breastfeeding was predominant (>84%) in both groups. The dietary intake of vitamin E was equivalent to 8.7 mg/day in the control, which was below the recommended intake (16 mg/day) [30] and there was no difference between the groups in terms of dietary intake of vitamin E ($p = 0.901$).

3.2. Effect of Vitamin E Supplementation on Serum and Breast Milk

At collection 1, the maternal serum alpha-tocopherol concentrations were similar between the control and supplemented groups, at 26.37 (4.6) μmol/L and 26.38 (5.4) μmol/L, respectively ($p = 0.996$). In the control group, there was no difference in the alpha-tocopherol concentrations between collection 1 and collection 2 ($p > 0.05$). Neither group contained cases of VED (<12 μmol/L). In addition, the lipid profiles were similar between the collections and between the groups ($p > 0.05$) (Table 2).

After supplementation with 800 IU RRR-alpha-tocopherol, a 183% increase in serum alpha-tocopherol was observed in the supplemented group (collection 2), reaching 48.27 μmol/L ($p < 0.001$) (Table 2).

For the alpha-tocopherol content in mature milk, the control group presented 6.91 (1.81) μmol/L and the supplemented group presented 6.98 (2.18) μmol/L ($p = 0.883$). One day after supplementation (collection 2), milk from the supplemented group presented higher levels of alpha-tocopherol (15 μmol/L) compared with that in the control group (6.94 μmol/L) ($p < 0.001$), an increase equivalent to 124% in the post-supplementation milk.

3.3. Factors Associated with Alpha-Tocopherol in Breast Milk after Supplementation

In the supplemented group, after Pearson correlation analysis, milk from collection 1, dietary intake of vitamin E, and alpha-tocopherol in serum from collection 2 were identified as positively related to alpha-tocopherol levels in milk from collection 2 (Figure 2). These variables were included in the multiple linear regression analysis to evaluate the factors associated with the alpha-tocopherol concentration in breast milk after supplementation. Only alpha-tocopherol in the milk before supplementation was a determinant for the increase in the vitamin content in the milk after administration of 800 IU alpha-tocopherol ($\beta = 0.927$, $p < 0.001$, 95% CI 1.925–2.396). Thus, the higher the vitamin concentration in milk, the greater the transfer of the vitamin to the mammary gland.

When dividing the participants of the supplemented group according to the effect of supplementation (quartile 1 and quartiles 2–4), where quartile 1 is equivalent to 83% of the vitamin E increase percentage in milk after supplementation, we observed that the dietary intake of vitamin E was a determinant that caused a greater response to supplementation ($p = 0.020$, 95% CI 0.209–0.877), which suggested that the higher the intake, the greater the effect of supplementation (Table 3). The characteristics of the participants divided by the effect of supplementation are described in Table 4, which showed that the consumption of calories, alpha-tocopherol and total fat was higher in the group showing a higher effect of supplementation ($p = 0.001$, $p = 0.013$, $p = 0.033$, respectively).

Table 1. Characterization of the 79 lactating women randomized into the control and supplemented groups of the study. Natal, Rio Grande do Norte, Brazil, 2017–2018.

Characteristics	**Control Group** *n* = 40	**Supplemented Group** *n* = 39	***p*-Value**
Maternal age (years), mean (SD)	27 (6.8)	27 (6.8)	0.833 *
Postpartum age (days), mean (SD)	57 (25.8)	56 (23.7)	0.833 *
Education level *n*, (%)			
Incomplete primary education	4 (10.0)	5 (12.8)	
Complete primary education	3 (7.5)	2 (5.1)	
Incomplete secondary education	14 (35.0)	6 (15.4)	0.149
Complete secondary education	16 (40.0)	22 (56.4)	
Complete higher education	3 (7.5)	4 (10.3)	
Family income level *n*, (%) [a]			
<1 Minimum wage	16 (40.0)	23 (59.0)	0.092
>1 Minimum wage	24 (60.0)	16 (41.0)	
Type of delivery *n*, (%)			
Vaginal	15 (37.5)	13 (33.3)	0.699
Caesarian	25 (62.5)	26 (66.7)	
Parity status *n*, (%)			
Primiparous	21 (52.5)	17 (43.6)	0.405
Multtiparou	19 (47.5)	22 (56.4)	
BMI classification (kg/m^2), (%) [b]			
Low weight	1 (2.5)	0 (0)	
Normal	15 (37.5)	18 (46.2)	0.735
Overweight	16 (40.0)	13 (33.3)	
Obese	8 (20.0)	8 (20.5)	
Type of maternal breastfeeding *n*, (%)			
Exclusive maternal breastfeeding	35 (87.5)	33 (84.6)	0.711
Maternal breast milk and other milks	5 (12.5)	6 (15.4)	
Calorie intake (Kcal/day), mean (SD)	3248.4 (711.2)	3270.7 (868.4)	0.970 *
Intake of alpha-tocopherol (mg/day), mean (SD)	8.7 (3.4)	8.8 (3.5)	0.901 *
Intake of total fat (g/dia), mean (SD)	69.2 (23.6)	69.9 (25.8)	0.905 *

n: number; BMI: Body Mass Index; SD: Standard deviation; Chi-square test. * Student's *t*-test for independent samples used for the variables maternal age, postpartum age, calorie consumption, alpha-tocopherol and total fat; [a] Brazilian minimum wage per month = US$ 291.5; [b] WHO classification, 2000. *p*-value = level of significance ($p < 0.05$ = statistically significant).

Table 2. Maternal biochemical indicators of the control and supplemented groups in collections 1 and 2, performed in the study. Natal, Rio Grande do Norte, Brazil, 2017–2018.

Biochemical Indicators Evaluated	**Control Group**				**Supplemented Group**				**Differences between Control Group and Supplemented Group**	
									p*-Value *	
	Collection 1	**Collection 2**	**Change**	***p*-Value ***	**Collection 1**	**Collection 2**	**Change**	***p*-Value ***	**Collection 1 CG × SG**	**Collection 2 CG × SG**
Serum alpha-tocopherol (µmol/L)	26.37 (4.6)	26.34 (4.92)	0.03 (2.5)	0.876	26.38 (5.4)	48.27 (10.5)	21.89 (7.4)	0.001	0.996	<0.001
Alpha-tocopherol in breast milk (µmol/L)	6.91 (1.8)	6.94 (2.0)	0.03 (1.2)	0.935	6.98 (2.2)	15.00 (5.1)	8.02 (4.2)	<0.001	0.883	<0.001
Serum cholesterol (mg/dL)	177 (41.0)	178 (42.0)	1.70 (33.5)	0.750	179 (44.0)	173 (36.0)	6.28 (16.0)	0.190	0.834	0.498
Serum triglycerides (mg/dL)	143 (99.0)	130 (86.0)	13.38 (57.8)	0.151	129 (66.0)	109 (51.0)	19.23 (32.9)	0.08	0.439	0.195
HDL (mg/dL)	40 (14.0)	41 (15.0)	0.25 (12.9)	0.903	42 (11.0)	42 (10.0)	0.31 (8.0)	0.811	0.574	0.724
LDL (mg/dL)	111 (35.0)	114 (40.0)	3.28 (34.4)	0.535	113 (43.0)	110 (35.0)	3.74 (14.7)	0.129	0.762	0.603

HDL: High-density lipoprotein; LDL: Low-density lipoprotein; ( ) Standard deviation; * Student's *t*-test for dependent samples; ** Student's *t*-test for independent samples. CG: Control group; SG: Supplemented group.

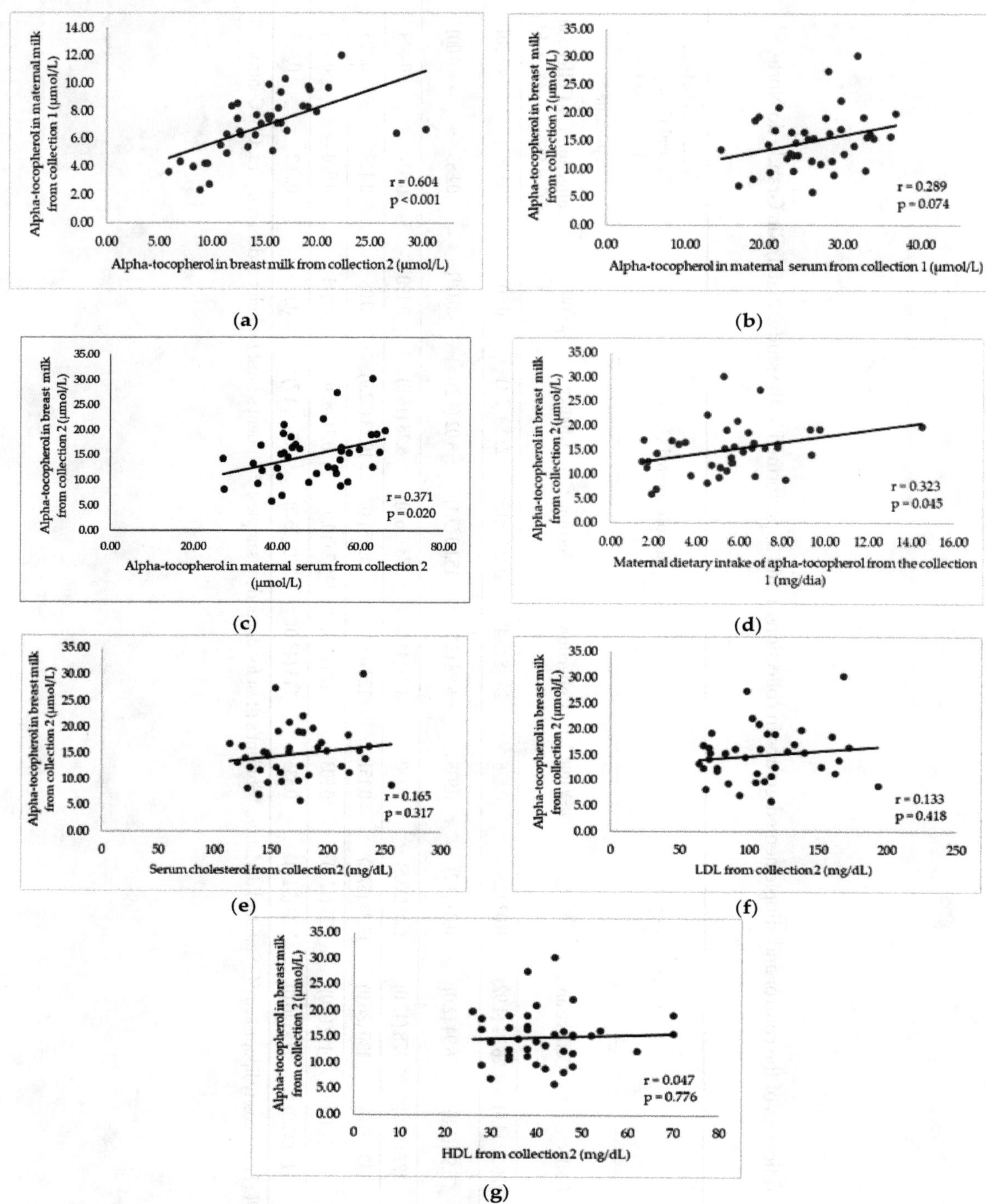

Figure 2. Correlations between alpha-tocopherol in breast milk obtained in collection 2 and maternal variables of the supplemented group. Natal, Rio Grande do Norte, Brazil, 2017–2018. (**a**) Correlation between alpha-tocopherol in breast milk from collection 1 and 2; (**b**) correlation between alpha-tocopherol in breast milk from collection 2 and serum from collection 1; (**c**) correlation between alpha-tocopherol in breast milk in serum from collection 2; (**d**) correlation between alpha-tocopherol in breast milk of collection 2 and the vitamin E intake of collection 1; (**e**) correlation between alpha-tocopherol in breast milk from collection 2 and serum cholesterol from collection 2; (**f**) correlation between alpha-tocopherol in breast milk from collection 2 and low-density lipoprotein (LDL) from collection 2; (**g**) correlation between alpha-tocopherol in breast milk from collection 2 and high-density lipoprotein (HDL) from collection 2. r = Pearson's correlation coefficient; *p* value = level of significance ($p < 0.05$ = statistically significant).

Table 3. Binary logistic regression model for variables associated with greater effect of 800 IU alpha-tocopherol supplementation in breast milk in the supplemented group.

Variables	Greater Effect of Supplementation (Quartiles 2–4) *	
	95% CI	*p*-Value
Alpha-tocopherol in milk collection 1 (µmol/L)	0.998–1.024	0.104
Alpha-tocopherol in serum collection 1 (µmol/L)	0.991–1.005	0.565
Alpha-tocopherol in serum collection 2 (µmol/L)	0.995–1.002	0.387
Dietary intake of vitamin E collection 1 (mg/day)	0.209–0.877	0.020 **
Serum cholesterol collection 1 (mg/dL)	0.937–1.163	0.431
LDL collection 1 (mg/dL)	0.846–1.051	0.289

* Above 83% of the vitamin E increase percentage in milk after supplementation. LDL: Low-density lipoprotein. *p*-value = level of significance. ** Significant difference.

Table 4. Characterization of the 39 lactating women randomized into the supplemented group, divided by the effect of milk supplementation (lower effect: quartile 1, equivalent to 83% of the vitamin increase percentage in the milk, and greater effect: quartiles 2–4). Natal, Rio Grande do Norte, Brazil, 2017–2018.

Characteristics	Quartile 1 $n = 9$	Quartiles 2–4 $n = 30$	*p*-Value
Maternal age (years), mean (SD)	27 (6.5)	27 (6.9)	0.922 *
Postpartum age (days), mean (SD)	58 (30.0)	55 (22.1)	0.749 *
Education level *n*, (%)			
Incomplete primary education	2 (22.2)	3 (10.0)	
Complete primary education	1 (11.1)	1 (3.3)	
Incomplete secondary education	1 (11.1)	5 (16.7)	0.343
Complete secondary education	3 (33.3)	19 (63.3)	
Complete higher education	2 (22.2)	2 (6.7)	
Family income level *n*, (%) [a]			
<1 Minimum wage	4 (44.4)	19 (63.3)	0.312
>1 Minimum wage	5 (55.6)	11 (36.7)	
Type of delivery *n*, (%)			
Vaginal	2 (22.2)	11 (36.7)	0.420
Caesarian	7 (77.8)	19 (63.3)	
Parity status *n*, (%)			
Primiparous	6 (66.7)	11 (36.7)	0.111
Multiparous	3 (33.3)	19 (63.3)	
BMI classification (kg/m^2), (%) [b]			
Low weight	0 (0)	0 (0)	
Normal	3 (33.3)	14 (46.7)	0.754
Overweight	4 (44.5)	10 (33.3)	
Obese	2 (22.2)	6 (20.0)	
Type of maternal breastfeeding *n*, (%)			
Exclusive maternal breastfeeding	8 (88.9)	25 (83.3)	0.685
Maternal breast milk and other milks	1 (11.1)	5 (16.7)	
Calory intake (Kcal/day), mean (SD)	2624.6 (453.7)	3464.5 (873.4)	0.001 *
Intake of alpha-tocopherol (mg/day), mean (SD)	6.8 (2.1)	9.3 (3.6)	0.013 *
Intake of total fat (g/dia), mean (SD)	58.5 (12.8)	73.3 (27.8)	0.033 *

n: number. BMI: Body Mass Index; SD: Standard deviation; Chi-square test. * *t*-test for independent samples used for the variables maternal age, postpartum age, calorie consumption, alpha-tocopherol and total fat; [a] Brazilian minimum wage per month = US$ 291.5; [b] WHO classification, 2000. *p*-value = level of significance ($p < 0.05$ = statistically significant).

4. Discussion

Mature milk is the most stable stage of lactation, in which the content of alpha-tocopherol is not influenced by pregnancy-related factors, as occurs in the colostrum [2,7]. It should be emphasized that the mature milk presents a higher concentration of lipids and in contrast, there is a lower secretion of alpha-tocopherol, suggesting that there are distinct mechanisms involved in the transfer of this vitamin into breast milk [2,35,36].

In the present study, the lactating women had adequate vitamin E status, in accordance with other studies considering the same stage of lactation [8,21]. However, a low dietary intake of vitamin E was noted (Table 1), which could trigger the mobilization of alpha-tocopherol from maternal reserves, such as the adipose tissue, into breast milk [15,19]. This low consumption of vitamin E was also reported in other populations in Brazil, Greece and Poland [21,25,36], which suggests a frequent inadequacy in vitamin E consumption during lactation.

Even in situations of inadequate consumption, the vitamin E concentration in milk was not influenced by diet and circulating maternal levels [8,20,21,37–40]. However, this present study was the first to identify a positive association between alpha-tocopherol levels in milk and ingested vitamin E (diet + supplementation) and with serum alpha-tocopherol (Figure 2d,c). This suggested that in high-consumption situations, the ingested and circulating maternal levels are the main factors responsible for the vitamin level in milk. It is likely that in situations of low vitamin E consumption (as found in the studies cited), milk vitamin E might originate from other sources, such as the body's reserve [4], explaining the absence of a relationship between those variables.

To prevent of VED in infants, it is necessary for breast milk to contain adequate levels of vitamin E, so that children can obtain the benefits of the micronutrient, through the creation of vitamin reserves in the body and its antioxidant action [4,19]. Some studies that evaluated this vitamin in mature milk observed values below the nutritional requirements of infants [20,23,36,37], which suggested that maternal vitamin E supplementation could be an important strategy to increase milk vitamin contents [17,20,21].

In this study, supplementation with 800 IU of alpha-tocopherol caused a 183% increase in serum alpha-tocopherol, and a 124% increase in breast milk alpha-tocopherol (Table 2). Other clinical trials using a lower dose (400 IU alpha-tocopherol) found an increase of 60% to 80% in the vitamin content in milk after supplementation [18,20–22], showing a reduced effect compared with that shown in the present study. These findings suggested that the response to supplementation might be influenced by both the dosage used and the determinant factors. However, trials have not evaluated the factors associated with the different responses to large vitamin E doses [17,20], being important to understand how this vitamin is transferred into the mammary gland.

When analyzing the factors associated with a better response in milk after supplementation, it is important to highlight that only the content of this vitamin in the basal milk (before supplementation) and the dietary intake were demonstrated to increase the levels of this micronutrient in milk (Table 3), which suggested that the higher the consumption of vitamin E and its levels in milk, the greater the transfer of alpha-tocopherol from the supplement to the mammary gland.

Assessment of the profile of lactating women in the supplemented group, showed that the participants with the highest supplementation effect (quartiles 2–4) had a higher intake of calories, alpha-tocopherol and total fat (Table 4). These findings suggested that the amount of fat available in the diet may improve the bioavailability of the vitamin in the body, such as its absorption and distribution to tissues, and in this case, to the mammary gland, as reported in [41–43].

Such evidence also demonstrated that in mature milk, the Michaelis–Menten kinetic theory could not be applied, as it proposes that the transfer of vitamin to milk occurs through active transport, characterized by a saturation of the lipoprotein receptors in the breast tissue in situations of large contents of vitamin E, which would prevent the continuous transfer of the vitamin into the breast milk after supplementation [38,44]. Notably, in a study of dairy cows, Weiss and Wyatt (2003) [45] suggested that the ability of lipoproteins to carry alpha-tocopherol could determine the uptake of this vitamin by the breast tissue, and that the limiting factor for this mechanism would be the maximum content of vitamin E in the lipoproteins.

To further investigate this relationship between lipoproteins and vitamin E transport, we determined the circulating lipoproteins and the serum cholesterol and triglycerides profiles; however, no relation between them and the response to supplementation was found (Table 2). In fact, the mechanism of transport of vitamin E to the mammary gland is poorly understood [2,46,47]. Circulating lipoproteins are responsible for this transfer, with LDL being the main carrier [44,48]; however, transport may occur in the presence or absence of its receptors in the mammary gland [2,44]. Other receptors are found in breast tissue, such as Scavenger Receptor B-1 (SR-B1), which has binding sites for both LDL and HDL, and CD36, which has high affinity binding sites for HDL, LDL, and very low-density lipoprotein (VLDL) [2,48]. It has also been suggested the participation of lipoprotein lipase (LPL), which may show increased activity during lactation, contributes to the greater circulation of alpha-tocopherol and its uptake [49].

These findings provide important information to understand the mechanisms by which vitamin E is transferred into the mammary gland, demonstrating that, in situations of supplementation with 800 IU of vitamin E and its effect in mature milk, the better the vitamin E status (considering the milk and dietary intake), the more effective uptake into the mammary gland will be, regardless of receptor saturation. Further investigation into how this transport occurs is required, by means of in vitro and in vivo studies and using labeled isotopes of alpha-tocopherol, for example, to investigate its biotransformation. Notably, in populations with dietary inadequacy and low contents of vitamin E in milk, supplementation with higher doses of the vitamin, such as 800 IU alpha-tocopherol, might be required to obtain a more effective intervention. The analysis of a single dose during the day allowed us to investigate possible factors that could interfere with the response to supplementation; however, it is necessary to analyze how long the effect of this supplementation could be sustained, its contribution to maternal and infant nutritional status, and the use of smaller daily doses.

Therefore, supplementation associated with an adequate intake of vitamin E is an effective strategy to increase vitamin E levels in breast milk and prevent cases of vitamin E deficiency in infants, especially premature infants [2,4,11].

5. Conclusions

Vitamin E supplementation increased vitamin levels in milk and in maternal serum, and a positive relationship was found between alpha-tocopherol levels in milk, serum and dietary intake of vitamin E. Factors associated with the increase in alpha-tocopherol contents in milk after maternal supplementation with 800 IU of vitamin E were the basal levels of alpha-tocopherol in milk and the dietary intake of vitamin E.

Author Contributions: A.d.S.R. contributed to article writing, review and editing. A.G.C.L.d.S., A.F.d.O., L.T.P.d.S., V.d.F.F. contributed to data collection and analysis of the samples. M.S.C., V.N.S. contributed to the lipid profile analysis. K.D.d.S.R. contributed to selection of the journal and participated in the orientation, design, analysis and review of the study. R.D. contributed to the orientation and design of the study.

Acknowledgments: We thank the study participants and the nursing team of the Pediatric Ambulatory Care of the Onofre Lopes University Hospital (HUOL), Natal-RN, Brazil.

References

1. Victora, C.G.; Bahl, R.; Barros, A.J.D.; França, G.V.A.; Horton, S.; Krasevec, J.; Murch, S.; Sankar, M.J.; Walker, N.; Rollins, N.C. Breastfeeding in the 21st century: Epidemiology, mechanisms, and lifelong effect. *Lancet* **2016**, *387*, 475–490. [CrossRef]
2. Debier, C. Vitamin E during pre- and postnatal periods. In *Vitamins & Hormones*; Elsevier: Amsterdam, The Netherlands, 2007; Volume 76, pp. 357–373. ISBN 9780123735928.
3. Brasil. *Saúde da Criança: Aleitamento Materno e Alimentação Complementar*, 2rd ed.; Ministério da Saúde: Brasília, Brazil, 2015; ISBN 9788533422902.
4. Traber, M.G. Vitamin E. In *Present Knowledge in Nutrition*, 10th ed.; Erdman, J.W., Jr., Macdonald, I.A., Zeisel, S.H., Eds.; ILSI Press: Washington, DC, USA, 2012; pp. 214–229. ISBN 978-0-470-95917-6.
5. Schulpis, K.H.; Michalakakou, K.; Gavrili, S.; Karikas, G.A.; Lazaropoulou, C.; Vlachos, G.; Bakoula, C.; Papassotiriou, I. Maternal-neonatal retinol and alpha-tocopherol serum concentrations in Greeks and Albanians. *Acta Paediatr.* **2004**, *93*, 1075–1080. [CrossRef] [PubMed]
6. Fares, S.; Feki, M.; Khouaja-Mokrani, C.; Sethom, M.M.; Jebnoun, S.; Kaabachi, N. Nutritional practice effectiveness to achieve adequate plasma vitamin A, E and D during the early postnatal life in Tunisian very low birth weight infants. *J. Matern.-Fetal Neonatal Med.* **2015**, *28*, 1324–1328. [CrossRef] [PubMed]
7. Kositamongkol, S.; Suthutvoravut, U.; Chongviriyaphan, N.; Feungpean, B.; Nuntnarumit, P. Vitamin A and E status in very low birth weight infants. *J. Perinatol.* **2011**, *31*, 471–476. [CrossRef]
8. Rodrigues, K.D.S.R. Estado Nutricional em Vitamina E de Mães e Crianças Pré-Termo e Termo do Nascimento aos 3 Meses Pós-Parto. Ph.D. Thesis, Departamento de Bioquímica, Universidade Federal do Rio Grande do Norte, Natal, Brazil, June 2016; 148p.
9. Lima, M.S.R.; Dimenstein, R.; Ribeiro, K.D.S. Vitamin E concentration in human milk and associated factors: A literature review. *J. Pediatria* **2014**, *90*, 440–448. [CrossRef]
10. Hampel, D.; Shahab-Ferdows, S.; Islam, M.M.; Peerson, J.M.; Allen, L.H. Vitamin Concentrations in Human Milk Vary with Time within Feed, Circadian Rhythm, and Single-Dose Supplementation. *J. Nutr.* **2017**, *147*, 603–611. [CrossRef] [PubMed]
11. Debier, C.; Pottier, J.; Goffe, C.; Larondelle, Y. Present knowledge and unexpected behaviours of vitamins A and E in colostrum and milk. *Livest. Prod. Sci.* **2005**, *98*, 135–147. [CrossRef]
12. Tijerina-Sáenz, A.; Innis, S.; Kitts, D. Antioxidant capacity of human milk and its association with vitamins A and E and fatty acid composition. *Acta Paediatr.* **2009**, *98*, 1793–1798. [CrossRef] [PubMed]
13. Stuetz, W.; Carrara, V.; Mc Gready, R.; Lee, S.; Sriprawat, K.; Po, B.; Hanboonkunupakarn, B.; Grune, T.; Biesalski, H.; Nosten, F. Impact of Food Rations and Supplements on Micronutrient Status by Trimester of Pregnancy: Cross-Sectional Studies in the Maela Refugee Camp in Thailand. *Nutrients* **2016**, *8*, 66. [CrossRef]
14. Szlagatys-Sidorkiewicz, A.; Zagierski, M.; Jankowska, A.; uczak, G.; Macur, K.; Bączek, T.; Korzon, M.; Krzykowski, G.; Martysiak-Żurowska, D.; Kamińska, B. Longitudinal study of vitamins A, E and lipid oxidative damage in human milk throughout lactation. *Early Hum. Dev.* **2012**, *88*, 421–424. [CrossRef]
15. Olafsdottir, A.S.; Wagner, K.-H.; Thorsdottir, I.; Elmadfa, I. Fat-Soluble Vitamins in the Maternal Diet, Influence of Cod Liver Oil Supplementation and Impact of the Maternal Diet on Human Milk Composition. *Ann. Nutr. Metab.* **2001**, *45*, 265–272. [CrossRef] [PubMed]
16. Garcia, L.R.S.; Ribeiro, K.D.d.S.; de Araújo, K.F.; Azevedo, G.M.M.; Pires, J.F.; Batista, S.D.; Dimenstein, R. Níveis de alfa-tocoferol no soro e leite materno de puérperas atendidas em maternidade pública de Natal, Rio Grande do Norte. *Revista Brasileira de Saúde Materno Infantil* **2009**, *9*, 423–428. [CrossRef]
17. Clemente, H.A.; Ramalho, H.M.M.; Lima, M.S.R.; Grilo, E.C.; Dimenstein, R. Maternal Supplementation with Natural or Synthetic Vitamin E and Its Levels in Human Colostrum. *J. Pediatr. Gastroenterol. Nutr.* **2015**, *60*, 533–537. [CrossRef] [PubMed]
18. Gaur, S.; Kuchan, M.J.; Lai, C.-S.; Jensen, S.K.; Sherry, C.L. Supplementation with *RRR*- or *all-rac*-α-Tocopherol Differentially Affects the α-Tocopherol Stereoisomer Profile in the Milk and Plasma of Lactating Women. *J. Nutr.* **2017**, *147*, 1301–1307. [CrossRef] [PubMed]
19. Traber, M.G. Vitamin E Inadequacy in Humans: Causes and Consequences. *Adv. Nutr.* **2014**, *5*, 503–514. [CrossRef]

20. Medeiros, J.F.P.; da Silva Ribeiro, K.D.; Lima, M.S.R.; das Neves, R.A.M.; Lima, A.C.P.; Dantas, R.C.S.; da Silva, A.B.; Dimenstein, R. α-Tocopherol in breast milk of women with preterm delivery after a single postpartum oral dose of vitamin E. *Br. J. Nutr.* **2016**, *115*, 1424–1430. [CrossRef] [PubMed]
21. Lira, L.Q. Efeito de Dois Protocolos de Suplementação Materna com Alfa-Tocoferol Sobre o Soro e o Leite de Lactantes até 60 Dias Pós-Parto. Ph.D. Thesis, Departamento de Bioquímica, Universidade Federal do Rio Grande do Norte, Natal, Brazil, December 2017; 127p.
22. de Melo, L.R.M.; Clemente, H.A.; Bezerra, D.F.; Dantas, R.C.S.; Ramalho, H.M.M.; Dimenstein, R. Effect of maternal supplementation with vitamin E on the concentration of α-tocopherol in colostrum. *J. Pediatria* **2017**, *93*, 40–46. [CrossRef]
23. Cortês da Silva, A.L.; da Silva Ribeiro, K.D.; Miranda de Melo, L.R.; Fernandes Bezerra, D.; Carvalho de Queiroz, J.L.; Santa Rosa Lima, M.; Franco Pires, J.; Soares Bezerra, D.; Osório, M.M.; Dimenstein, R. Vitamina e no leite humano e sua relação com o requerimento nutricional do recém-nascido a termo. *Revista Paulista de Pediatria* **2017**, *35*, 158–164. [CrossRef]
24. Ma, D.; Ning, Y.; Gao, H.; Li, W.; Wang, J.; Zheng, Y.; Zhang, Y.; Wang, P. Nutritional Status of Breast-Fed and Non-Exclusively Breast-Fed Infants from Birth to Age 5 Months in 8 Chinese Cities. *Asia Pac. J. Clin. Nutr.* **2014**, *23*, 282–292. [CrossRef]
25. Antonakou, A.; Chiou, A.; Andrikopoulos, N.K.; Bakoula, C.; Matalas, A.-L. Breast milk tocopherol content during the first six months in exclusively breastfeeding Greek women. *Eur. J. Nutr.* **2011**, *50*, 195–202. [CrossRef]
26. GPower Software. Available online: http://www.gpower.hhu.de (accessed on 19 June 2017).
27. Faul, F.; Erdfelder, E.; Lang, A.-G.; Buchner, A. G*Power 3: A flexible statistical power analysis program for the social, behavioral, and biomedical sciences. *Behav. Res. Methods* **2007**, *39*, 175–191. [CrossRef] [PubMed]
28. de Lira, L.Q.; Lima, M.S.R.; de Medeiros, J.M.S.; da Silva, I.F.; Dimenstein, R. Correlation of vitamin A nutritional status on alpha-tocopherol in the colostrum of lactating women: Relationship of serum retinol and alpha-tocopherol in colostrum. *Matern. Child Nutr.* **2013**, *9*, 31–40. [CrossRef]
29. Nierenberg, D.W.; Nann, S.L. A method for determining concentrations of retinol, tocopherol, and five carotenoids in human plasma and tissue samples. *Am. J. Clin. Nutr.* **1992**, *56*, 417–426. [CrossRef]
30. *Dietary Reference Intakes for Vitamin C, Vitamin E, Selenium, and Carotenoids*; National Academies Press: Washington, DC, USA, 2000; ISBN 9780309069359.
31. Martin, S.S.; Blaha, M.J.; Elshazly, M.B. Comparison of a novel method vs. the Friedewald equation for estimating low-density lipoprotein cholesterol levels from the standard lipid profile. *JAMA* **2013**, *310*, 2061–2068. [CrossRef]
32. Araújo, M.O.D.; Guerra, T.M. *Alimentos per Capita*, 3rd ed.; Editora Universitária—UFRN: João Pessoa, Brazil, 2007; p. 323. ISBN 9788572733.
33. Tomita, L.Y.; Cardoso, M.A. *Relação de Medidas Caseiras, Composição Química e Receitas de Alimentos Nipo-Brasileiros*; Metha: São Paulo, Brazil, 2002; p. 85. ISBN 9788588888012.
34. Virtual Nutri Plus. Available online: http:/www.virtualnutriplus.com.br/ (accessed on 10 January 2018).
35. Schweigert, F.J.; Bathe, K.; Chen, F.; Boscher, U.; Dudenhausen, J.W. Effect of the stage of lactation in humans on carotenoid levels in milk, blood plasma and plasma lipoprotein fractions. *Eur. J. Nutr.* **2004**, *43*, 39–44. [CrossRef]
36. Didenco, S.; Gillingham, M.B.; Go, M.D.; Leonard, S.W.; Traber, M.G.; McEvoy, C.T. Increased vitamin E intake is associated with higher α-tocopherol concentration in the maternal circulation but higher α-carboxyethyl hydroxychroman concentration in the fetal circulation. *Am. J. Clin. Nutr.* **2011**, *93*, 368–373. [CrossRef] [PubMed]
37. Xue, Y.; Campos-Gimenez, E.; Redeuil, K.M.; Leveques, A.; Actis-Goretta, L.; Vinyes-Pares, G.; Zhang, Y.; Wang, P.; Thakkar, S.K. Concentrations of Carotenoids and Tocopherols in Breast Milk from Urban Chinese Mothers and Their Associations with Maternal Characteristics: A Cross-Sectional Study. *Nutrients* **2017**, *9*, 1229. [CrossRef] [PubMed]
38. Dimenstein, R.; Medeiros, A.C.P.; Cunha, L.R.F.; Araújo, K.F.; Dantas, J.C.O.; Macedo, T.M.S.; Stamford, T.L.M. Vitamin E in human serum and colostrum under fasting and postprandial conditions. *J. Pediatria* **2010**, *86*, 345–348. [CrossRef] [PubMed]
39. Jiang, J.; Xiao, H.; Wu, K.; Yu, Z.; Ren, Y.; Zhao, Y.; Li, K.; Li, J.; Li, D. Retinol and α-tocopherol in human milk and their relationship with dietary intake during lactation. *Food Funct.* **2016**, *7*, 1985–1991. [CrossRef]

40. Martysiak-Żurowska, D.; Szlagatys-Sidorkiewicz, A.; Zagierski, M. Concentrations of alpha- and gamma-tocopherols in human breast milk during the first months of lactation and in infant formulas: Tocopherols in human milk and infant formulas. *Matern. Child Nutr.* **2013**, *9*, 473–482. [CrossRef] [PubMed]
41. Leonard, S.W.; Good, C.K.; Gugger, E.; Traber, M.G. Vitamin E bioavailability from fortified breakfast cereal is greater than that from encapsulated supplements. *Am. J. Clin. Nutr.* **2004**, *79*, 86–92. [CrossRef] [PubMed]
42. Bruno, R.S.; Leonard, S.W.; Park, S.I.; Zhao, Y.; Traber, M.G. Human vitamin E requirements assessed with the use of apples fortified with deuteriumlabeled alpha-tocopheryl acetate. *Am. J. Clin. Nutr.* **2006**, *83*, 299–304. [CrossRef] [PubMed]
43. Traber, M.G.; Leonard, S.W.; Bobe, G.; Fu, X.; Saltzman, E.; Grusak, M.A.; Estande, S.L. α-Tocopherol Disappearance Rates from Plasma Depend on Lipid Concentrations: Studies Using Deuterium-Labeled Collard Greens in Younger and Older Adults. *Am. J. Clin. Nutr.* **2015**, *101*, 752–759. [CrossRef] [PubMed]
44. Jensen, S.K.; Johannsen, A.K.B.; Hermansen, J.E. Quantitative secretion and maximal secretion capacity of retinol, β-carotene and α-tocopherol into cows' milk. *J. Dairy Res.* **1999**, *66*, 511–522. [CrossRef] [PubMed]
45. Weiss, W.P.; Wyatt, D.J. Effect of Dietary Fat and Vitamin E on α-Tocopherol in Milk from Dairy Cows. *J. Dairy Sci.* **2003**, *86*, 3582–3591. [CrossRef]
46. Lauridsen, C.; Engel, H.; Jensen, S.K.; Craig, A.M.; Traber, M.G. Lactating Sows and Suckling Piglets Preferentially Incorporate RRR- over All-rac-alpha-Tocopherol into Milk Plasma and Tissues. *J. Nutr.* **2002**, *132*, 1258–1264. [CrossRef]
47. Wang, Y.; Tong, J.; Li, S.; Zhang, R.; Chen, L.; Wang, Y.; Zheng, M.; Wang, M.; Liu, G.; Dai, Y.; et al. Over-Expression of Human Lipoprotein Lipase in Mouse Mammary Glands Leads to Reduction of Milk Triglyceride and Delayed Growth of Suckling Pups. *PLoS ONE* **2011**, *6*, 208–295. [CrossRef]
48. Monks, J.; Huey, P.U.; Hanson, L.; Eckel, R.H.; Neville, M.C.; Gavigan, S.A. lipoprotein-containing particle is transferred from the serum across the mammary epithelium into the milk of lactating mice. *J. Lipid Res.* **2001**, *42*, 686–696.
49. Mardones, P.; Rigotti, A. Cellular mechanisms of vitamin e uptake: Relevance in α-tocopherol metabolism and potential implications for disease. *J. Nutr. Biochem.* **2004**, *15*, 252–260. [CrossRef]

4

Breastfeeding Status and Duration and Infections, Hospitalizations for Infections and Antibiotic Use in the First Two Years of Life in the ELFE Cohort

Camille Davisse-Paturet [1,*], Karine Adel-Patient [2], Amandine Divaret-Chauveau [3,4], Juliette Pierson [1], Sandrine Lioret [1], Marie Cheminat [5], Marie-Noëlle Dufourg [5], Marie-Aline Charles [1,5] and Blandine de Lauzon-Guillain [1,*]

1 Université de Paris, CRESS, INSERM, INRA F-75004 Paris, France
2 UMR Service de Pharmacologie et Immunoanalyse, CEA, INRA, Université Paris-Saclay, 91191 Gif-sur-Yvette, France
3 Unité d'allergologie pédiatrique, Hôpital d'enfants, CHRU de Nancy, 54500 Vandoeuvre-lès-Nancy, France
4 EA3450, DevAH-Department of Physiology, Faculty of Medicine, University of Lorraine, 54500 Vandoeuvre-lès-Nancy, France
5 Ined, Inserm, Joint Unit Elfe F-75020 Paris, France
* Correspondence: camille.davisse-paturet@inserm.fr (C.D.-P.); blandine.delauzon@inserm.fr (B.d.L.-G.)

Abstract: In low- and middle-income countries, the protective effect of breastfeeding against infections is well established, but in high-income countries, the effect could be weakened by higher hygienic conditions. We aimed to examine the association between breastfeeding and infections in the first 2 years of life, in a high-income country with relatively short breastfeeding duration. Among 10,349 young children from the nationwide Etude Longitudinale Française depuis l'Enfance (ELFE) birth cohort, breastfeeding and parent-reported hospitalizations, bronchiolitis and otitis events, and antibiotic use were prospectively collected up to 2 years. Never-breastfed infants were used as reference group. Any breastfeeding for <3 months was associated with higher risks of hospitalizations from gastrointestinal infections or fever. Predominant breastfeeding for <1 month was associated with higher risk of a single hospital admission while predominant breastfeeding for ≥3 months was associated with a lower risk of long duration (≥4 nights) of hospitalization. Ever breastfeeding was associated with lower risk of antibiotic use. This study confirmed the well-known associations between breastfeeding and hospitalizations but also highlighted a strong inverse association between breastfeeding and antibiotic use. Although we cannot infer causality from this observational study, this finding is worth highlighting in a context of rising concern regarding antibiotic resistance.

Keywords: breastfeeding; infections; birth cohort; hospitalizations; antibiotic use

---

1. Introduction

In 2013, infectious diseases were in the four main categories of leading causes of death among children under 5 years of age worldwide [1]. Nonetheless, disparities exist between countries. Infections are the leading causes of death in sub-Saharan African countries but not in high-income countries. The good hygienic conditions and health care system available in some countries significantly reduce the prevalence and fatal issue of such diseases but do not fully prevent them.

The World Health Organization (WHO) recommends exclusive breastfeeding for 6 months, or at least the first 4 months of life [2]. These recommendations were mainly based on the protective effect of breastfeeding against infectious morbidity and mortality [3]. In fact, breast milk components, such as immunoglobulin A (IgA) or maternal leukocytes, can both supplement and promote the newborn's immature immune system [4] and therefore lead to protective effect against infections.

More precisely, recent literature has shown that breastfeeding is related to a reduced rate of hospital admission for diarrhea and respiratory infections as well as a protective effect on otitis media in children up to 2 years old [3,5]. Of note, otitis media studies were mostly from high-income countries, whereas results on diarrhea and respiratory infection studies were mostly found in settings from low- and middle-income countries [6,7]. In high-income countries, the preventive effect of breastfeeding on respiratory tract infections is less consistent across studies [7]. In the cluster-randomized trial on promotion of breastfeeding (PROBIT), which took place in Belarus in the 1990s, breastfeeding was related to a reduced risk of gastrointestinal infections in the first year of life [8].

The aim of this study was to assess the association between breastfeeding duration and several indicators of infectious morbidity, in France, a high-income country with the specificity of low breastfeeding initiation rate (69.7%) and median duration below the guidelines (17 weeks among breastfeeding mothers) [3,9].

2. Materials and Methods

2.1. Study Population

This analysis was based on data from the ELFE (Etude Longitudinale Française depuis l'Enfance) study, a multidisciplinary nationwide birth cohort including 18,329 children born in 2011 in France [10]. The inclusion criteria were as follows: singleton or twins born after 33 weeks of gestation, to mothers aged 18 years or older. Participating mothers had to provide written consent for their own and their child's participation. Fathers signed the consent form for the child's participation when present at inclusion or were informed about their rights to oppose it. The ELFE study was approved by the Advisory Committee for Treatment of Health Research Information (Comité Consultatif sur le Traitement des Informations pour la Recherche en Santé), the National Data Protection Authority (Commission Nationale Informatique et Libertés), and the National Statistics Council.

2.2. Breastfeeding

The feeding method was prospectively collected up to 2 years and the calculation of breastfeeding duration was detailed in a previous paper [11]. As previously described, two breastfeeding definitions were used in the present study: any breastfeeding and predominant breastfeeding. Any breastfeeding was defined as the infant receiving breastmilk. Predominant breastfeeding was defined as the only milk given to the infant being human milk (no animal milk or infant formula).

For each breastfeeding definition, infants were first categorized as ever or never breastfed and then according to their breastfeeding duration (never, <1 month, 1 month to <3 months, 3 months to <6 months, ≥6 months).

2.3. Parental Report of Infections

In the present study, infections were assessed with several indicators: hospitalizations; frequency of bronchiolitis and otitis events; and antibiotic use.

At the 1- and 2-year phone interviews, parents reported hospitalizations in the previous year (date, duration, and main cause). Infants with at least one hospitalization for infectious disease were identified (mainly fever, gastrointestinal infection, and bronchiolitis). Hospitalizations from infectious diseases between birth and 2 years of age were characterized by the number of events (none, 1, ≥2) and cumulative duration (never, 1–3 nights, ≥4 nights).

At the 1-year phone interview, parents both reported whether the child ever had a bronchiolitis event and if the child had had at least 3 bronchiolitis events since birth. At the 2-year phone interview, parents reported whether the child had had 3 bronchiolitis episodes or more since birth. A mixed variable was computed from both interviews resulting in a 3-category variable assessing bronchiolitis events in the first 2 years of life (never, 1 or 2 events, ≥3 events).

At the 2-year phone interview, parents reported otitis events since birth (<3 events, ≥3 events). Unfortunately, it was not possible to distinguish infant with no otitis event from those having 1 or 2 events.

At the 1- and 2-year phone interviews, parents reported the frequency of antibiotic use for their child in the previous 12 months. These frequencies were then combined into a 4-category variable (never, once, 2 or 3 times, >3 times).

2.4. Other Variables

Maternal and household data were collected using face-to-face interviews at the maternity unit and then by phone interview at the 2-month follow-up. Because these data were more thoroughly assessed during the 2-month interview and only marginally changed during these 2 months, we used the data collected at 2 months in our analyses. Socio-demographic characteristics collected during the maternity stay were used only when the 2-month values were missing.

Maternal socio-demographic characteristics included age at the birth of her first child (<25, 25–29, 30–34, ≥35 years), education level (below secondary school, secondary school, high school, 2-year university degree, 3-year university degree, 5-year university degree or higher), place of birth (France, abroad), and employment status (unemployed, employed). Household characteristics included income per consumption unit (≤€750, €751 to 1111, €1112 to 1500, €1501 to 1944, €1945 to 2500, >€2500 /month) and composition (couple with children, single parenthood, step family).

Maternal health-related characteristics included smoking status during pregnancy (never smoked, smoked only before pregnancy, smoked only in early pregnancy, smoked throughout pregnancy) and pre-pregnancy body mass index (BMI) (<18.5 kg/m^2, 18.5 to 24.9 kg/m^2, 25.0 to 29.9 kg/m^2, ≥30.0 kg/m^2).

Infant's birth order (first born, second, third, fourth, or higher), caesarean-section delivery, sex, twin birth, and gestational age were collected at birth from medical records. Infant's age at first attendance at a shared childcare facility was computed from the 1-year phone interview as a 5-category variable (≤2 months, >2 to ≤4 months, >4 to ≤6 months, >6 to ≤12 months, never attended in the first year).

2.5. Sample Selection

Infants whose parents withdrew consent during the first year (n = 57) and not meeting eligibility criteria (n = 1) were excluded, resulting in 17,984 eligible infants. In twin pregnancies, one twin was randomly selected (n = 287 exclusions) to avoid family clusters.

We excluded infants without any follow-up at 2 years (n = 4705). We then excluded infants with missing data on breastfeeding (n = 147) and those with missing data on infections or antibiotic use (n = 1894). We also excluded infants with incomplete information for potential confounding variables (n = 889). These exclusions lead to a sample of 10,349 infants for the complete case analysis regarding parental reports of infections and antibiotic use (Figure 1).

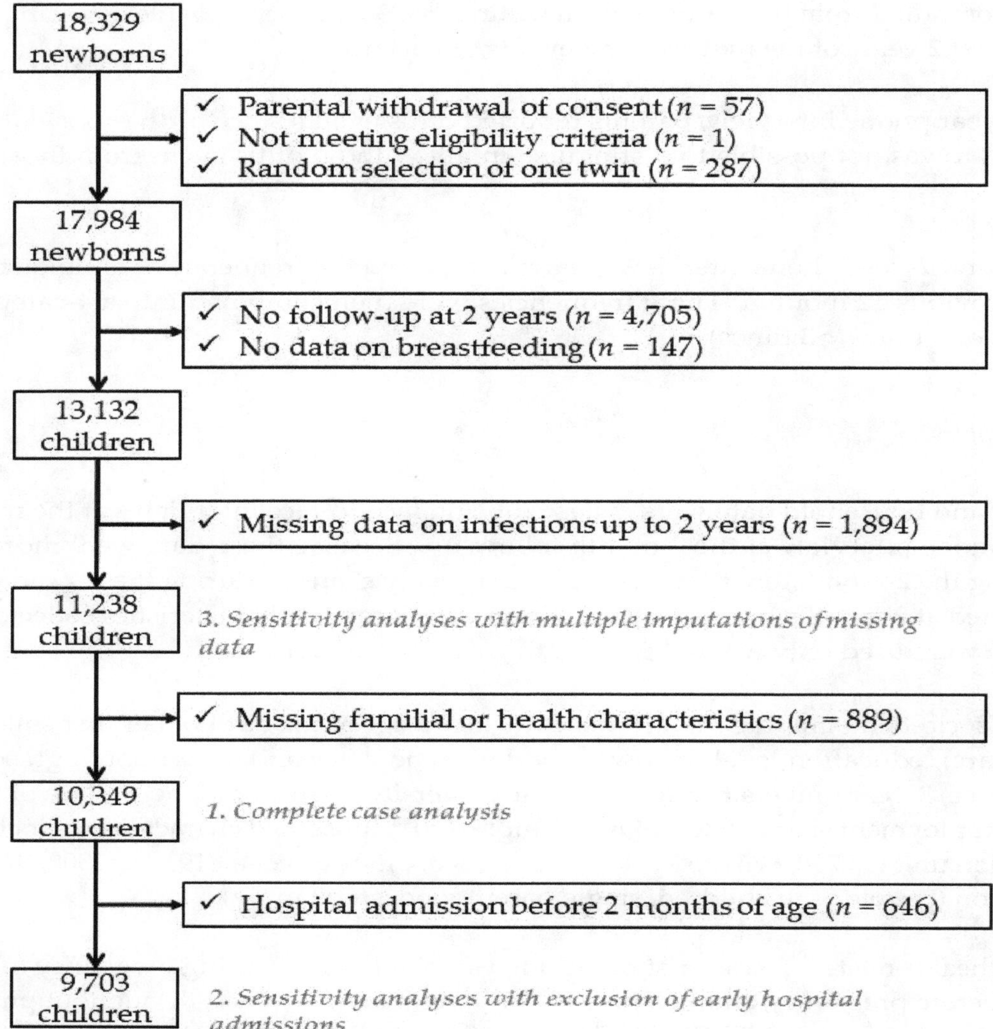

Figure 1. Sample selection.

2.6. *Analyses*

2.6.1. Main Analyses

To compare selected families to their non-selected ELFE counterparts, we used chi-squared tests for categorical variables and Student *t*-tests for continuous variables.

Associations between breastfeeding and parental reports of infections or antibiotic use were assessed with multinomial logistic regression models. Never-breastfed infants were systematically used as the reference group. In all analyses, we adjusted for potential confounding factors (maternal age at first child, education level, employment status, smoking status during pregnancy and pre-pregnancy BMI, household monthly income per consumption unit, household composition, caesarean section and infant's sex, gestational age, birth order, and age at first attendance at a shared childcare facility), and variables related to study design (recruitment wave, maternity unit size, and mother's region of residence).

2.6.2. Sensitivity Analyses

As early hospitalizations may lead to early breastfeeding cessation, we repeated the main analyses after excluding infants with hospitalizations occurring before the age of 2 months, leading to a sample of 9703 infants.

To deal with missing data for potential confounding factors, we first conducted our analyses on complete cases (Figure 1, n = 10,349). Secondly, we used multiple imputations to deal with these missing data. This method assigned data to missing measurements based on the measurement of infants with similar profiles. We assumed that data were missing at random and generated five independent datasets with the fully conditional specification method (MI procedure, FCS statement, NIMPUTE option), and then calculated pooled effect estimates (SAS MIANALYSE procedure). Further details are available in Table S1, Supplementary Materials. This method allowed us to assess again the association between breastfeeding duration and infections up to 2 years on a sample of 11,238 infants (Figure 1). The model used for these analyses was the same as in our main analysis.

All analyses were carried out with SAS software version 9.4 (SAS Institute, Cary, NC, USA). Statistical significance was defined as $p < 0.05$.

3. Results

The comparison between selected families and their non-selected ELFE counterparts is available in Table S2, Supplementary Materials. Briefly, selected mothers were older, less likely to be single parents, born in France, with a higher education level, and employed and they breastfed longer than non-selected mothers.

The sample's characteristics according to any breastfeeding duration are described in Table 1.

Table 1. Included families' characteristics according to any breastfeeding duration (n = 10,349).

Family Characteristics	Breastfeeding Duration				
	Never (*n* = 2489)	**<1 Month** (*n* = 1704)	**1 to <3 Months** (*n* = 1629)	**3 to <6 Months** (*n* = 1964)	**≥6 Months** (*n* = 2563)
Maternal age at birth (years)	30.4 (4.9)	30.0 (5.0)	30.4 (4.5)	30.9 (4.3)	31.6 (4.6)
Maternal place of birth (France)	96.6% (2405)	94.5% (1611)	92.4% (1505)	90.3% (1774)	82.7% (2120)
Pre-pregnancy body mass index (kg/m^2)	23.9 (5.2)	23.8 (4.9)	23.4 (4.5)	22.8 (4.1)	23.0 (4.3)
Education level					
Below secondary school	7.2% (178)	5.4% (92)	3.8% (62)	3.6% (71)	5.1% (131)
Secondary school	17.2% (428)	15.8% (269)	9.7% (158)	7.3% (143)	7.9% (202)
High school	21.6% (537)	21.4% (365)	18.4% (300)	15.1% (297)	13.7% (352)
2-year university degree	24.5% (611)	25.5% (434)	26.2% (427)	23.7% (465)	21.2% (543)
3-year university degree	15.8% (394)	18.2% (310)	19.6% (320)	22.3% (437)	22.8% (584)
5-year university degree or higher	13.7% (341)	13.7% (234)	22.2% (362)	28.1% (551)	29.3% (751)
Employed before pregnancy	77.9% (1938)	75% (1278)	79.7% (1299)	80.2% (1576)	71.4% (1829)
Traditional household composition	87.9% (2188)	87.9% (1498)	91.3% (1487)	91.6% (1799)	90.2% (2311)
Household monthly income (€)	3379 (3171)	3276 (2750)	3665 (4608)	3738 (3671)	3506 (2663)
Smoking status during pregnancy					
Never smoker	51.9% (1292)	50.1% (853)	57.5% (936)	60.7% (1193)	66.1% (1694)
Only before pregnancy	24% (598)	27.4% (467)	25.9% (422)	25.1% (492)	23.6% (604)
Only in early pregnancy	3.5% (88)	4.7% (80)	3.4% (56)	3.8% (74)	2.9% (75)
Throughout pregnancy	20.5% (511)	17.8% (304)	13.2% (215)	10.4% (205)	7.4% (190)
Caesarean section	19.2% (478)	18% (307)	18% (294)	15.7% (309)	15.2% (389)
Gestational age (weeks)	39.5 (1.5)	39.7 (1.4)	39.7 (1.4)	39.7 (1.4)	39.7 (1.4)
Boys	48.8% (1215)	49.4% (841)	51.6% (841)	50.1% (984)	48.7% (1249)
First born	42.9% (1069)	50.5% (861)	49.7% (809)	45.7% (897)	37.6% (963)
Age at first attendance at a shared childcare facility					
≤2 months	55.7% (1386)	54.2% (924)	48.4% (788)	46.4% (912)	61.6% (1580)
>2 months to 4 months	7.4% (183)	5.8% (99)	8% (130)	3.6% (70)	2.1% (53)
>4 months to 6 months	18.8% (469)	20.4% (347)	26.3% (429)	24.3% (477)	11.2% (286)
>6 months to 12 months	9.1% (227)	9.2% (157)	8.2% (133)	13.7% (269)	10.7% (273)
Never attended in the first year	9% (224)	10.4% (177)	9.1% (149)	12% (236)	14.5% (371)
% (n) or mean (± SD)					

3.1. *Hospitalizations from Infectious Diseases*

Breastfeeding status considered as a binary variable (ever vs. never) was related neither to the number of events (0, 1, ≥2) nor to the cumulative duration of hospitalizations or infectious causes of hospitalizations, whatever the definition of breastfeeding used (any or predominant) (Table 2).

Table 2. Association between breastfeeding and parent reports of hospitalizations from infection: multivariate analyses (n = 10,349).

Breastfeeding Status and Duration	Parental Report of Hospitalizations from Infection											
	Number of Events (Ref = None)			Total Duration (Ref = Never)					Causes			
	1	≥2	*p*	1–3 Nights	≥4 Nights	*p*	Fever	*p*	Gastroint. Inf.	*p*	Bronchiolitis	*p*
Number of infants in each group	842	413		470	429		282		397		475	
Any breastfeeding status			0.52			0.33		0.11		0.40		0.98
Never	1 (Ref)	1 (Ref)		1 (Ref)	1 (Ref)		1 (Ref)		1 (Ref)		1 (Ref)	
Ever	1.10 (0.93; 1.31)	1.04 (0.82; 1.32)		1.16 (0.92; 1.46)	0.92 (0.73; 1.16)		1.28 (0.95; 1.74)		1.11 (0.87; 1.42)		1.00 (0.80; 1.24)	
Any breastfeeding duration			0.29			0.25		0.17		0.08		0.10
Never	1 (Ref)	1 (Ref)		1 (Ref)	1 (Ref)		1 (Ref)		1 (Ref)		1 (Ref)	
<1 month	1.13 (0.90; 1.42)	1.20 (0.89; 1.62)		1.21 (0.90; 1.63)	1.02 (0.76; 1.38)		1.38 (0.94; 2.02)		1.42 (1.05; 1.91)		0.92 (0.68; 1.24)	
1 to <3 months	1.22 (0.97; 1.53)	1.15 (0.84; 1.58)		1.17 (0.86; 1.60)	1.08 (0.79; 1.46)		1.55 (1.06; 2.28)		0.91 (0.64; 1.29)		1.24 (0.93; 1.65)	
3 to <6 months	1.13 (0.91; 1.42)	0.94 (0.68; 1.29)		1.28 (0.96; 1.71)	0.85 (0.63; 1.17)		1.13 (0.76; 1.68)		1.03 (0.75; 1.43)		1.07 (0.80; 1.42)	
≥6 months	0.96 (0.77; 1.20)	0.89 (0.65; 1.21)		1.00 (0.74; 1.34)	0.77 (0.57; 1.04)		1.13 (0.78; 1.65)		1.04 (0.76; 1.42)		0.82 (0.62; 1.10)	
Number of infants in each group	839	413		468	428		281		395		474	
Predominant breastfeeding status			0.42			0.27		0.65		0.73		0.59
Never	1 (Ref)	1 (Ref)		1 (Ref)	1 (Ref)		1 (Ref)		1 (Ref)		1 (Ref)	
Ever	1.10 (0.94; 1.29)	0.96 (0.77; 1.19)		1.12 (0.91; 1.39)	0.88 (0.72; 1.09)		1.06 (0.82; 1.39)		1.04 (0.83; 1.30)		1.06 (0.86; 1.30)	
Predominant breastfeeding duration			0.24			0.08		0.25		0.14		0.24
Never	1 (Ref)	1 (Ref)		1 (Ref)	1 (Ref)		1 (Ref)		1 (Ref)		1 (Ref)	
<1 month	1.24 (1.01; 1.52)	1.09 (0.82; 1.44)		1.27 (0.97; 1.65)	1.07 (0.81; 1.40)		1.13 (0.80; 1.59)		1.28 (0.97; 1.68)		1.25 (0.96; 1.62)	
1 to <3 months	1.13 (0.92; 1.39)	0.99 (0.74; 1.32)		1.05 (0.79; 1.38)	1.00 (0.76; 1.31)		1.28 (0.92; 1.79)		1.02 (0.76; 1.37)		1.04 (0.79; 1.37)	
3 to <6 months	1.02 (0.82; 1.27)	0.79 (0.57; 1.08)		1.08 (0.81; 1.44)	0.67 (0.49; 0.93)		0.85 (0.58; 1.24)		0.84 (0.61; 1.17)		1.00 (0.75; 1.32)	
≥6 months	0.90 (0.68; 1.19)	0.92 (0.63; 1.34)		1.05 (0.74; 1.50)	0.67 (0.45; 1.00)		0.88 (0.56; 1.40)		0.89 (0.60; 1.34)		0.81 [0.56; 1.18)	

OR (CI 95%) multinomial logistic regressions adjusted for maternal age at first child, education level, employment status, smoking status during pregnancy and pre-pregnancy BMI, household monthly income per consumption unit, household composition, caesarean section and infant's sex, gestational age, birth order, and age at first attendance at a shared childcare facility, recruitment wave, maternity unit size and level, and mother's region of residence. Analyses were performed separately for each breastfeeding definition.

Compared to never-breastfed infants, infants who were predominantly breastfed for <1 month were at higher risk of being hospitalized once, which justifies our sensitivity analysis excluding early infections. The association remained consistent after the exclusion of infants with early hospitalizations (before the age of 2 months) (Table S3, Supplementary Materials).

Compared to never-breastfed infants, infants who were predominantly breastfed for at least 3 months were at lower risk of long duration (≥4 nights) of hospitalizations. These associations remained consistent after the exclusion of infants with early hospitalizations (before the age of 2 months).

Compared to never-breastfed infants, any breastfed for 1 to <3 months infants were at higher risk of hospitalization from fever and any breastfed for <1 month infants were at higher risk of hospitalization from gastrointestinal infections. The first association disappeared after the exclusion of early hospitalization, whereas the second one remained consistent.

3.2. Bronchiolitis Events

Overall, the number of bronchiolitis events was significantly related neither to ever breastfeeding nor to breastfeeding duration. However, ever any breastfeeding tended to be related to a higher risk of 1 or 2 bronchiolitis events but not to frequent bronchiolitis events. In contrast, predominant breastfeeding duration tended to be negatively related to the risk of frequent bronchiolitis events (Table 3). These tendencies remained after the exclusion of early hospitalization events (Table S4, Supplementary Materials).

Table 3. Association between breastfeeding and parent reports of bronchiolitis events, otitis events, and antibiotic use: multivariate analyses (n = 10,349).

Breastfeeding Status and Duration		Parental Report								
		Bronchiolitis Events (Ref = None)			Otitis Events (Ref ≤ 3)		Antibiotic Use (Ref = Never)			
		1 or 2	≥3	p	≥3	p	Once	2 or 3 Times	>3 Times	p
Number of infants in each group		6340	1264		2606		1944	1860	4411	
Any breastfeeding status				0.17		0.32				0.02
	Never	1 (Ref)	1 (Ref)		1 (Ref)		1 (Ref)	1 (Ref)	1 (Ref)	
	Ever	1.11 (0.99; 1.24)	1.09 (0.92; 1.28)		1.06 (0.95; 1.18)		0.94 (0.80; 1.09)	0.84 (0.72; 0.98)	0.83 (0.73; 0.94)	
Any breastfeeding duration				0.05		0.37				0.00
	Never	1 (Ref)	1 (Ref)		1 (Ref)		1 (Ref)	1 (Ref)	1 (Ref)	
	<1 month	1.07 (0.93; 1.24)	1.19 (0.96; 1.48)		1.08 (0.94; 1.25)		0.99 (0.80; 1.22)	1.02 (0.83; 1.26)	1.09 (0.92; 1.30)	
	1 to <3 months	1.09 (0.94; 1.26)	1.08 (0.87; 1.35)		1.12 (0.97; 1.29)		1.04 (0.84; 1.28)	0.95 (0.77; 1.18)	0.98 (0.82; 1.17)	
	3 to <6 months	1.15 (1.00; 1.33)	1.20 (0.97; 1.48)		1.06 (0.92; 1.22)		1.00 (0.82; 1.22)	0.78 (0.64; 0.95)	0.79 (0.67; 0.94)	
	≥6 months	1.12 (0.98; 1.29)	0.90 (0.73; 1.12)		0.98 (0.86; 1.13)		0.79 (0.66; 0.95)	0.71 (0.59; 0.85)	0.61 (0.52; 0.71)	
Number of infants in each group		6335	1263		2605		1940	1857	4410	
Predominant breastfeeding status				0.30		0.92				0.00
	Never	1 (Ref)	1 (Ref)		1 (Ref)		1 (Ref)	1 (Ref)	1 (Ref)	
	Ever	1.08 (0.98; 1.19)	1.04 (0.90; 1.21)		0.99 (0.90; 1.10)		0.96 (0.83; 1.10)	0.84 (0.73; 0.96)	0.79 (0.71; 0.89)	
Predominant breastfeeding duration				0.06		0.98				0.00
	Never	1 (Ref)	1 (Ref)		1 (Ref)		1 (Ref)	1 (Ref)	1 (Ref)	
	<1 month	1.09 (0.95; 1.24)	1.19 (0.98; 1.45)		1.02 (0.89; 1.16)		1.11 (0.92; 1.33)	1.05 (0.87; 1.26)	0.97 (0.83; 1.14)	
	1 to <3 months	1.13 (0.99; 1.30)	1.08 (0.89; 1.32)		1.01 (0.88; 1.15)		0.95 (0.79; 1.14)	0.82 (0.68; 0.99)	0.87 (0.74; 1.01)	
	3 to <6 months	1.10 (0.96; 1.270)	0.99 (0.81; 1.22)		0.97 (0.85; 1.11)		0.88 (0.73; 1.06)	0.71 (0.59; 0.85)	0.65 (0.56; 0.76)	
	≥6 months	0.94 (0.80; 1.110)	0.77 (0.59; 1.00)		0.97 (0.82; 1.15)		0.89 (0.71; 1.10)	0.75 (0.60; 0.93)	0.62 (0.51; 0.75)	

OR (CI 95%) multinomial logistic regressions adjusted for maternal age at first child, education level, employment status, smoking status during pregnancy and pre-pregnancy BMI, household monthly income per consumption unit, household composition, caesarean section and infant's sex, gestational age, birth order, and age at first attendance at a shared childcare facility, recruitment wave, maternity unit size and level, and mother's region of residence. Analyses were performed separately for each breastfeeding definition.

3.3. Otitis Events

Both any and predominant breastfeeding were not related to frequent otitis events (at least 3 in the first 2 years) (Table 3).

3.4. Antibiotic Use

Ever breastfeeding was related to a lower risk of frequent antibiotic use (at least 2 times in the first 2 years of life), whatever the definition of breastfeeding used (Table 3).

Compared to no breastfeeding, breastfeeding durations (any and predominant) of at least 3 months were associated with a lower risk of frequent antibiotic use.

All these associations remained after the exclusion of infants with early hospitalizations (Table S4, Supplementary Materials).

3.5. Analyses after Multiple Imputations

Compared to never-breastfed infants, predominantly breastfed for <1 month infants were no longer at higher risk of a single hospitalization event (OR (95% CI) = 1.17 (0.96; 1.42)) (Table S5, Supplementary Materials). Any breastfed for <1 month infants were also no longer at higher risk of hospitalization from gastrointestinal infections (1.32 (0.99; 1.75)).

Compared to never-breastfed infants, any breastfed for ≥6 months infants were at lower risk of longer hospitalizations (≥4 nights) (0.71 (0.53; 0.95)).

Other previously highlighted results remained consistent (Tables S5 and S6, Supplementary Materials).

4. Discussion

In the ELFE study, predominant breastfeeding for over 3 months was related to lower risk of at least 4 nights of hospitalization up to 2 years, while any breastfeeding for over 3 months was related to higher risk of 1 or 2 bronchiolitis events in the first 2 years of age. Finally, both any and predominant breastfeeding durations were negatively associated with frequency of antibiotic use.

We first examined infectious morbidity through common infectious diseases such as bronchiolitis and otitis. Unfortunately, data on diarrhea occurrence were not collected. Contrary to a previous meta-analysis conducted in industrialized countries [12], a lower risk of otitis has not been related to breastfeeding duration. A possible explanation may be the restrictive classification (<3 or ≥3 events) applied in the ELFE questionnaires, not allowing the distinguishing of absence of event from low frequency of events (1 or 2). Consistent with an Italian cohort specifically designed to study respiratory infections [13], we found that, in the main analyses, long duration of predominant breastfeeding (at least 6 months) was associated with a lower risk of frequent bronchiolitis events. Similarly, in the Generation R population-based study, exclusive breastfeeding was related to a lower risk of low respiratory tract infections and, to a lesser extent, upper respiratory tract infections up to 4 years of age [14].

Infections with higher concern can be approximated with hospitalizations. A recent meta-analysis highlighted a protective effect of breastfeeding against hospitalizations from diarrhea and respiratory infections, including lower respiratory tract infection and pneumonia [7]. More recently, the Norwegian MoBa study highlighted a higher risk of hospitalization up to 18 months among infants breastfed for ≤6 months than among those breastfed for at least 12 months [15], but matched sibling analyses, enabled to account for shared maternal characteristics, showed weaker and non-significant associations. We have not observed such associations within the ELFE cohort. Regarding hospitalizations from diarrhea, the meta-analysis included two studies from Europe, highlighting protective associations between breastfeeding and diarrhea [16,17]. Both studies provided data on infants born in the 1990s. Regarding hospitalizations from respiratory infection, the meta-analysis included two studies from Europe, highlighting protective associations between breastfeeding and respiratory infections [18,19], both published before 1995. As infants from the ELFE were born in 2011, they might differ from infants included in these studies. Moreover, in the present analyses only hospitalizations for bronchiolitis could be considered and not all respiratory infections. The low number of hospitalizations for bronchiolitis in our results might prevent any potential association with breastfeeding to arise.

We are unable to provide a biological explanation for the higher risk of 1 or 2 bronchiolitis events in the first 2 years of life related to any breastfeeding but not to predominant breastfeeding. An additional sensitivity analysis adjusting for family history of allergy (parental and/or sibling history of asthma, eczema, and hay fever) did not modify the results (data not shown). A similar unexpected association was found in an Italian case–control study, with a higher breastfeeding rate among infants hospitalized for bronchiolitis than among their control counterparts [20].

Reverse causation bias is a probable hypothesis for the highlighted higher risk of parental reported hospital admission from infection or gastrointestinal infection related to short breastfeeding duration (<1 month) compared to never breastfeeding. As early adverse health events, including hospital admission, can lead to early breastfeeding cessation, the exclusion of early cases of hospitalization allowed us to control this reverse causation bias but not fully as not all adverse health events lead to hospitalization.

Finally, in the present study, antibiotic use was considered as a proxy for bacterial infections. This indicator was strongly related to breastfeeding, a longer duration being related to a lower use of antibiotics up to 2 years of age. Similar results were found in a Czech cross-sectional survey, with lower risk of early exposure to antibiotics among breastfed infants [21]. Likewise, in a Finnish cohort, 1-year breastfed infants were less likely to have been provided with antibiotics during the first year of life than their non-breastfed counterparts [22], and a negative association between breastfeeding duration and antibiotic use was found in a cross-sectional anthropometric and questionnaire study [23]. However, we cannot exclude that health-seeking behaviors could be different among breastfeeding parents and non-breastfeeding parents, leading to the differential use of antibiotics. Moreover, as both breastfeeding and antibiotic use could influence the infant's microbiome [22], microbiome was suggested as a potential mechanism in the association between breastfeeding and lower rates of infections from hospitalization. It would be of great interest to examine these potential mechanisms from stool samples collected in the first months of life.

The ELFE study is a recent nationwide birth cohort aimed at assessing the development of healthy-born children from birth to adulthood from a broad and interdisciplinary point of view. The prospective design limits recall bias for both exposure and outcomes assessment. However, we have to acknowledge the inability to consider exclusive breastfeeding in the present study according to the WHO definition, because the use of water, water-based drinks, and fruit juice in the 0–2-month period were not collected in the ELFE study. While the study may lack specificity when assessing particular outcomes (e.g., antibiotic types), the strength of our approach is the use of complementary indicators of infectious morbidity, with the occurrence of common infectious diseases, hospitalizations, and antibiotic use. Hospitalizations could reflect the most severe cases and allowed for controlling bias due to parental reporting. It is interesting to note that breastfeeding was more related to the duration of hospitalization than to the number of events. When matching with the national health system database will be available, it would be of great interest to conduct similar analyses based on medical care use rather than parental report. The use of antibiotics would be more specific for bacterial infections, but it remains difficult to distinguish a lower need for antibiotics from the reluctance to such use. The very large sample and the collection of detailed socio-demographic or economic data ensure good statistical power and favor control for potential confounders. Exclusion rates due to missing data for these analyses were high, but multiple imputations did not change the results.

5. Conclusions

Even in the context of a high-income country with short breastfeeding duration, we highlighted a lower risk of infectious morbidity related to breastfeeding duration, especially for duration of hospitalization and antibiotic use. The strong association highlighted for antibiotic use would be of great interest in the context of rising concerns regarding antibiotic resistance.

Supplementary Materials:
Table S1: Details regarding variables used for the multiple imputations, Table S2: Comparison of included and excluded families (Chi-squared and Student *t*-tests, Table S3: Multivariate adjusted analyses assessing breastfeeding and parent reports of hospitalizations from infection among infants without hospitalization events before 2 months of age (n = 9,703), Table S4: Multivariate adjusted analyses assessing breastfeeding and parent reports of bronchiolitis events, otitis events, and antibiotic use among infants without hospitalization events before 2 months of age (n = 9,703), Table S5: Multivariate adjusted analyses assessing breastfeeding and parent reports of hospitalizations from infection using multiple imputations to deal with missing measurements on familial or health characteristics (n = 11,238), Table S6: Multivariate adjusted analyses assessing breastfeeding and parent reports of bronchiolitis events, otitis events, and antibiotic use using multiple imputations to deal with missing measurements on familial or health characteristics (n = 11,238).

Author Contributions: The corresponding author affirms that all listed authors meet authorship criteria and that no others meeting these criteria have been omitted. C.D.-P. conducted the statistical analyses, interpreted the results, drafted the initial manuscript, and approved the final manuscript as submitted. K.A.-P., A.D.-C., J.P. and S.L. contributed to the interpretation of the results, critically reviewed the manuscript, and approved the final version submitted. M.C. and M.-N.D. contributed to the data acquisition, critically reviewed the manuscript, and approved the final version submitted. M.-A.C. and B.d.L.-G. conceptualized and designed the study, contributed to the interpretation of the results, reviewed and revised the manuscript, and approved the final manuscript as submitted.

Funding: The ELFE survey is a joint project between the French Institute for Demographic Studies (INED) and the National Institute of Health and Medical Research (INSERM), in partnership with the French blood transfusion service (Etablissement français du sang, EFS), Santé publique France, the National Institute for Statistics and Economic Studies (INSEE), the Direction générale de la santé (DGS, part of the Ministry of Health and Social Affairs), the Direction générale de la prévention des risques (DGPR, Ministry for the Environment), the Direction de la recherche, des études, de l'évaluation et des statistiques (DREES, Ministry of Health and Social Affairs), the Département des études, de la prospective et des statistiques (DEPS, Ministry of Culture), and the Caisse nationale des allocations familiales (CNAF), with the support of the Ministry of Higher Education and Research and the Institut national de la jeunesse et de l'éducation populaire (INJEP). Via the RECONAI platform, it received a government grant managed by the National Research Agency under the "Investissements d'avenir" program (ANR-11-EQPX-0038). The funders had no role in the study design, data collection and analysis, decision to publish, or preparation of the manuscript. This research received no external funding.

Acknowledgments: We would like to thank the scientific coordinators (Marie-Aline Charles, Bertrand Geay, Henri Léridon, Corinne Bois, Marie-Noëlle Dufourg, Jean-Louis Lanoé, Xavier Thierry, Cécile Zaros), IT and data managers, statisticians (A. Rakotonirina, R. Kugel, R. Borges-Panhino, M. Cheminat, H. Juillard), administrative and family communication staff, and study technicians (C. Guevel, M. Zoubiri, L. Gravier, I. Milan, R. Popa) of the ELFE coordination team as well as the families who gave their time for the study.

References

1. Kyu, H.H.; Pinho, C.; Wagner, J.A.; Brown, J.C.; Bertozzi-Villa, A.; Charlson, F.J.; Coffeng, L.E.; Dandona, L.; Erskine, H.E.; Ferrari, A.J.; et al. Global and National Burden of Diseases and Injuries Among Children and Adolescents Between 1990 and 2013: Findings From the Global Burden of Disease 2013 Study. *JAMA Pediatr.* **2016**, *170*, 267–287.
2. World Health Organization. *Feeding and Nutrition of Infants and Young Children, Guidelines for the WHO European Region, with Emphasis on the Former Soviet Countries*; WHO: Geneva, Switzerland, 2003.
3. Victora, C.G.; Bahl, R.; Barros, A.J.; Franca, G.V.; Horton, S.; Krasevec, J.; Murch, S.; Sankar, M.J.; Walker, N.; Rollins, N.C.; et al. Breastfeeding in the 21st century: Epidemiology, mechanisms, and lifelong effect. *Lancet* **2016**, *387*, 475–490. [CrossRef]
4. Field, C.J. The immunological components of human milk and their effect on immune development in infants. *J. Nutr.* **2006**, *135*, 1–4. [CrossRef]
5. Korvel-Hanquist, A.; Djurhuus, B.D.; Homoe, P. The Effect of Breastfeeding on Childhood Otitis Media. *Curr. Allergy Asthma Rep.* **2017**, *17*, 45. [CrossRef]
6. Bowatte, G.; Tham, R.; Allen, K.J.; Tan, D.J.; Lau, M.; Dai, X.; Lodge, C.J. Breastfeeding and childhood acute otitis media: A systematic review and meta-analysis. *Acta Paediatr.* **2015**, *104*, 85–95. [CrossRef]
7. Horta, B.L.; Victora, C.G. *Short-Term Effects of Breastfeeding: A Systematic Review of the Benefits of Breastfeeding on Diarrhoea and Pneumonia Mortality*; World Health Organization: Geneva, Switzerland, 2013.
8. Kramer, M.S.; Chalmers, B.; Hodnett, E.D.; Sevkovskaya, Z.; Dzikovich, I.; Shapiro, S.; Collet, J.P.; Vanilovich, I.;

Mezen, I.; Ducruet, T.; et al. Promotion of Breastfeeding Intervention Trial (PROBIT). *JAMA* **2001**, *285*, 413–420. [CrossRef]

9. Wagner, S.; Kersuzan, C.; Gojard, S.; Tichit, C.; Nicklaus, S.; Geay, B.; Humeau, P.; Thierry, X.; Charles, M.A.; Lioret, S.; et al. Breastfeeding duration in France according to parents and birth characteristics. Results from the ELFE longitudinal French Study, 2011. *Bull. Epidemiol. Hebd.* **2015**, *29*, 522–532.
10. Vandentorren, S.; Bois, C.; Pirus, C.; Sarter, H.; Salines, G.; Leridon, H.; Elfe, T. Rationales, design and recruitment for the Elfe longitudinal study. *BMC Pediatr.* **2009**, *9*, 58. [CrossRef]
11. Wagner, S.; Kersuzan, C.; Gojard, S.; Tichit, C.; Nicklaus, S.; Thierry, X.; Charles, M.A.; Lioret, S.; De Lauzon-Guillain, B. Breastfeeding initiation and duration in France: The importance of intergenerational and previous maternal breastfeeding experiences—results from the nationwide ELFE study. *Midwifery* **2019**, *69*, 67–75. [CrossRef]
12. Lodge, C.J.; Bowatte, G.; Matheson, M.C.; Dharmage, S.C. The Role of Breastfeeding in Childhood Otitis Media. *Curr. Allergy Asthma Rep.* **2016**, *16*, 68. [CrossRef]
13. Lanari, M.; Prinelli, F.; Adorni, F.; Di Santo, S.; Faldella, G.; Silvestri, M.; Musicco, M. Maternal milk protects infants against bronchiolitis during the first year of life. Results from an Italian cohort of newborns. *Early Hum. Dev.* **2013**, *89*, 51–57. [CrossRef]
14. Tromp, I.; Kiefte-De Jong, J.; Raat, H.; Jaddoe, V.; Franco, O.; Hofman, A.; De Jongste, J.; Moll, H. Breastfeeding and the risk of respiratory tract infections after infancy: The Generation R Study. *PLoS ONE* **2017**, *12*, e0172763. [CrossRef]
15. Stordal, K.; Lundeby, K.M.; Brantsaeter, A.L.; Haugen, M.; Nakstad, B.; Lund-Blix, N.A.; Stene, L.C. Breast-feeding and Infant Hospitalization for Infections: Large Cohort and Sibling Analysis. *J. Pediatr. Gastroenterol. Nutr.* **2017**, *65*, 225–231. [CrossRef]
16. Quigley, M.A.; Kelly, Y.J.; Sacker, A. Breastfeeding and hospitalization for diarrheal and respiratory infection in the United Kingdom Millennium Cohort Study. *Pediatrics* **2007**, *119*, e837–e842. [CrossRef]
17. Kramer, M.S.; Guo, T.; Platt, R.W.; Sevkovskaya, Z.; Dzikovich, I.; Collet, J.P.; Shapiro, S.; Chalmers, B.; Hodnett, E.; Vanilovich, I.; et al. Infant growth and health outcomes associated with 3 compared with 6 mo of exclusive breastfeeding. *Am. J. Clin. Nutr.* **2003**, *78*, 291–295. [CrossRef]
18. Pisacane, A.; Graziano, L.; Zona, G.; Granata, G.; Dolezalova, H.; Cafiero, M.; Coppola, A.; Scarpellino, B.; Ummarino, M.; Mazzarella, G. Breast feeding and acute lower respiratory infection. *Acta Paediatr.* **1994**, *83*, 714–718. [CrossRef]
19. Howie, P.W.; Forsyth, J.S.; Ogston, S.A.; Clark, A.; Florey, C.D. Protective effect of breast feeding against infection. *BMJ* **1990**, *300*, 11–16. [CrossRef]
20. Nenna, R.; Cutrera, R.; Frassanito, A.; Alessandroni, C.; Nicolai, A.; Cangiano, G.; Petrarca, L.; Arima, S.; Caggiano, S.; Ullmann, N.; et al. Modifiable risk factors associated with bronchiolitis. *Ther. Adv. Respir. Dis.* **2017**, *11*, 393–401. [CrossRef]
21. Parizkova, P.; Dankova, N.; Fruhauf, P.; Jireckova, J.; Zeman, J.; Magner, M. Associations between breastfeeding rates and infant disease: A survey of 2338 Czech children. *Nutr. Diet. J. Dietit. Assoc. Aust.* **2019**. [CrossRef]
22. Korpela, K.; Salonen, A.; Virta, L.J.; Kekkonen, R.A.; De Vos, W.M. Association of Early-Life Antibiotic Use and Protective Effects of Breastfeeding: Role of the Intestinal Microbiota. *JAMA Pediatr.* **2016**, *170*, 750–757. [CrossRef]
23. Krenz-Niedbala, M.; Koscinski, K.; Puch, E.A.; Zelent, A.; Breborowicz, A. Is the Relationship Between Breastfeeding and Childhood Risk of Asthma and Obesity Mediated by Infant Antibiotic Treatment? *Breastfeed. Med.* **2015**, *10*, 326–333. [CrossRef]

5

The Concentration of Omega-3 Fatty Acids in Human Milk is Related to their Habitual but Not Current Intake

Agnieszka Bzikowska-Jura [1], Aneta Czerwonogrodzka-Senczyna [1], Edyta Jasińska-Melon [2], Hanna Mojska [2], Gabriela Olędzka [3], Aleksandra Wesołowska [4,*] and Dorota Szostak-Węgierek [1]

1 Department of Clinical Dietetics, Faculty of Health Sciences, Medical University of Warsaw, E Ciolka Str. 27, 01-445 Warsaw, Poland
2 Department of Metabolomics Food and Nutrition Institute, 61/63 Powsińska Str., 02-903 Warsaw, Poland
3 Department of Medical Biology, Faculty of Health Sciences, Medical University of Warsaw, Litewska Str. 14/16, 00-575 Warsaw, Poland
4 Laboratory of Human Milk and Lactation Research at Regional Human Milk Bank in Holy Family Hospital, Faculty of Health Sciences, Department of Neonatology, Medical University of Warsaw, Zwirki i Wigury Str. 63A, 02-091 Warsaw, Poland
* Correspondence: aleksandra.wesolowska@wum.edu.pl

Abstract: This study determined fatty acid (FA) concentrations in maternal milk and investigated the association between omega-3 fatty acid levels and their maternal current dietary intake (based on three-day dietary records) and habitual dietary intake (based on intake frequency of food products). Tested material comprised 32 samples of human milk, coming from exclusively breastfeeding women during their first month of lactation. Milk fatty acids were analyzed as fatty acid methyl ester (FAME) by gas chromatography using a Hewlett-Packard 6890 gas chromatograph with MS detector 5972A. We did not observe any correlation between current dietary intake of omega-3 FAs and their concentrations in human milk. However, we observed that the habitual intake of fatty fish affected omega-3 FA concentrations in human milk. Kendall's rank correlation coefficients were 0.25 ($p = 0.049$) for DHA, 0.27 ($p = 0.03$) for EPA, and 0.28 ($p = 0.02$) for ALA. Beef consumption was negatively correlated with DHA concentrations in human milk ($r = -0.25$; $p = 0.046$). These findings suggest that current omega-3 FA intake does not translate directly into their concentration in human milk. On the contrary, their habitual intake seems to markedly influence their milk concentration.

Keywords: human milk; omega-3 fatty acids; docosahexaenoic acid; eicosapentaenoic acid; α-linolenic acid; dietary intake; food frequency questionnaire

---

1. Introduction

Human milk is universally recognized as the optimal food for infants. Many studies have shown the role of fat in human milk as the main source of energy, selected fatty acids (FAs), crucial fat-soluble vitamins, and key nutrients for the infant development [1–3]. Among FAs, polyunsaturated fatty acids (PUFAs) are of principal importance. The two major classes of PUFAs are those of omega-3 and omega-6 families. Omega-3 fatty acids have a carbon–carbon double bond located in the third position from the methyl end of the chain. There are several different omega-3 FAs, but the majority of human milk research focuses on three: docosahexaenoic acid (DHA), α-linolenic acid (ALA), and eicosapentaenoic acid (EPA). ALA contains 18 carbon atoms, whereas EPA and DHA are considered "long-chain" (LC) omega-3 FAs, because EPA contains 20 carbons and DHA contains 22 [4]. Omega-3 FAs, mainly DHA, are important components of retinal photoreceptors and brain cell membranes. Therefore, DHA is essential for infant visual and cognitive development [5–7]. The European Food Safety Authority (EFSA) recommends 100 mg/day as the adequate intake of DHA for infants [8].

Fatty acids in human milk may originate either from the maternal dietary FAs, from FAs released from maternal adipose tissue, or from *de novo* synthesis in maternal tissues [5]. The human fatty acid desaturase can form only carbon–carbon double bonds located in the ninth position from the methyl end of a fatty acid. ALA may be endogenously converted to EPA and then to DHA. Therefore, ALA is considered an essential fatty acid, which means that it must be obtained from the diet [9,10]. However, the results of the studies show that the ability to convert ALA to DHA in humans is low, as less than 10% of ALA is converted to DHA [11]. For that reason, DHA from the maternal diet is a much more efficient source of DHA for neural tissue than an equivalent amount of ALA [10,12]. Therefore, consuming EPA and DHA directly from food and/or supplements is the only practical way to increase the levels of these fatty acids in the body.

Many national health authorities [13,14], including the Polish Society for Pediatric Gastroenterology, Hepatology, and Nutrition [15] recommend that maternal intake of DHA should be at least 200 mg per day. Women can meet the recommendation by consuming one to two portions of fatty fish (e.g., salmon, sardines) per week (equivalent of 150–300 g). Although the maternal intake of DHA is crucial for infant brain and retina development, studies carried out in the United States [16], Canada [17,18], and Europe [19] have reported that breastfeeding women do not meet dietary recommendations. This probably results from low fatty fish consumption [20], and is partly related to concerns of methylmercury fish contamination [21], as well as low DHA supplements use [16–18].

The tissue levels of FAs in a woman during lactation are directly related to her reserve capacity and the metabolic utilization of fatty acids (synthesis, oxidation and transport). Hence, the maternal diet and metabolism of FAs of women during lactation seem to be the most important factors affecting DHA concentration in human milk. Human milk FA composition changes continuously as dietary FAs are rapidly transported from chylomicrons into human milk with a peak between six and 12 h after dietary DHA intake [21,22].

To investigate the relationship between maternal diet and human milk composition, several dietary assessment methods have been developed and evaluated. The most common are food frequency questionnaires (FFQs) and multiple-day food records. Since food records do not rely on memory, they have been used as a reference method to validate other dietary assessment methods. On the other hand, day-to-day variations and seasonal variations in food consumption may decrease their objectivity. Furthermore, individuals are not always able to recall all the foods consumed or the specific components of the food (especially when dining out), and have difficulty in determining accurate portion sizes and typically underreport dietary intake. This is in contrast to FFQs, which often overestimate the intake of energy and nutrients [23]. Nonetheless, the FFQ has been suggested as an optimal tool in estimating dietary intake of omega-3 fatty acids as it evaluates long-term diet rather than food records [24]. Most of the FFQs available in the literature were designed to assess a wide range of nutrients; however, they were not appropriate for dietary assessment focusing specifically on fatty acids. Given that omega-3 FAs are contained in a particular range of foods, we used a tailored omega-3 FA FFQ. Serra-Majem et al. [25] suggested that its validity is comparable to the whole diet-based FFQs. (0.42–0.52 versus 0.19–0.54). We hypothesize that the concentration of omega-3 fatty acids in human milk is related to their habitual but not current intake; for this reason, in this study, we aimed to determine FA concentrations in maternal milk and assess the association between omega-3 fatty acids levels and their maternal dietary intake evaluated with two methods: dietary intake based on the three-day dietary record, and intake frequency of food products (FFQ, or food frequency questionnaire).

2. Materials and Methods

2.1. Subjects and Study Session Design

The Ethics Committee of the Medical University of Warsaw (KB/172/115) approved the study protocol, and all the participating women signed informed consents. A convenience sample of exclusively breastfeeding women (n = 32) was recruited from the Holy Family Hospital in Warsaw. Participants were enrolled during their first month of lactation (weeks two to four). Inclusion criteria comprised: age ≥18 years, singleton pregnancy, and full-term delivery (gestational age ≥37 weeks). Exclusion criteria were as follows: pre-existing chronic or gestational diseases, smoking during pregnancy and/or breastfeeding, low birth weight of the newborn, and low milk supply. The survey consisted of two parts. Firstly, we collected data about socio-demographic and other maternal characteristics, such as: age, education level, material status, pre-pregnancy anthropometric parameters (weight and height), and total weight gain during pregnancy. Then, we collected dietary information involving three-day dietary record and intake frequency of food products. During the study session, the actual body weight and height of every mother were measured using a Seca 799 measurement station and column scales (±0.1 kg/cm; Seca, Chino, CA, USA). The pre-pregnancy and actual body mass index (BMI) was calculated as the ratio of the body weight to the height squared (kg/m^2). Interpretation of these results followed the international classification proposed by the World Health Organization (WHO): below 18.5 kg/m^2, underweight; 18.5–24.9 kg/m^2, normal weight; 25.0–29.9 kg/m^2, overweight; 30.0 kg/m^2 and above, obese [26].

2.2. Human Milk Collection

Twenty-four-hour human milk samples (n = 32) were collected by women at home after they had been given detailed instructions on taking, storing, and transporting samples to the Holy Family Hospital in Warsaw. Foremilk and hindmilk samples were collected from all the participants from four time periods (06:00–12:00, 12:00–18:00, 18:00–24:00, and 24:00–06:00) to minimize possible circadian influences on the milk fatty acid composition. The term foremilk refers to the milk at the beginning of a feeding, and hindmilk refers to milk at the end of a feeding, which has a higher fat content than the milk at the beginning of that particular feeding. A total of 5 to 10 mL of foremilk and hindmilk samples were obtained from the breast(s) from which the infant was fed. Samples were collected into pre-labeled polypropylene containers provided to each woman. Participants were instructed to store milk in the refrigerator (~4 °C) during the 24-h collection process. Then, milk samples were stored at −20 °C for later analysis.

2.3. Lipid Concentration and Fatty Acid Analysis of Human Milk

Tested material comprised 32 samples of human milk. The lipid concentration in human milk was analyzed using the Miris human milk analyzer (HMA) (Miris, Uppsala, Sweden) with a validated protocol, as discussed in a previous study [27]. Collected milk samples for fatty acids analysis were immediately frozen in plastic test tubes at a temperature of −20 °C and delivered to the Department of Metabolomics (Food and Nutrition Institute, Warsaw, Poland) into thermic bags. Samples were stored at −80 °C until analysis. Frozen samples were thawed only once at room temperature, without light. After thawing, samples were shaken at room temperature (3–5 min) to obtain a homogeneous mixture. Aliquots were extracted and analyzed for fatty acid (FA) composition and content.

2.3.1. Fat Extraction

Milk samples were extracted from 1 mL of sample with chloroform-methanol (2:1) (Avantor Performance Materials S.A., Warsaw, Poland) containing 0.02% butyl-hydroxytoluene (2,6-tert-butyl-4-methylphenol, BHT, ≥99.0%, GC, powder) (Sigma-Aldrich CHEMIE GmbH, CA, USA) as an antioxidant, according to Folch et al. [28].

2.3.2. Gas Chromatography-Mass Spectrometry Analysis

Milk fatty acids were analyzed as fatty acid methyl ester (FAME) by gas chromatography using a Hewlett-Packard 6890 gas chromatograph with MS detector 5972 A. The methylation procedure was as follows: organic extracts were evaporated at 40 °C in a gentle nitrogen stream, and then were saponified with 0.5 mL of potassium hydroxide in methanol (0.5 N) (Avantor Performance Materials S.A., Poland) for 10 min at 80 °C in an electric multiblock heater and subsequently methylated with 1 mL of hydrochloric acid in methanol (3 N) (Sigma-Aldrich CHEMIE GmbH, USA) for 15 min at 85 ± 2 °C. After cooling to room temperature, fatty acid methyl esters were extracted with 1 mL of isooctane (2,2,4 trimethylopentane) (Avantor Performance Materials S.A., Poland). One microliter of the sample was injected into the GC column. The GC-MS analysis has been used with a split injector (1:100 ratio), injector and detector temperatures of −250 °C, and carrier gas helium (20 mL/s; the pressure of 43.4 psi). The chromatography oven was programmed to 175 °C for 40 min; thereafter, it was increased by 5 °C per min until the temperature reached 220 °C, and was held at this temperature for 16 min. FAMEs separations were performed on a CP Sil 88 fused silica capillary column (100 m × 0.25 mm i.d., film thickness: 0.20 μm; Agilent J & W GC Columns, CA, USA). Peak identification was verified by comparison with authentic standards (Supelco FAME Mix 37 Component; Sigma-Aldrich, CA, USA) and by mass spectrometry. The obtained results were expressed as a percentage by weight (% *wt/wt*) of all the fatty acids detected with a chain length between eight and 24 carbon atoms. The method was validated and accredited by the Polish Centre of Accreditation (accreditation certificate AB 690). Quality control was also implemented by the use of certified reference materials: BCR-163 (Beef-Pork FAT blend; ABP cat. 3; 8 g; Sigma-Aldrich, CA, USA).

2.4. Fatty Acids Dietary Intake and Intake Frequency of Food Products

The assessment of women's fatty acids intake was based on a three-day dietary record. Mothers were asked to note each food and dietary supplement they had consumed in the tree consecutive days prior to the human milk sampling day. No dietary recommendation was given before the study; participants were allowed to consume self-chosen diets. To verify the sizes of declared food portions, we used the "Album of Photographs of Food Products and Dishes" developed by the National Food and Nutrition Institute [29]. Fatty acids dietary intake was calculated using Dieta 5.0 nutritional software (National Food and Nutrition Institute, Warsaw, Poland). Additionally, the habitual intake of fatty acids was assessed using a FFQ containing 19 items. The FFQ provided information about the consumption frequency of DHA sources in the last three months, such as fish, seafood, meat (poultry, turkey, pork, beef), and eggs. We also collected information about the consumption frequency of other fatty acids sources, including vegetable oils (e.g., canola oil, olive oil, linseed oil, coconut oil), butter, milk and dairy products, nuts, and seeds. The response options were arranged in five categories, from "never", "less than once a week", "once or twice a week", "more than twice a week but not every day", to "every day".

2.5. Statistical Analysis

Statistical analyses were performed using Statistica 12PL, Tulusa, USA and IBM Statistics 21, New York, NY, USA. A p-value below 0.05 was adopted as statistically significant. Variables distributions were evaluated with a Shapiro–Wilk test and descriptive statistics. Data were presented as means and standard deviations as well as medians and interquartile ranges. Correlations between the intake of fatty acids and fatty acids concentrations in human milk were estimated with Pearson's r correlation coefficient. Correlations between omega-3 fatty acids (DHA, EPA, ALA) concentrations in human milk, and food consumption frequency were estimated with Kendall's tau correlation coefficients.

3. Results

3.1. Maternal Characteristics

The mean maternal age was 30.9 ± 6.5 years and most of them were primiparous (75%; n = 24). Detailed anthropometric data are shown in Table 1. Before pregnancy and during the first month postpartum, none of the participants was classified as being underweight (BMI <18.5 kg/m^2). In both periods of time, most of them (n = 23, 72%) had normal body mass, and 28% (n = 9) were classified as being overweight or obese. All the participants declared high university education and high material status. We do not observed statistically significant differences between pre-pregnancy and postpartum BMI values (t-test was 1.13; $p = 0.26$).

Table 1. Characteristics of the mothers.

Characteristic	Mean ± SD	Range
Age (years)	30.9 ± 6.5	27–44
Height (cm)	1.66 ± 0.1	1.54–1.8
Pre-pregnancy weight (kg)	62.2 ± 11.8	44–90
Pre-pregnancy body mass index (kg/m^2)	22.6 ± 3.4	18.6–30.9
Weight gain during pregnancy (kg)	15.1 ± 4.8	7–30
Weight at first month postpartum (kg)	65.5 ± 13.2	45.6–95
Body mass index at first month postpartum (kg/m^2)	23.6 ± 3.8	18.5–32.1

3.2. Fatty Acids Concentrations in Human Milk

The fatty acids profile of human milk is shown in Table 2. The relative proportion of saturated, monounsaturated, and polyunsaturated fatty acids was 41.9 ± 4.9%, 39.6 ± 3.1%, and 15.1 ± 3.4%, respectively. The predominant fatty acids in human milk were oleic acid (35.4 ± 3.1%), palmitic acid (19.7 ± 2.5%), and linoleic acid (11.1 ± 2.6%). No significant correlation was found between DHA concentrations, palmitic (r = −0.24; $p = 0.2$) and oleic (r = 0.13; $p = 0.48$) FAs; however, we found correlation with linoleic acid (r = 0.44; $p = 0.013$). Also, a significant negative correlation was found between DHA concentration and the omega-6:omega-3 ratio in human milk (r = −0.45; $p = 0.012$). When only the milk of mothers supplementing their diet with DHA were considered (n = 22), the mean concentration of DHA was 0.78% of total fatty acids. The difference between the concentration of DHA in supplementing and not supplementing mothers was not statistically significant (r = 0.29; $p = 0.37$).

Table 2. Fatty acids composition (%) of human milk [1].

Fatty Acids	Mean ± SD	Median (Interquartile Range)
Saturated fatty acids (SFA)	41.9 ± 4.9	42.3 (38.0–45.7)
C4:0 (butanoic acid)	0.0 ± 0.0	0.0 (0.0–0.0)
C6:0 (caproic acid)	0.0 ± 0.0	0.0 (0.0–0.0)
C8:0 (caprylic acid)	0.1 ± 0.0	0.1 (0.1–0.1)
C10:0 (capric acid)	1.1 ± 0.3	1.1 (1.0–1.4)
C12:0 (lauric acid)	3.5 ± 1.1	3.3 (2.5–4.1)
C13:0 (tridecanoic acid)	0.1 ± 0.0	0.1 (0.0–0.1)
C14:0 (myristic acid)	9.5 ± 2.5	9.3 (7.9–11.1)
C15:0 (pentadecanoic acid)	0.8 ± 0.2	0.7 (0.7–0.8)
C16:0 (palmitic acid)	19.7 ± 2.5	19.9 (17.4–22.0)
C17:0 (margaric acid)	0.5 ± 0.1	0.5 (0.4–0.6)
C18:0 (stearic acid)	6.4 ± 1.5	6.0 (5.4–7.3)
C20:0 (arachidic acid)	0.2 ± 0.1	0.2 (0.1–0.2)
C21:0 (henicosanoic acid)	0.0 ± 0.0	0.0 (0.0–0.0)
C22:0 (behenic acid)	0.1 ± 0.0	0.1 (0.1–0.1)
C23:0 (tetracosanoic acid)	0.0 ± 0.0	0.0 (0.0–0.0)

Table 2. *Cont.*

Fatty Acids	Mean ± SD	Median (Interquartile Range)
Monounsaturated fatty acids (MUFA)	39.6 ± 3.1	39.0 (38.0–42.0)
C14:1 (myristoleic acid)	0.2 ± 0.1	0.2 (0.2–0.3)
C15:1 (pentadecenoic acid)	0.0 ± 0.0	0.0 (0.0–0.0)
C16:1 trans	0.4 ± 0.1	0.4 (0.3–0.4)
C16:1 cis	2.6 ± 0.5	2.6 (2.3–2.9)
C17:1 (heptadecenoic acid)	0.2 ± 0.0	0.2 (0.2–0.3)
C18:1 cis (oleic acid)	35.4 ± 3.1	34.9 (33.6–37.6)
C18:1 trans (vaccenic acid)	1.2 ± 0.5	1.2 (0.8–1.5)
C20:1 (gadoleic acid)	0.8 ± 0.2	0.7 (0.7–0.9)
C22:1 (erucic acid)	0.2 ± 0.1	0.1 (0.1–0.2)
C24:1 (lignoceric acid)	0.2 ± 0.0	0.2 (0.1–0.2)
Polyunsaturated fatty acids (PUFA)	15.1 ± 3.4	15.3 (12.7–16.8)
n-3 polyunsaturated	2.7 ± 0.9	2.6 (2.1–3.1)
C18:3 (α-linolenic acid, ALA)	1.5 ± 0.6	1.4 (1.0–1.8)
C20:3 (eicosatrienoic acid)	0.1 ± 0.0	0.1 (0.0–0.1)
C20:5 (eicosapentaenoic acid, EPA)	0.2 ± 0.1	0.2 (0.2–0.3)
C22:6 (docosahexaenoic acid, DHA)	0.7 ± 0.3	0.7 (0.5–1.0)
n-6 polyunsaturated	12.1 ± 2.7	12.1 (10.4–13.4)
C18:2 (linoleic acid, LA)	11.1 ± 2.6	11.1 (9.5–12.3)
C18:3 (γ-linoleic acid)	0.1 ± 0.0	0.1 (0.1–0.1)
C20:3 (dihomo-γ-linoleic acid)	0.3 ± 0.1	0.3 (0.2–0.4)
C20:4 (arachidonic acid, ARA)	0.5 ± 0.1	0.5 (0.4–0.6)
Ratio		
n-6:n-3	4.6 ± 1.0	4.8 (4.1–5.1)
DHA:LA [2]	0.1 ± 0.0	0.1 (0.0–0.1)
ARA [3]:DHA [4]	0.9 ± 0.4	0.7 (0.5–1.1)
LA:ALA [5]	8.1 ± 2.4	7.8 (6.4–9.6)
Total fat concentration [6]	3.49 ± 1.0	3.5 (3.0–4.2)

[1] Data are presented as the relative proportion of each fatty acid (% of total fatty acids). [2] LA linoleic acid; [3] ARA arachidonic acid; [4] DHA docosahexaenoic acid; [5] ALA α-linolenic acid. [6] Total fat concentration is presented as grams per 100 mL.

3.3. Fatty Acids Dietary Intake and Its Association with Concentration in Human Milk

The fatty acids dietary intake is shown in Table 3. Mean energy intake was 1752 kcal ± 228.3 kcal, which was lower than the recommended level (EER, estimated energy requirement = 2555 kcal per day). The risk of deficient energy intake was observed in 100% of the participants. According to the Polish nutritional standards, the recommended intake for ALA is 0.5% of total energy, which in our participants it corresponded to 0.97 g per day. The mean dietary intake of ALA (1.5 ± 0.8% of total fatty acids) was higher than recommended levels; nevertheless, 22% of participants did not meet the recommendation. When only dietary sources were considered, the mean intake of DHA (243 mg ± 333.5) (Table 4) reached the Polish [15] and European [13,14] recommendation of 200 mg of DHA daily, whereas among 59% of the women, we observed insufficient DHA intake. Including taken supplements, the percentage of deficient DHA intake decreased, and was 16%. The majority of the participants (69%; n = 22) reported taking DHA supplements, and 10% (n = 3) of women declared taking supplements containing DHA and EPA.

Table 5 presents correlation coefficients (Pearson's r) between human milk fatty acids concentrations and maternal fatty acids dietary intake, as well as maternal dietary intake together with supplementation. We did not observe any statistically significant correlation between these factors ($p > 0.05$).

Table 3. Fatty acids content in mothers' diet.

Fatty Acids	Mean ± SD (g)	Median (Interquartile Range) (g)
Saturated fatty acids (SFA)	23.9 ± 10.3	20.9 (7.3–69.5)
C4:0 (butanoic acid)	0.4 ± 0.3	0.5 (0–1.1)
C6:0 (caproic acid)	0.3 ± 0.2	0.3 (0–0.8)
C8:0 (caprylic acid)	0.2 ± 0.2	0.2 (0–1.0)
C10:0 (capric acid)	0.5 ± 0.3	0.5 (0–1.6)
C12:0 (lauric acid)	0.9 ± 0.9	0.7 (0.2–5.5)
C14:0 (myristic acid)	2.8 ± 1.4	2.7 (0.7–7.9)
C15:0 (pentadecanoic acid)	0.3 ± 0.2	0.3 (0–0.9)
C16:0 (palmitic acid)	12.6 ± 5.2	11.6 (4.5–35.0)
C17:0 (margaric acid)	0.2 ± 0.1	0.2 (0–0.7)
C18:0 (stearic acid)	5.2 ± 2.8	5.1 (1.2–18.3)
C20:0 (arachidic acid	0.1 ± 0.1	0.1 (0–0.3)
Monounsaturated fatty acids (MUFA)	24.7 ± 8.9	24.8 (13.2–55.0)
C14:1 (myristoleic acid)	0.2 ± 0.2	0.2 (0–0.8)
C15:1 (pentadecenoic acid)	0.1 ± 0.1	0.1 (0–0.2)
C16:1	1.3 ± 0.4	1.2 (0.6–2.4)
C17:1 (heptadecenoic acid)	0.1 ± 0.1	0.1 (0–0.5)
C18:1 (oleic and vaccenic acids)	22.1 ± 8.3	21.7 (11.5–50.3)
C20:1 (gadoleic acid)	0.3 ± 0.2	0.2 (0.1–0.9)
C22:1 (erucic acid)	0.3 ± 0.3	0.1 (0–1.1)
Polyunsaturated fatty acids (PUFA)	10.7 ± 4.0 13.5 ± 14.2 [s]	11.2 (4.9–22.9) 11.3 (4.9–88.4) [s]
C18:2 (linoleic acid, LA)	8.5 ± 3.4	8.5 (4.1–21.1)
C18:3 (α-linolenic acid, ALA)	1.5 ± 0.8	1.4 (0.5–4.3)
C20:5 (eicosapentaenoic acid, EPA)	0.1 ± 0.2 0.1 ± 0.2 [s]	0 (0–0.5) 0.1 (0–0.5) [s]
C22:6 (docosahexaenoic acid, DHA)	0.2 ± 0.3 0.6 ± 0.6 [s]	0.1 (0–1.2) 0.4 (0–1.8) [s]

[s] Diet + supplementation.

Table 4. Estimated daily intake of EPA and DHA from food, supplement, and food + supplement in lactating women.

	EPA (mg)	DHA (mg)
Food	104.4 ± 152.0 (18, 0–190)	243.3 ± 333.5 (50, 37–411)
Supplement [1]	29.7 ± 43.6 (0, 0–43)	370.6 ± 465.1 (250, 8–549)
Food + supplement	134.1 ± 153.9 (85, 1–215)	614.0 ± 574.6 (354, 202–905)

Data are presented as means ± SD (median, interquartile range). [1] Participants who did not take supplements or those who took supplements that did not contain EPA/DHA were considered as 0 mg supplement on EPA and DHA.

Table 5. Correlations between human milk fatty acids and fatty acids in the mother's diet and supplementation.

Concentration in Human Milk	Dietary Intake, Sole or Together with Supplementation					
	SFA	MUFA	PUFA	ALA	EPA	DHA
SFA [1]	0.26	0.16	−0.20	−0.13	−0.18 −0.19 [s]	−0.10 −0.16 [s]
MUFA [2]	−0.14	−0.04	0.14	0.26	0.21	0.19
PUFA [3]	−0.20	−0.14	0.20	0.01	0.08	−0.01
ALA [4]	−0.19	−0.09	0.04	0.32	0.20	−0.06
EPA [5]	−0.16	0.05	0.05	−0.11	0.20 0.17 [s]	−0.02 0.17 [s]
DHA [6]	−0.24	−0.18	−0.04	−0.26	0.16 0.23 [s]	0.04 0.24 [s]

Data are presented as Pearson's r coefficients.; [1] SFA, Saturated fatty acids; [2] MUFA, Monounsaturated fatty acids; [3] PUFA, Polyunsaturated fatty acids; [4] ALA, α-linolenic acid; [5] EPA, eicosapentaenoic acid; [6] DHA, docosahexaenoic acid; [s] Pearson's r coefficients diet + supplementation.

3.4. Association between Intake Frequency of Food Products and DHA Concentrations in Human Milk

Table 6 presents Kendall's rank correlation coefficients between the intake frequency of food products and DHA concentrations in human milk. According to the FFQ, almost half of the participants (~47%) declared fatty fish consumption once or twice a week. On the other hand, almost 43% of the women consumed fish less than once a week or never. Based on the three-day dietary record, the most frequently consumed fatty fish species were salmon and mackerel, which were reported by seven (22%) and six women (19%), respectively. Butter and milk were the most frequently used foods, which were consumed by approximately ~44% and ~38% of participants, respectively.

Table 6. Intake frequency (%) of food products and correlations with DHA concentrations in human milk [1].

Food	Never	Less than Once a Week	Once or Twice a Week	More than Twice a Week but Not Every Day	Every Day	Correlation [1] with Concentrations in Human Milk		
						DHA [2]	EPA [3]	ALA [4]
Fatty fish (e.g., salmon, herring)	12.50	31.25	46.88	9.38	0.00	0.25 *	0.27 *	0.28 *
Lean fish (e.g., cod, sole)	21.88	31.25	43.75	3.13	0.00	0.14	0.08	0.21
Seafood	31.25	43.75	25.17	0.00	0.00	0.21	0.13	0.19
Poultry and turkey	3.13	3.13	43.75	40.63	9.38	0.09	0.13	0.08
Pork	6.25	40.63	37.50	15.63	0.00	0.02	0.29 *	0.18
Beef	9.38	50.00	34.38	6.25	0.00	−0.25 *	−0.14	0.11
Meat products (e.g., sausages, sliced meats)	6.25	12.50	37.50	18.75	25.00	0.24	−0.11	−0.10
Eggs	15.63	6.25	34.38	34.38	9.38	−0.14	−0.06	−0.00
Milk	31.25	15.63	9.38	6.25	37.50	0.02	0.05	0.26 *
Fermented dairy products	37.50	28.13	21.88	12.50	0.00	0.17	0.10	0.29 *
Cheese	25.00	28.13	15.63	18.75	12.50	−0.02	−0.02	0.00
Cottage cheese	21.88	12.50	43.75	15.63	6.25	0.22	0.06	0.17
Milk desserts	46.88	28.13	9.38	15.63	0.00	0.11	−0.12	−0.18
Butter	15.63	9.38	12.50	18.75	43.75	−0.14	−0.11	0.10
Canola oil	18.75	28.13	21.88	25.00	6.25	0.09	−0.0	0.13
Olive oil	12.50	18.75	25.00	43.75	0.00	0.08	0.02	0.03
Linseed oil	62.50	15.63	9.38	9.38	3.13	0.01	0.10	0.30 *
Coconut oil	56.25	25.00	15.63	3.13	0.00	−0.12	−0.07	0.29 *
Nuts and seeds	6.25	18.75	21.88	28.13	25.00	−0.03	0.02	0.01

[1] Data are presented as Kendall's rank correlation coefficients. * $p < 0.05$. [2] DHA, docosahexaenoic acid; [3] EPA, eicosapentaenoic acid; [4] ALA, α-linolenic acid.

We found a significant positive correlation between fatty fish consumption and all the omega-3 fatty acids concentrations in human milk. Kendall's rank correlation coefficients were 0.25 ($p = 0.049$) for DHA, 0.27 ($p = 0.03$) for EPA, and 0.28 ($p = 0.02$) for ALA. The ALA content in maternal milk was also positively correlated with the intake frequency of linseed oil (r = 0.30; $p = 0.01$), coconut oil (r = 0.29; $p = 0.02$), milk (r = 0.26; $p = 0.04$), and fermented dairy products (r = 0.29; $p = 0.02$), whereas EPA concentration was positively correlated with intake frequency of pork (r = 0.29; $p = 0.02$). Beef consumption, by contrast, was negatively correlated with DHA concentration in human milk (r = −0.25; $p = 0.046$). No other significant correlations between intake frequency of food products and DHA concentration in human milk were found.

The major food contributor of total omega-3 FAs intake was fatty fish (45%) and lean fish (17%) (Figure 1). Seafood (mainly shrimps) (10%), poultry products (8%), and meat products (6%) also made significant contributions to the estimated intake of omega-3 FAs. Within seafood and fish categories, salmon was found to be the main source of all omega-3 FAs, DHA (67%), EPA (53%), and ALA (59%).

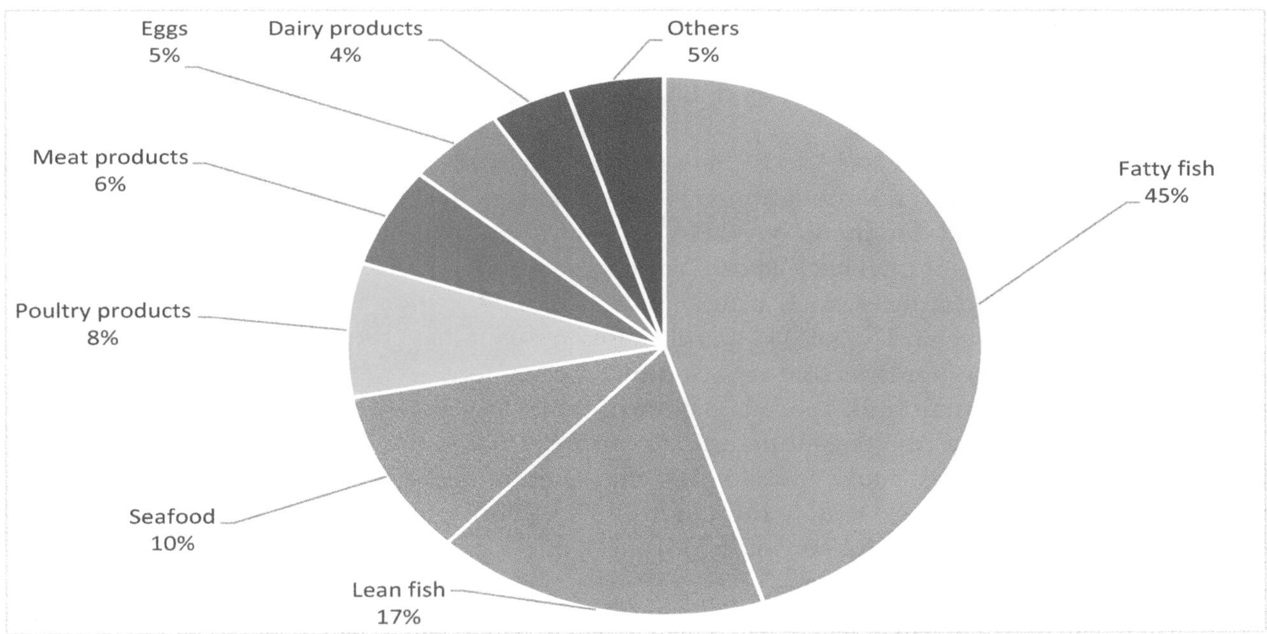

Figure 1. The relative contribution of food groups to total omega-3 FAs intake from the three-day dietary record.

Food items were divided into groups based on the Dieta 5.0 nutritional software database. Food items that contributed to less than 1% of total omega-3 FAs intake were categorized as "others". This included fats and vegetable oils, mixed dishes, and sauces.

4. Discussion

Our study has revealed three primary findings concerning the studied population. First, the mother's dietary intake of omega-3 FAs met Polish and European standards. Secondly, milk DHA concentration averaged about 0.70% of total fatty acids, which was twofold higher than the worldwide average (WWA) [30]. The third finding of this study is that there were no correlations between dietary intake of omega-3 FAs measured with three-day dietary records and their concentrations in human milk, whereas the intake frequency of food products—mainly fatty fish—was positively correlated with the concentration of ALA, EPA, and DHA in human milk.

In our study, the average maternal dietary DHA and ALA intakes (including taken supplements) were 613 ± 575 mg and 152 ± 0.81 mg, respectively. For DHA, this value was threefold higher than Polish [15] and European [13,14] recommendations (200 mg DHA per day). Our finding is not consistent with previous studies conducted in the United States [31,32], Canada [17,33], and Europe [34], which reported that the majority of breastfeeding women in the Alberta Pregnancy Outcomes and Nutrition (APrON) cohort were not meeting any of the various authorities' omega-3 FAs recommendations [35]. Similarly, in the Latvian study (Latvia and Poland are situated in the same geographic region, both countries have access to the Baltic Sea), DHA daily intake was lower than recommended, and was only 136 ± 26 mg [36]. It is widely reported that supplementation increases mother's milk DHA concentrations [37,38], and our results confirmed these findings. DHA concentration in the milk of mothers who supplemented their diet with DHA was higher than in the whole group, and was 0.78% of total fatty acids. However, we did not observe statistically significant differences between DHA concentrations in the milk of mothers who supplemented and did not supplement their diet with DHA ($r = 0.29$; $p = 0.37$). When only dietary sources were considered, the insufficient intake of DHA was observed among 59% of participants, whereas including taken supplements, the percentage decreased to 16%.

Based on the three-day dietary record, we observed that the largest contributor of omega-3 FAs intake was fatty fish, lean fish, and seafood, which was consumed once or twice a week by 47%, 44%, and 25% of participants, respectively. Other foods significantly contributing to total omega-3 FAs intake were poultry, red meat (pork and beef), and eggs. These findings were consistent with other studies [18,19], which reported that seafood, fish, poultry, meat, and eggs were the primary dietary sources of total omega-3 FAs.

The mean concentration of DHA in human milk in our study (0.7 ± 0.3% of total fatty acids) was higher than those reported in the meta-analysis based on 106 studies published between 1986–2006 year [30]. The authors found that the WWA DHA concentration in human milk was 0.32 ± 0.22% with a wide range of 0.06% to 1.4% of total fatty acids. We observed that our result was twofold compared to the data from Mediterranean countries, such as Italy (0.28–0.35%) [39,40], Spain (0.31–0.38) [41,42], and also Nordic countries such as Iceland (0.30%) [43] and Denmark (0.35%) [44]. Our mean DHA concentration in human milk was also higher than that reported by Jackson and Harris [45]. They suggested that the target of DHA level in human milk should be 0.3% of total fatty acids, emphasizing however that the optimal DHA level remains to be established. An approximate DHA concentration in human milk may be achieved when DHA intake exceeds 200 mg. Brenna and Lapillonne [14] have developed a regression analysis equation to calculate human milk DHA concentration depending on dietary DHA intake, based on the data from Gibbson et al. [46]:

$$\text{human milk DHA concentration (\% of total fatty acids)} = 0.72 \times \text{maternal DHA intake (g per day)} + 0.20.$$

Inserting our mean maternal DHA intake into this equation, we obtain a value of 0.63%, which is similar to the mean DHA concentration in human milk from our analysis (0.7%). In our study, the daily DHA intake was significantly higher than recommended, which may explain that the target DHA level in human milk was reached.

In our study, the mean concentration of ALA in human milk was 1.5 ± 0.8%, which was higher than those reported by Presa-Owens et al. (0.79%) [47] and Kotelzko et al. (0.81%) [48]. Some oils, such as soybean oil and canola oil, and legumes such as soybeans contain large amounts of ALA. Our findings suggest that women in our study consume these types of products to a greater extent than those in other Western countries [49]. However, in our study, the ratio of LA to ALA in maternal milk was higher than recommended (2.8:1) [50], and was 8:1. As LA and ALA compete for the same key enzymes in long-chain polyunsaturated fatty acids (LCPUFAs) biosynthesis, and ALA has a higher affinity than LA for ð-6-desaturase, the dietary ratio of LA:ALA is more relevant for proper LCPUFAs production than the intake of each fatty acid individually [49]. Furthermore, there is evidence that the DHA concentration in maternal milk has a positive correlation with the intelligence quotient of the child, whereas LA concentration has a negative correlation. It indicates that the FA profile during the lactation period is of particular significance [51–53]. In our study, the ratio of DHA:LA (0.1:1) was higher than the mean ratio from 28 countries [54]. Lassek and Gaulin [54] reported that the DHA:LA ratio at the level of ~0.04:1–0.07:1 is linked to higher cognitive test score results. It is worth noting that in our study, the majority of women (94%, n = 30) had the DHA:LA ratio in their milk of at least 0.04:1. Further, their mean ratio of omega-6:omega-3 FAs (4.6:1) was three times lower than the value reported by Silva et al. (14:1) [55], and nearly two times lower than that in the Latvian study (7:1) [36]. Silva et al. [52] and Nishimura et al. [56] suggested that a diet low in fish and high in vegetable oils, mainly soybean oil, facilitated a higher omega-6:omega-3 ratio (>10:1). However, we did not observe a significant correlation between fish or vegetable oils consumption and the omega-6:omega-3 ratio in human milk. The EFSA recommended a 4:1 proportion for dietary omega-6:omega-3 FAs [8]. It has been suggested that a very high omega-6:omega-3 ratio (~15:1) may promote cardiovascular diseases and cancers [57].

We found a significant positive correlation ($r = 0.25$; $p = 0.049$) between habitual fatty fish consumption and DHA concentration in human milk, which is consistent with results from other studies [36,49,56,58]. A Danish observational study reported a higher proportion of DHA concentration in the milk of mothers who consumed fish than in those who did not consume fish (0.63% compared with 0.41%; $p = 0.018$) and in women who consumed fatty fish compared with those who did not consume fish (0.73% compared with 0.41%; $p < 0.01$) [59]. Contrary to these findings, Juber et al. [59] reported that intake of fish did not correlate with mother's milk DHA levels. The results may depend on fish breeding (farmed or wild) and the fish species that are most commonly consumed in a specific region. For instance, when consuming 100 g of wild salmon, the total DHA intake is lower (0.31% of total fatty acids) compared to eating the same quantity of farmed salmon (0.88% of total fatty acids). It is caused by the higher total fat content in farmed salmon (12.3 g/100 g) than in wild salmon (2.07 g/100 g) [60]. In our study, the most commonly consumed fish were salmon and mackerel, but we did not have information about breeding, so the dietary intake of DHA based on three-day dietary record may be overestimated on underestimated in some cases. Using Dieta 5.0 nutritional software, we based our analysis on its nutritional database, which did not have distinctions between wild and farmed fish. However, Qiunn and Kuawa [61] concluded that an additional portion of fish (no information about breeding) per week led to a 0.014% increase of DHA concentration in human milk. We also observed that the DHA levels in human milk were negatively correlated ($r = -0.25$; $p = 0.046$) with beef consumption, the fat of which consists mainly of saturated fatty acids (SFA) (~52.3 g/100 g) and contains low amounts of PUFA (3.8 g/100 g) [62].

We noted that similarly to DHA, the ALA and EPA concentrations in human milk were also significantly positively correlated with the frequency of fatty fish consumption ($r = 0.27$; $p = 0.02$ for ALA and $r = 0.28$; $p = 0.03$ for EPA). ALA concentration in human milk was also positively correlated with the frequency of consuming linseed oil, coconut oil, milk, and milk products. Milk fat consists mainly of SFA (59.4 g/100 g) with the dominating palmitic acid (~30.6% of total FAs) [63], which was predominant SFA in human milk in our study. However, no significant correlation between milk consumption and palmitic acid concentration in human milk was found ($r = 0.13$; $p = 0.29$).

We did not find a correlation between dietary intake of DHA based on the three-day dietary record and any omega-3 FAs (ALA, EPA, and DHA) concentrations in human milk. It confirmed the results of Nishimura et al. [55], who did not observe any association between dietary EPA and DHA intake during the postpartum period and their concentrations in human milk. However, they noted that the dietary EPA and DHA content during the third trimester of pregnancy was directly related to the content of these fatty acids in mature human milk. These results suggest that maternal body stocks of fatty acids have a greater influence on breast milk fatty acid composition than the estimated dietary intake during the postpartum period, validating previously reported results [2,64]. An additional possible explanation would be also the increased weight gain and body fat storage observed in women mainly during late pregnancy [65]. Fiddler et al. [66] reported that about 20% of the supplemented 0.2 g of DHA per day was secreted into milk and observed a pronounced increase in DHA content in human milk (% of total FAs), with a peak between 6–12 h after dietary DHA intake. Although 24-h human milk samples were collected in our study, these findings may explain the lack of correlation between the intake of omega-3 FAs measured with the three-day dietary record and its concentration in human milk. Further, while the synthesis of DHA from ALA may be sufficient for the healthy breastfeeding women, some non-physiological conditions, such as non-alcoholic fatty liver, which reduces the activity of ð-6-desaturase enzymes, could contrary affect the synthesis of DHA, decreasing the levels of omega-3 FAs in erythrocytes and then in human milk [67]. Moreover, the endogenous synthesis of PUFAs is mediated by genes controlling the elongation of very long chain fatty acids protein 2 and 5 (ELOVL2 and ELOVL5) [68]. It is also suggested that the genes encoding fatty acids desaturases 1 and 2 (FADS1 FADS2 gene cluster) were reported to be associated with omega-3 and omega-6 FA proportions in human plasma, tissues, and milk [69]. Moltó-Puigmartí et al. [69] found that DHA proportions were lower in women homozygous for the minor allele than in women who were homozygous for the major allele (DHA proportions in plasma phospholipids: $p < 0.01$; DHA proportions in milk: $p < 0.05$). Contrary to our and previous citied studies, a Greek observational study reported that human milk omega-3 PUFA content was positively correlated with maternal dietary intakes of total PUFAs ($r = 0.26$; $p < 0.05$), inversely correlated with maternal carbohydrates intake ($r = -0.29$; $p < 0.05$), and unrelated to maternal energy, total fat, SFA, MUFA, and protein intakes [37].

Bravi et al. [70] carried out a systemic review searching studies investigating the impact of maternal diet on their milk composition. Considering fatty acid profiles, most of the studies were based on supplements intervention or assessed maternal nutritional status with a food frequency questionnaire. As the authors concluded, the gathered results were scarce and diversified.

The time of incorporation of omega-3 FAs into plasma lipids is quite long, and similar to their half-life. The longest time of incorporation is in adipose tissue, which is an important source of plasma lipids. As the content of omega-3 FAs in human milk depends on its availability from the plasma [71], dietary intake assessment methods studying habitual intake are more appropriate to exhibit the discussed correlation. Thus, the survey based solely on a three-day dietary record, especially in this case, does not work. This is not only because of the described omega-3 FAs kinetics, but also because omega-3 FAs food sources (mainly fish) are not consumed every day, and whether they happen to occur in the three-day period is a matter of chance.

The strengths of this study are the use of milk collection protocol, which enabled minimizing possible errors in the measurement of human milk composition, and also an assessment of maternal diet with two techniques (food frequency questionnaire and three-day dietary record). Additionally, contrary to other authors [56], we assayed α-linolenic acid that can convert to DHA; therefore, a correlation between dietary intake of DHA and its concentration in human milk is more reliable. Our study has also limitations. First, there were the issues of convenience sampling and the modest number of participants, resulting from the complex nutrition questionnaire and milk collection protocol. Second, this study was conducted in a large city (the capital of Poland); all the participants had a university education and high material status. Third, genetic polymorphisms that influence the use of PUFAs from the diet have not been studied. These factors may limit the generalization of our findings to a broader population, because the availability and consumption patterns of food products (e.g., fish and seafood) is strongly related to the place of living and material status.

5. Conclusions

To summarize, this study shows that the women under study during breastfeeding had an adequate intake of foods that are natural sources of omega-3 FAs (fatty fish, seafood, vegetable oils), which resulted in a high concentration of DHA in their milk. However, it should be stressed that we did not observe a correlation between dietary intake of omega-3 FAs and their concentrations in human milk. On the other hand, we observed that the intake frequency of some food products affected omega-3 FAs concentrations in human milk. Considering these findings and the highest content of DHA in human milk being observed between 6–12 h after dietary DHA intake, a short-term assessment of omega-3 FAs intake (based on three-day dietary record) may be unreliable. A FFQ assessing nutritional habits in the last three months prior to the study seems to the more reliable tool, reflecting the habitual intake of omega-3 FAs.

Author Contributions: A.B.-J., A.C.-S., A.W., G.O. and D.S.-W. were responsible for the conception and design of this study. A.W. was involved in the funding acquisition. A.B.-J. was responsible for the data collection and statistical analysis. E.J.-M. and H.M. were responsible for fatty acids analysis of human milk (fat extraction and gas chromatography-mass spectrometry analysis). A.B.-J. was responsible for writing the manuscript. A.C.-S., A.W., G.O. and D.S.-W. were responsible for revising the manuscript critically for important intellectual content. The manuscript has been revised by all co-authors.

Acknowledgments: All the authors have reviewed and approved the final manuscript. This study was supported by a Polish Society of Clinical Child Nutrition research grant obtained in 2015 for the project entitled "Association between human milk composition and the nutritional status and body composition of lactating women". We thank all the mothers from the Holy Hospital in Warsaw who participated in this study.

References

1. Innis, S.M. Impact of maternal diet on human milk composition and neurological development of infants. *Am. J. Clin. Nutr.* **2014**, *99*, 734–741. [CrossRef] [PubMed]
2. Koletzko, B.; Rodriguez-Palmero, M.; Demmelmair, H.; Fidler, N.; Jensen, R.; Sauerwald, T. Physiological aspects of human milk lipids. *Early Hum. Dev.* **2001**, *65*, 3–18. [CrossRef]
3. Birch, E.E.; Castaneda, Y.S.; Wheaton, D.H.; Birch, D.G.; Uauy, R.D.; Hoffman, D.R. Visual maturation of term infants fed long-chain polyunsaturated fatty acid-supplemented or control formula for 12 mo. *Am. J. Clin. Nutr.* **2005**, *81*, 871–879. [CrossRef] [PubMed]
4. Jones, P.J.H.; Rideout, T. Lipids, sterols, and their metabolites. In *Modern Nutrition in Health and Disease*, 11st ed.; Ross, A.C., Caballero, B., Cousins, R.J., Tucker, K.L., Ziegler, T.R., Eds.; Lippincott Williams & Wilkins: Baltimore, MD, USA, 2014.
5. Innis, S.M. Human milk: Maternal dietary lipids and infant development. *Proc. Nutr. Soc.* **2007**, *66*, 397–404. [CrossRef] [PubMed]
6. Weiser, M.J.; Butt, C.M.; Mohajeri, M.H. Docosahexaenoic acid and cognition throughout the lifespan. *Nutrients* **2016**, *8*, 99. [CrossRef] [PubMed]
7. Innis, S.M. Metabolic programming of long-term outcomes due to fatty acid nutrition in early life. *Matern. Child Nutr.* **2011**, *7*, 112–123. [CrossRef] [PubMed]
8. European Food Safety Authority (EFSA). Scientific Opinion on Nutrient Requirements and Dietary Intakes of Infants and Young Children in the European Union. 2013. Available online: https://efsa.onlinelibrary.wiley.com/doi/pdf/10.2903/j.efsa.2013.3408 (accessed on 1 October 2018).
9. Goyens, P.L.; Spilker, M.E.; Zock, P.L.; Katan, M.B.; Mensink, R.P. Conversion of alpha-linolenic acid in humans is influenced by the absolute amounts of alpha-linolenic acid and linoleic acid in the diet and not by their ratio. *Am. J. Clin. Nutr.* **2006**, *84*, 44–53. [CrossRef] [PubMed]
10. Pawlosky, R.J.; Hibbeln, J.R.; Novotny, J.A.; Salem, N. Physiological compartmental analysis of alpha-linolenic acid metabolism in adult humans. *J. Lipid Res.* **2001**, *42*, 1257–1265. [PubMed]
11. Arterburn, L.M.; Hall, E.B.; Oken, H. Distribution, interconversion, and dose response of n-3 fatty acids in humans. *Am. J. Clin. Nutr.* **2006**, *83*, 1467–1476. [CrossRef] [PubMed]
12. Greiner, R.C.; Winter, J.; Nathanielsz, P.W.; Brenna, J.T. Brain docosahexaenoate accretion in fetal baboons: Bioequivalence of dietary alpha-linolenic and docosahexaenoic acids. *Pediatr. Res.* **1997**, *42*, 826–834. [CrossRef] [PubMed]
13. Koletzko, B.; Lien, E.; Agostoni, C.; Bohles, H.; Campoy, C.; Cetin, I.; Decsi, T.; Dudenhausen, J.W.; Dupont, C.; Forsyth, S.; et al. The roles of long-chain polyunsaturated fatty acids in pregnancy, lactation and infancy: Review of current knowledge and consensus recommendations. *J. Perinat. Med.* **2008**, *36*, 5–14. [CrossRef]
14. Brenna, J.T.; Lapillonne, A. Background paper on fat and fatty acid requirements during pregnancy and lactation. *Ann. Nutr. Metab.* **2009**, *55*, 97–122. [CrossRef] [PubMed]
15. Szajewska, H.; Horvath, A.; Rybak, A.; Socha, P. Breastfeeding. A Position Paper by the Polish Society for Paediatric Gastroenterology, Hepatology and Nutrition. *Med. Standards/Ped.* **2016**, *13*, 9–24.
16. Oken, E.; Kleinman, K.P.; Olsen, S.F.; Rich-Edwards, J.W.; Gillman, M.W. Associations of seafood and elongated n-3 fatty acid intake with fetal growth and length of gestation: Results from a US pregnancy cohort. *Am. J. Epidemiol.* **2004**, *160*, 774–783. [CrossRef] [PubMed]
17. Friesen, R.W.; Innis, S.M. Dietary arachidonic acid to EPA and DHA balance is increased among Canadian pregnant women with low fish intake. *J. Nutr.* **2009**, *139*, 2344–2350. [CrossRef] [PubMed]
18. Denomme, J.; Stark, K.D.; Holub, B.J. Directly quantitated dietary (n-3) fatty acid intakes of pregnant Canadian women are lower than current dietary recommendations. *J. Nutr.* **2005**, *135*, 206–211. [CrossRef] [PubMed]
19. Sioen, I.; Devroe, J.; Inghels, D.; Terwecoren, R.; De Henauw, S. The influence of n-3 PUFA supplements and n-3 PUFA enriched foods on the n-3 LC PUFA intake of Flemish women. *Lipids* **2010**, *45*, 313–320. [CrossRef] [PubMed]
20. Coletto, D.; Morrison, J. Seafood Survey: Public Opinion on Aquaculture and a National Aquaculture Act. 2011. Available online: http://www.aquaculture.ca/files/CAIA-PUBLIC-REPORT-May-2011.pdf (accessed on 2 October 2018).

21. Oken, E.; Kleinman, K.P.; Berland, W.E.; Simon, S.R.; Rich-Edwards, J.W.; Gillman, M.W. Decline in fish consumption among pregnant women after a national mercury advisory. *Obstet. Gynecol.* **2003**, *102*, 346–351. [CrossRef] [PubMed]
22. Amaral, Y.N.; Marano, D.; Silva, L.M.; Guimarães, A.C.; Moreira, M.E. Are There Changes in the Fatty Acid Profile of Breast Milk with Supplementation of Omega-3 Sources? A Systematic Review. *Rev. Bras. Ginecol. Obstet.* **2017**, *39*, 128–141. [CrossRef] [PubMed]
23. Yang, Y.J.; Kim, M.K.; Hwang, S.H.; Ahn, Y.; Shim, J.E.; Kim, D.H. Relative validities of 3-day food records and the food frequency questionnaire. *Nutr. Res. Pract.* **2010**, *4*, 142–148. [CrossRef] [PubMed]
24. Liu, M.J.; Li, H.T.; Yu, L.X.; Xu, G.S.; Ge, H.; Wang, L.L.; Zhang, Y.L.; Zhou, Y.B.; Li, Y.; Bai, M.X.; et al. A correlation study of DHA dietary intake and plasma, erythrocyte and breast milk DHA concentrations in lactating women from coastland, Lakeland, and inland areas of China. *Nutrients* **2016**, *8*, 312. [CrossRef] [PubMed]
25. Serra-Majem, L.; Nissensohn, M.; Øverby, N.C.; Fekete, K. Dietary methods and biomarkers of omega 3 fatty acids: A systematic review. *Br. J. Nutr.* **2012**, *107*, 64–76. [CrossRef] [PubMed]
26. Euro Who. Available online: http://www.euro.who.int/en/health-topics/disease-prevention/nutrition/ahealthy-lifestyle/body-mass-index-bmi (accessed on 14 May 2019).
27. Bzikowska-Jura, A.; Czerwonogrodzka-Senczyna, A.; Olędzka, G.; Szostak-Węgierek, D.; Weker, H.; Wesołowska, A. Maternal Nutrition and Body Composition During Breastfeeding: Association with Human Milk Composition. *Nutrients* **2018**, *10*, 1379. [CrossRef] [PubMed]
28. Folch, J.; Lees, M.; Sloane, G.H.S. A simple method for the isolation and purification of total lipides from animal tissues. *J. Biol. Chem.* **1957**, *226*, 497–509. [PubMed]
29. Szponar, L.; Wolnicka, K.; Rychlik, E. *Album of Photographs of Food Products and Dishes*; National Food and Nutrition Institute: Warsaw, Poland, 2011.
30. Brenna, J.T.; Varamini, B.; Jensen, R.G.; Diersen-Schade, D.A.; Boettcher, J.A.; Arterburn, L.M. Docosahexaenoic and arachidonic acid concentrations in human breast milk worldwide. *Am. J. Clin. Nutr.* **2007**, *85*, 1457–1464. [CrossRef] [PubMed]
31. Nochera, C.L.; Goossen, L.H.; Brutus, A.R.; Cristales, M.; Eastman, B. Consumption of DHA + EPA by low-income women during pregnancy and lactation. *Nutr. Clin. Pract.* **2011**, *26*, 445–450. [CrossRef]
32. Hibbeln, J.R.; Davis, J.M.; Steer, C.; Emmett, P.; Rogers, I.; Williams, C.; Golding, J. Maternal seafood consumption in pregnancy and neurodevelopmental outcomes in childhood (ALSPAC study): An observational cohort study. *Lancet* **2007**, *369*, 578–585. [CrossRef]
33. Sontrop, J.; Avison, W.R.; Evers, S.E.; Speechley, K.N.; Campbell, M.K. Depressive symptoms during pregnancy in relation to fish consumption and intake of n-3 polyunsaturated fatty acids. *Paediatr. Perinat. Epidemiol.* **2008**, *22*, 389–399. [CrossRef]
34. Rodriguez-Bernal, C.L.; Ramon, R.; Quiles, J.; Murcia, M.; Navarrete-Munoz, E.M.; Vioque, J.; Ballester, F.; Rebagliato, M. Dietary intake in pregnant women in a Spanish Mediterranean area: As good as it is supposed to be? *Public Health Nutr.* **2013**, *16*, 1379–1389. [CrossRef]
35. Jia, X.; Pakseresht, M.; Wattar, N.; Wildgrube, J.; Sontag, S.; Andrews, M.; Begum Subhan, F.; McCargar, F.; Field, C. Women who take n-3 long-chain polyunsaturated fatty acid supplements during pregnancy and lactation meet the recommended intake. *Appl. Physiol. Nutr. Metab.* **2015**, *40*, 474–481. [CrossRef]
36. Aumeistere, L.; Ciprovica, I.; Zavadska, D.; Volkovs, V. Fish intake reflects DHA level in breast milk among lactating women in Latvia. *Int. Breastfeed. J.* **2018**, *13*. [CrossRef] [PubMed]
37. Antonakou, A.; Skenderi, K.P.; Chiou, A.; Anastasiou, C.A.; Bakoula, C.; Matalas, A.L. Breast milk fat concentration and fatty acid pattern during the first six months in exclusively breastfeeding Greek women. *Eur. J. Nutr.* **2013**, *52*, 963–973. [CrossRef] [PubMed]
38. Makrides, M.; Gibson, R.A.; McPhee, A.J.; Collins, C.T.; Davis, P.G.; Doyle, L.W.; Simmer, K.; Colditz, P.B.; Morris, S.; Smithers, L.G.; et al. Neurodevelopmental outcomes of preterm infants fed high-dose docosahexaenoic acid: A randomized controlled trial. *JAMA* **2009**, *301*, 175–182. [CrossRef] [PubMed]
39. Marangoni, F.; Agostoni, C.; Lammardo, A.M.; Bonvissuto, M.; Giovannini, M.; Galli, C.; Riva, E. Polyunsaturated fatty acids in maternal plasma and in breast milk. *Prostaglandins Leukot. Essent. Fat. Acids* **2002**, *66*, 535–540. [CrossRef]

40. Marangoni, F.; Agostoni, C.; Lammardo, A.M.; Giovannini, M.; Galli, C.; Riva, E. Polyunsaturated fatty acid concentrations in human hindmilk are stable throughout 12-months of lactation and provide a sustained intake to the infant during exclusive breastfeeding: An Italian study. *Br. J. Nutr.* **2000**, *84*, 103–109. [PubMed]
41. Rueda, R.; Ramirez, M.; Garcia-Salmeron, J.L.; Maldonado, J.; Gil, A. Gestational age and origin of human milk influence total lipid and fatty acid contents. *Ann. Nutr. Metab.* **1998**, *42*, 12–22. [CrossRef] [PubMed]
42. Sala-Vila, A.; Campoy, C.; Castellote, A.I.; Garrido, F.J.; Rivero, M.; Rodríguez-Palmero, M.; López-Sabater, M.C. Influence of dietary source of docosahexaenoic and arachidonic acids on their incorporation into membrane phospholipids of red blood cells in term infants. *Prostaglandins Leukot. Essent. Fat. Acids* **2006**, *74*, 143–148. [CrossRef] [PubMed]
43. Olafsdottir, A.S.; Thorsdottir, I.; Wagner, K.H.; Elmadfa, I. Polyunsaturated fatty acids in the diet and breast milk of lactating icelandic women with traditional fish and cod liver oil consumption. *Ann. Nutr. Metab.* **2006**, *50*, 270–276. [CrossRef]
44. Kovacs, A.F.S.; Marosvolgyi, T.; Burus, I.; Decsi, T. Fatty acids in early human milk after preterm and full-term delivery. *J. Pediatr. Gastroenterol. Nutr.* **2005**, *41*, 454–459. [CrossRef]
45. Jackson, K.H.; Harris, W.S. Should there be a target level of docosahexaenoic acid in breast milk? *Curr. Opin. Clin. Nutr. Metab. Care* **2016**, *19*, 92–96. [CrossRef]
46. Gibson, R.A.; Neumann, M.A.; Makrides, M. Effect of increasing breast milk docosahexaenoic acid on plasma and erythrocyte phospholipid fatty acids and neural indices of exclusively breast fed infants. *Eur. J. Clin. Nutr.* **1997**, *51*, 578–584. [CrossRef] [PubMed]
47. Presa-Owens, S.D.; Lopez-Subater, M.C.; Rivero-Urgell, M. Fatty acid composition of human milk in Spain. *J. Pediatr. Gastroenterol. Nutr.* **1996**, *22*, 180–185. [CrossRef] [PubMed]
48. Koletzko, B.; Thiel, I.; Abiodun, P.O. The fatty acid composition of human milk in Europe and Africa. *J. Pediatr.* **1992**, *120*, 62–70. [CrossRef]
49. Wu, T.C.; Lau, B.H.; Chen, P.H.; Wu, L.T.; Tang, R.B. Fatty acid composition of Taiwanese Human Milk. *J. Chin. Med Assoc.* **2010**, *73*, 581–588. [CrossRef]
50. ISSFAL. Recommendations for Intake of Polyunsaturated Fatty Acids in Healthy Adults. 2004. Available online: http://www.issfal.org/ (accessed on 31 May 2019).
51. Lassek, W.D.; Gaulin, S.J.C. Maternal milk DHA concentration predicts cognitive performance in a sample of 28 nations. *Matern. Child Nutr.* **2015**, *11*, 773–779. [CrossRef] [PubMed]
52. Bernard, J.Y.; Armand, M.; Peyre, H.; Garcia, C.; Forhan, A.; De Agostini, M.; Charles, M.A.; Heude, B. Breastfeeding, polyunsaturated fatty acid levels in colostrum and child intelligence quotient at age 5–6 years. *J. Pediatr.* **2017**, *183*, 43–50. [CrossRef] [PubMed]
53. Zielinska, M.; Hamulka, J.; Wesolowska, A. Carotenoid Content in Breastmilk in the 3rd and 6th Month of Lactation and Its Associations with Maternal Dietary Intake and Anthropometric Characteristics. *Nutrients* **2019**, *11*, 193. [CrossRef] [PubMed]
54. Lassek, W.D.; Gaulin, S.J. Linoleic and docosahexaenoic acids in human milk have opposite relationships with cognitive test performance in a sample of 28 countries. *Prostaglandins Leukot. Essent. Fat. Acids* **2014**, *91*, 195–201. [CrossRef] [PubMed]
55. Silva, M.H.L.; Silva, M.T.C.; Brandão, S.C.C.; Gomes, J.C.; Peternelli, L.A.; Franceschini, S.C.C. Fatty acid composition of mature breast milk in Brazilian women. *Food Chem.* **2005**, *93*, 297–303. [CrossRef]
56. Nishimura, R.Y.; de Castro, G.S.F.; Junior, A.A.J.; Sartorelli, D.S. Breast milk fatty acid composition of women living far from the coastal area in Brazil. *J. Pediatr.* **2013**, *89*, 263–268. [CrossRef]
57. Simopoulos, A.P. The importance of the ratio of omega-6/omega-3 essential fatty acids. *Biomed. Pharmacother.* **2002**, *56*, 365–379. [CrossRef]
58. Lauritzen, L.; Jorgensen, M.H.; Hansen, H.S.; Michaelsen, K.F. Fluctuations in human milk long-chain PUFA levels in relation to dietary fish intake. *Lipids* **2002**, *37*, 237–244. [CrossRef] [PubMed]
59. Juber, B.A.; Jackson, K.H.; Johnson, K.B.; Harris, W.S.; Baack, M.L. Breast milk DHA levels may increase after informing women: A community-based cohort study from South Dakota USA. *Int. Breastfeed. J.* **2016**, *12*, 7. [CrossRef] [PubMed]
60. Strobel, C.; Jahreis, G.; Kuhnt, K. Survey of n-3 and n-6 polyunsaturated fatty acids in fish and fish products. *Lipids Health Dis.* **2012**, *11*, 144. [CrossRef] [PubMed]

61. Quinn, E.A.; Kuzawa, C.W. A dose-response relationship between fish consumption and human milk DHA concentration among Filipino women in Cebu City. *Philippines Acta Paediatr.* **2012**, *101*, 439–445. [CrossRef] [PubMed]
62. United States Department of Agriculture (USDA). Available online: https://ndb.nal.usda.gov/ndb/search/list (accessed on 30 October 2018).
63. Kunachowicz, H.; Nadolna, I.; Przygoda, B.; Iwanow, K. *Food Composition Tables*; PZWL: Warsaw, Poland, 2005.
64. Torres, A.G.; Ney, J.G.; Meneses, F.; Trugo, N.M. Polyunsaturated fatty acids and conjugated linoleic acid isomers in breast milk are associated with plasma non-esterified and erythrocyte membrane fatty acid composition in lactating women. *Br. J. Nutr.* **2006**, *95*, 517–524. [CrossRef]
65. Haggarty, P. Fatty acid supply to the human fetus. *Annu. Rev. Nutr.* **2010**, *30*, 237–255. [CrossRef]
66. Fidler, N.; Sauerwald, T.; Pohl, A.; Demmelmair, H.; Koletzko, B. Docosahexaenoic acid transfer into human milk after dietary supplementation: A randomized clinical trial. *J. Lipid Res.* **2000**, *41*, 1376–1383.
67. Valenzuela, R.; Videla, L.A. The importance of the long-chain polyunsaturated fatty acid n-6/n-3 ratio in development of non-alcoholic fatty liver associated with obesity. *Food Funct.* **2011**, *2*, 644–648. [CrossRef]
68. Wu, Y.; Wang, Y.; Tian, H.; Lu, T.; Yu, M.; Xu, W.; Liu, G.; Xie, L. DHA intake interacts with ELOVL2 and ELOVL5 genetic variants to influence polyunsaturated fatty acids in human milk. *J. Lipid. Res.* **2019**, *60*, 1043–1049. [CrossRef]
69. Moltó-Puigmartí, C.; Plat, J.; Mensink, R.P.; Müller, A.; Jansen, E.; Zeegers, M.P.; Thijs, C. FADS1 FADS2 gene variants modify the association between fish intake and the docosahexaenoic acid proportions in human milk. *Am. J. Clin. Nutr.* **2010**, *91*, 1368–1376. [CrossRef] [PubMed]
70. Bravi, F.; Wiens, F.; Decarli, A.; Dal Pont, A.; Agostoni, C.; Ferraroni, M. Impact of maternal nutrition on breast-milk composition: A systematic review. *Am. J. Clin. Nutr.* **2016**, *104*, 646–662. [CrossRef] [PubMed]
71. Van, R.M.; Hunter, D. Biochemical Indicators of Dietary Intake. In *Nutritional Epidemiology*, 3rd ed.; Oxford University Press: Oxford, UK, 2013; pp. 150–212. ISBN -13: 978-0199754038.

6

No Association between Glucocorticoid Diurnal Rhythm in Breastmilk and Infant Body Composition at 3 Months

Jonneke Hollanders [1,†,*], Lisette R. Dijkstra [1,†], Bibian van der Voorn [2], Stefanie M.P. Kouwenhoven [3], Alyssa A. Toorop [1], Johannes B. van Goudoever [3], Joost Rotteveel [1] and Martijn J.J. Finken [1]

1 Emma Children's Hospital, Amsterdam UMC, Pediatric Endocrinology, Vrije Universiteit Amsterdam, 1000-1183 Amsterdam, The Netherlands; l.dijkstra@amsterdamumc.nl (L.R.D.); a.toorop@amsterdamumc.nl (A.A.T.); j.rotteveel@amsterdamumc.nl (J.R.); m.finken@amsterdamumc.nl (M.J.J.F.)

2 Department of Paediatric Endocrinology, Obesity Center CGG, Sophia Children's Hospital, 3000-3099 Rotterdam, The Netherlands; b.vandervoorn@erasmusmc.nl

3 Emma Children's Hospital, Amsterdam UMC, Department of Pediatrics, Vrije Universiteit Amsterdam, 1000-1183 Amsterdam, The Netherlands; s.kouwenhoven@amsterdamumc.nl (S.M.P.K.); h.vangoudoever@amsterdamumc.nl (J.B.v.G.)

* Correspondence: j.hollanders@amsterdamumc.nl

† Both authors contributed equally to the article.

Abstract: Objective: Glucocorticoids (GCs) in breastmilk have previously been associated with infant body growth and body composition. However, the diurnal rhythm of breastmilk GCs was not taken into account, and we therefore aimed to assess the associations between breastmilk GC rhythmicity at 1 month and growth and body composition at 3 months in infants. Methods: At 1 month postpartum, breastmilk GCs were collected over a 24-h period and analyzed by LC-MS/MS. Body composition was measured using air-displacement plethysmography at 3 months. Length and weight were collected at 1, 2, and 3 months. Results: In total, 42 healthy mother–infant pairs were included. No associations were found between breastmilk GC rhythmicity (area-under-the-curve increase and ground, maximum, and delta) and infant growth trajectories or body composition (fat and fat free mass index, fat%) at 3 months. Conclusions: This study did not find an association between breastmilk GC rhythmicity at 1 month and infant's growth or body composition at 3 months. Therefore, this study suggests that previous observations linking breastmilk cortisol to changes in infant weight might be flawed by the lack of serial cortisol measurements and detailed information on body composition.

Keywords: cortisol; cortisone; growth; circadian rhythm; human milk

---

1. Introduction

Growing attention is focused on the etiology of obesity, and it has been hypothesized that part of its origin can be traced back to events occurring in early life (i.e., the Developmental Origins of Health and Disease (DOHaD) hypothesis) [1].

Given its effects on fat disposition and metabolism, the hypothalamus-pituitary-adrenal (HPA) axis has been implicated to play a role in the pathway leading to obesity [2,3]. Not only endogenous but also maternal glucocorticoids (GCs) appear to be involved. Evidence from animal experiments indicates that increased transplacental supply of maternal GCs may be associated with a lower birth weight and cardiovascular correlates, such as hypertension and hyperglycemia [4]. In humans, fetal exposure to excess maternal cortisol, e.g., due to maternal anxiety or depression, has been associated with a higher risk of childhood adiposity [5].

After birth, small amounts of maternal GCs appear to be transferred to the developing infant through breastmilk. Maternal GCs in breastmilk have been shown to cross the intestinal barrier in animals [6], and have been associated with growth and body composition. Hinde et al. (2015) [7] found that cortisol in the breastmilk of rhesus macaques was positively associated with weight gain in offspring. In humans, Hahn-Holbrook et al. (2016) [8] showed that cortisol in breastmilk at the age of 3 months was inversely associated with body mass index (BMI) percentile gains in the first 2 years of life. Whether the findings from these studies are contradictory is unclear, since length was not taken into account by Hinde et al. [7]. Moreover, the effect of GCs on growth might change between the ages of 3 months and 2 years.

Our group has previously shown that GCs in breastmilk follow maternal HPA-axis activity, with a peak in the morning and a nadir at night [9]. Although previous studies have found associations between cortisol in breastmilk and growth of offspring, none of them took GC rhythmicity into account. However, obesity has previously been associated with a flatter diurnal cortisol slope in adults [10], and there is also some evidence that a blunted GC rhythm is associated with obesity in children [11,12]. Both Hinde et al. (2015) [7] and Hahn-Holbrook et al. (2016) [8] did not collect samples around peak GC levels, while Hahn-Holbrook et al. (2016) also had a wide time window during which samples could be collected (11:30–16:00).

We therefore aimed to assess the associations between breastmilk GC rhythmicity and infant growth and body composition. We measured cortisol and cortisone in breastmilk at 1 month of age over a 24-hour period, measured body composition using air-displacement plethysmography at 3 months of age, and collected length and weight data monthly up to that age. Due to associations found between a blunted endogenous GC rhythm and obesity in both children and adults [10–12], we hypothesized that less GC variability in breastmilk could be associated with a higher fat mass in the infants.

2. Materials and Methods

2.1. *Population*

Healthy mother–infant pairs were recruited at the maternity ward of the Amsterdam UMC, location VUMC (a tertiary hospital) in the Netherlands between March 2016 and July 2017. Subjects were eligible for inclusion when infants were born at term age (37–42 weeks) with a normal birth weight (−2 to +2 SDS), and when mothers had the intention to breastfeed for a minimum of three months. Exclusion criteria were: (1) Major congenital anomalies, (2) multiple pregnancy, (3) pre-eclampsia or HELLP, (4) medication use other than "over the counter" drugs, (5) maternal alcohol consumption of >7 IU/week, and/or 6) a maternal temperature of >38.5 °C at the time of sampling. Approval of the Medical Ethics Committee of the VUMC was obtained (protocol number 2015.524), and written informed consent was obtained from all participating mothers.

2.2. *Data Collection*

2.2.1. Peripartum

Shortly after inclusion, within the first days postpartum, mothers filled in a questionnaire pertaining to their pregnancy and birth, as well as maternal and infant anthropometric and demographic data.

2.2.2. One Month Postpartum

At 30 days postpartum (±5 days), mothers collected a portion of breastmilk (1–2 mL) prior to each feeding moment, over a 24-h period (i.e., five to eight times). Although only foremilk was collected through this method, previous research has shown that GC concentrations are similar in fore- and hindmilk [13]. Mothers could follow their own feeding schedule and were therefore asked to report the exact time of sampling. Milk was collected manually or with a breast pump; we requested that mothers used the same method for all samples. Milk was stored in the mother's freezer, and subsequently in the laboratory at −20 °C for less than 3 months prior to analysis.

At the time of sampling, maternal distress was quantified with the Hospital Anxiety and Depression Scale (HADS) [14]. This questionnaire contains 14 questions scored from 0 to 3, which assess self-reported levels of depression and anxiety symptoms. Seven questions concern depressive symptoms (HDS) and seven questions assess anxiety symptoms (HAS). A score of ≥8 on a subscale is indicative of clinically relevant depression and/or anxiety symptoms.

2.2.3. Three Months Postpartum

At 3 months postpartum (±2 weeks), the body composition of the infants was assessed with the Pea Pod, an air-displacement plethysmography (ADP) system (COSMED USA, Inc., Concord, CA, USA) [15]. It is based on a bi-compartmental model, which uses pressure and volume changes in the chamber through which body density was determined. Age- and sex-specific fat and fat free mass density values were subsequently used to calculate fat mass (FM) and fat free mass (FFM) [15].

As part of the national standard care, weight and length at 1, 2, and 3 months of age were measured by the staff of the child health clinic and were obtained through a questionnaire. Weight was measured fully undressed on a balance scale with an accuracy of 1 g. Length was measured in the supine position to the nearest 0.1 cm. Additionally, all mothers were asked if their infants were still breastfed for >80% at the age of 3 months.

2.3. Laboratory Analysis

Cortisol and cortisone concentrations in breastmilk were determined by isotope dilution liquid chromatography–tandem mass spectrometry (LC–MS/MS), as previously described [16]. In brief, internal standards (13C3-labeled cortisol and 13C3-labeled cortisone) were added to 200 μL of the samples. Then, breastmilk was washed 3 times with 2 mL of hexane to remove lipids. Finally, samples were extracted and analyzed using Isolute plates (Biotage, Uppsala, Sweden) and analyzed by LC-MS/MS (Acquity with Quattro Premier XE, Milford MA, USA, Waters Corporation). The intra-assay coefficients of variation (CV%) were 4 and 5% for cortisol levels of 7 and 23 nmol/L, and 5% for cortisone levels of 8 and 33 nmol/L for LC-MS/MS measurements. The inter-assay CV% was <9% for both cortisol and cortisone. The lower limit of quantitation (LLOQ) was 0.5 nmol/L for both cortisol and cortisone. All samples were measured in duplicate.

2.4. Statistics

First, data of GC concentrations in breastmilk were converted into the following rhythm parameters, in order to provide a full overview of GC rhythmicity:

- The maximum GC concentration, as a proxy for peak concentrations;
- The delta between maximum and minimum GC concentrations, as a measure of rhythm variability; and
- Area under the curve (AUC) ground (g) and increase (i), using the trapezoid rule [17].Calculations were corrected for total sampling time, since this differed between mothers. AUCg is a measure of total GC exposure, while AUCi provides information on GC variability.

Mother–infant pairs were excluded from analyses when no valid GC data was available around the time of the expected morning peak (5:00–10:00) and/or when the total sample collection was <8 h.

Fat% was determined from the FM and FFM values. The fat mass index (FMI) and fat free mass index (FFMI) were calculated by dividing FM and FFM values (in kg), respectively, by infant length squared (m^2), since fat mass and fat free mass are known to change with length [18]. Length and weight data were converted to SDS [19,20]. Body mass index (BMI) was only calculated at 3 months of age, and converted to SDS [19].

Linear regressions were used to assess the associations between GC rhythm parameters at 1 month of age and length SDS, weight SDS, BMI SDS, FMI, and FFMI at 3 months of age. First, unadjusted regression analyses were performed. Next, the following potential confounders were tested: Sex, HADS-score (HAS and/or HDS ≥ 8), pre-pregnancy BMI, ethnicity (Caucasian vs. non-Caucasian), socio-economic status, birth weight SDS, gestational age, weight gain during pregnancy, parity (1 vs. >1), mode of delivery (vaginal vs. caesarian section), and % breastmilk at 3 months of age (< or >80%). Due to our sample size, the three variables with the largest confounding effect (i.e., largest change in β of the independent variable) were used for the multiple linear regression analyses. Thus, weight gain during pregnancy, % breastmilk at 3 months of age, and ethnicity were included in the final model assessing the association between GC rhythm parameters and body composition outcomes. No effect modification was found for infant sex, and analyses were therefore not stratified.

Lastly, length and weight SDS growth trajectories between 1 and 3 months of age were plotted against AUCi and AUCg values by using generalized estimating equations (GEEs), and 95% confidence intervals were calculated according to the method described by Figueiras et al. [21]. AUCi and AUCg outcomes for cortisol and cortisone were categorized as ≤p25, p25–75, and ≥p75.3.

3. Results

3.1. Population

Forty-four mother–infant pairs were included in the study. One mother–infant pair was lost to follow-up, three mother–infant pairs returned the growth questionnaires but did not consent to the Pea Pod measurement, and one pair was excluded because no samples were collected between 5:00 and 10:00 and/or because the total sampling time was <8 h. Therefore, a total of 42 mother–infant pairs were included in the growth trajectory analyses, whereas 39 mother-infant pairs were included in the body composition analyses at 3 months of age. Of the included mother–infant pairs, 59.5% were mother–son pairs. Table 1 shows the characteristics of the population. Supplementary Table S1 shows the cortisol and cortisone concentrations in breastmilk in 4-h intervals.

Table 1. Characteristics of the study population (n = 42).

	Unit	Mean ± SD or n (%)
Gestational Age	Weeks	39.9 ± 1.3
Birth weight	grams	3561 ± 498
	SDS	0.2 ± 1.0
Birth length *	cm	52.0 ± 2.6
	SDS	1.0 ± 1.6
Male sex		25 (59.5)
Primiparity		23 (54.8)
Caesarian section		21 (51.2)
HAS and/or HDS ≥ 8 at 1-month pp		6 (14.6)
Pre-pregnancy maternal BMI	kg/m^2	22.3 ± 2.8
Weight gain during pregnancy	kg	13.1 ± 3.2
Maternal age	years	36.0 ± 4.7
Non-Caucasian ethnicity		8 (20.0)
Socioeconomic status	SDS	0.6 ± 1.2
>80% breastfed at 3 months of age		35 (87.5)
Age at breastmilk sampling	days	30.8 ± 2.6
Age at Pea Pod measurement **	days	90.5 ± 7.0

Values represent Mean ± SD or n (%); pp = postpartum. HAS, Hospital Anxiety Score; HDS, Hospital Depression Score. * n = 31, ** n = 39.

3.2. Linear Regression Analyses

No associations were found between the GC rhythm parameters (AUCi, AUCg, maximum, and delta) and body composition in the unadjusted analyses. Adjusting the analyses for weight gain during pregnancy, % breastmilk at 3 months of age, and ethnicity did not change the results (Table 2).

Table 2. Adjusted associations between breastmilk glucocorticoid rhythmicity at 1 month of age and infant body composition at 3 months of age ($n = 39$).

		Length		Weight		BMI		FMI		FFMI		Fat %	
		B	95% CI	B	95% CI	B	95% CI	B	95% CI	B	95% CI	B	95% CI
Cortisol	Maximum	0.006	(−0.04 to 0.05)	0.022	(−0.02 to 0.07)	0.022	(−0.02 to 0.06)	0.003	(−0.04 to 0.05)	−0.006	(−0.04 to 0.03)	0.048	(−0.17 to 0.27)
	Delta	0.006	(−0.04 to 0.05)	0.024	(−0.02 to 0.07)	0.025	(−0.02 to 0.07)	0.003	(−0.04 to 0.05)	−0.004	(−0.04 to 0.03)	0.043	(−0.18 to 0.26)
	AUCi	0.025	(−0.15 to 0.20	0.101	(−0.07 to 0.28)	0.1	(−0.06 to 0.26)	0.06	(−0.10 to 0.23)	−0.095	(−0.23 to 0.04)	0.53	(−0.34 to 1.39)
	AUCg	0.029	(−0.13 to 0.19)	0.06	(−0.11 to 0.23)	0.046	(−0.11 to 0.20)	0.06	(−0.10 to 0.22)	−0.107	(−0.24 to 0.02)	0.53	(−0.28 to 1.33)
Cortison	Maximum	−0.002	(−0.04 to 0.03)	0.01	(−0.03 to 0.05)	0.014	(−0.02 to 0.05)	-0.006	(−0.04 to 0.03)	-0.006	(−0.04 to 0.02)	-0.007	(−0.19 to 0.18)
	Delta	−0.002	(−0.04 to 0.04)	0.018	(−0.02 to 0.06)	0.024	(−0.01 to 0.06)	-0.003	(−0.04 to 0.03)	-0.001	(−0.03 to 0.03)	0.005	(−0.19 to 0.20)
	AUCi	−0.005	(−0.09 to 0.08)	0.042	(−0.05 to 0.13)	0.055	(−0.02 to 0.14)	0.002	(−0.08 to 0.09)	-0.008	(−0.08 to 0.06)	0.034	(−0.41 to 0.48)
	AUCg	−0.001	(−0.07 to 0.07)	0.003	(−0.07 to 0.07)	0.004	(−0.06 to 0.07)	-0.013	(−0.08 to 0.05)	-0.02	(−0.08 to 0.04)	-0.02	(−0.37 to 0.33)

Values represent β (95% CI) as analyzed with linear regression. Analyses were adjusted for weight gain during pregnancy, % breastmilk at 3 months of age, and ethnicity. AUCi or g, area under the curve increase or ground; FMI, fat mass index; FFMI, fat free mass index.

3.3. Growth Trajectories

Figure 1 shows the growth trajectories for length and weight SDS according to breastmilk cortisone AUCi and AUCg outcomes. No differences were found between the categories ≤p25, p25–75, and ≥p75. Results for breastmilk cortisol AUCi and AUCg were similar (data not shown).

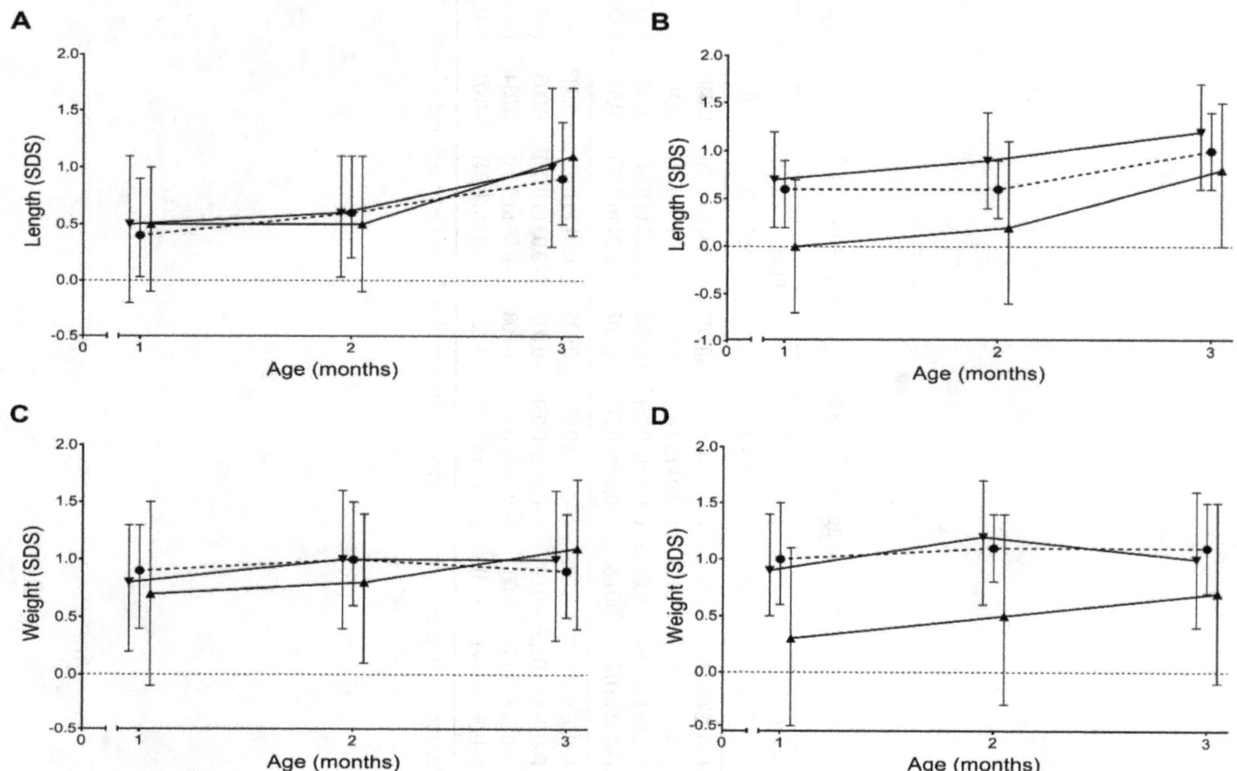

Figure 1. Growth trajectories between 1 and 3 months of age for length and weight, according to breastmilk cortisone AUC outcomes (n = 42). Results for breastmilk cortisol AUCi and AUCg were similar (data not shown). A = length for AUCi, B = weight for AUCg, C = weight for AUCi, D = weight for AUCg; ▼ = AUCi or g < p25, ● = AUCi or g = p25–75, ▲ = AUCi or g > p75, AUCi or g, area under the curve increase or ground.

4. Discussion

In this study, despite increased evidence for associations between blunted endogenous GC rhythms and obesity in both children and adults [10–12], no associations were found between GC rhythmicity in breastmilk sampled at 1 month and infant body composition or growth at 3 months. Therefore, our study could not confirm previous observations in animals and humans. Hinde et al. (2015) [7] measured cortisol in breastmilk of 108 rhesus macaques at 1 month of age, and analyzed growth outcomes at 3.5 months of age. They found that higher cortisol concentrations were associated with greater weight gain over time. Hahn-Holbrook et al. (2016) [8] studied associations between breast-milk cortisol and BMI gains up until the age of 2 years in 51 mother-infant pairs. They found that higher milk cortisol concentrations were associated with smaller BMI gains in offspring.

The different results between this study and previous studies could have several explanations. First, cortisol sampling in the previous studies did not take the diurnal rhythm of breastmilk GCs into account. Hinde et al. [7] sampled between 11:30 and 13:00, which did not capture the peak GC concentration, since in Rhesus macaques, similar to humans, this occurs at around 8:00. Hahn-Holbrook et al. [8] collected a single breastmilk sample within a wide time window (11:30–16:00), which also did not capture peak concentrations. Analyses were corrected for time of collection, but it has previously been shown that correcting for the time of sampling cannot account for all the variability observed in cortisol levels [9,22]. Second, in our study, GC concentrations were determined by LC-MS/MS, which has been shown to be more sensitive and reliable than radioimmunoassay and chemiluminescent immunoassay [23], which were used by Hinde et al. and Hahn-Holbrook et al., respectively. Lastly, it has previously been shown that increases in fat mass are specifically associated with mid-childhood overweight and obesity [24]. Therefore, in this study, body composition was measured by ADP, which is able to differentiate between fat mass and fat free mass. In contrast, weight gain and changes in BMI were used as outcomes measured by Hinde et al. [7] and Hahn-Holbrook et al. [8], respectively, both of which are less precise methods to determine body composition. Our more detailed methods when measuring GC concentrations in breastmilk as well as when determining body composition might therefore have led to more accurate conclusions.

Alternatively, the absence of associations might be due to the small sample size in this study, especially compared to Hinde et al. [7], who included 108 mother–infant pairs, resulting in more power to detect small differences. However, this should be balanced against the use of air-displacement plethysmography in this study, which is superior to weight gain for the assessment of body composition. Additionally, our follow-up until the age of 3 months was rather short. In contrast, follow-up took place up to 2 years of age in Hahn-Holbrook et al.'s study [8]. It is therefore possible that effects of GCs in breastmilk might only be noticeable at a later age. On the other hand, an increasing number of nutritional, lifestyle, and family factors determine body composition with advancing age, and it is therefore progressively more difficult to determine to what extent breastmilk cortisol explains BMI gains.

This study has several strengths and limitations. This was the first study to assess the association between GC rhythmicity in breastmilk and body composition in offspring. Body composition and GC rhythmicity were analyzed in detail, respectively, by the use of ADP and by measuring both cortisol and cortisone in breastmilk using samples that were collected over a 24-h period. Cortisone concentrations have been shown to be more reliable than cortisol measurements, at least in saliva and hair [25,26]. This is possibly due to the local conversion of cortisol by 11β-hydroxysteroid dehydrogenase type 2, which leads to higher concentrations of cortisone [27]. However, this study also has its limitations. The sample size of this study was relatively small, and it is therefore possible that modest effects could not be detected. It was also not possible to correct for all potential confounders. However, many confounders were considered, and the three variables with the largest confounding effect were included in the final model, which did not change the results compared to unadjusted analyses. It is therefore unlikely that adjusting for more variables would have altered the results. Second, the follow-up in this study was relatively short, and it is therefore possible that breastmilk GC rhythmicity has an effect that is only noticeable at a later age. Additionally, selection bias cannot be ruled out, since we did not collect data on mothers who were eligible for inclusion but decided against participation and since we included mother–infant pairs at a (tertiary) hospital. The study population might therefore not reflect the general population; for example, 51% of the mothers gave birth via Caesarian section, compared to approximately 17% in the general population [28]. Lastly, the interplay between GCs and infant body composition is complex, and could be moderated by, for example, exposure to GCs and other conditions in utero, the number of feeds per day, and the extrauterine environment of the infants, including synchrony in mother–infant interactions as well as stressful events. Unfortunately, we were not able to take these factors into account.

5. Conclusions

This study did not find an association between breastmilk GC rhythmicity at 1 month of age and growth trajectories as well as body composition of the offspring at 3 months of age. Therefore, this study suggests that previous observations linking breastmilk cortisol to changes in infant weight might be flawed by the lack of serial cortisol measurements and detailed information on body composition.

Author Contributions: J.H. conceptualized the study, collected the data, performed the analyses and drafted and corrected the manuscript. L.R.D. conceptualized the study, collected the data, performed the analyses and drafted the manuscript. B.v.d.V. conceptualized the study, collected the data and reviewed the manuscript. S.M.P.K. helped with the study design and the body composition analyses, and reviewed the manuscript. A.A.T. conceptualized the study, collected the data and reviewed the manuscript. J.B.v.G. helped with the study design and reviewed the manuscript. J.R. conceptualized the study, helped with the data analyses and reviewed the manuscript. M.J.J.F. conceptualized the study, helped with the data analyses and reviewed the manuscript.

Acknowledgments: The study participants, for giving their time and energy to this study. D.L. for including mother-infant pairs and analyzing breastmilk and saliva samples. A.C.H., F.M., A.F. and other colleagues at the endocrinology laboratory for their contribution to the GC analyses.

References

1. Barker, D.J.; Osmond, C. Infant mortality, childhood nutrition, and ischaemic heart disease in England and Wales. *Lancet* **1986**, *1*, 1077–1081. [CrossRef]
2. Finken, M.J.; van der Voorn, B.; Heijboer, A.C.; de Waard, M.; van Goudoever, J.B.; Rotteveel, J. Glucocorticoid Programming in Very Preterm Birth. *Horm. Res. Paediatr.* **2016**, *85*, 221–231. [CrossRef] [PubMed]
3. Rosmond, R.; Bjorntorp, P. The hypothalamic-pituitary-adrenal axis activity as a predictor of cardiovascular disease, type 2 diabetes and stroke. *J. Intern. Med.* **2000**, *247*, 188–197. [CrossRef] [PubMed]
4. Drake, A.J.; Tang, J.I.; Nyirenda, M.J. Mechanisms underlying the role of glucocorticoids in the early life programming of adult disease. *Clin. Sci.* **2007**, *113*, 219–232. [CrossRef] [PubMed]
5. Entringer, S. Impact of stress and stress physiology during pregnancy on child metabolic function and obesity risk. *Curr. Opin. Clin. Nutr. Metab. Care* **2013**, *16*, 320–327. [CrossRef] [PubMed]
6. Angelucci, L.; Patacchioli, F.R.; Scaccianoce, S.; Di Sciullo, A.; Cardillo, A.; Maccari, S. A model for later-life effects of perinatal drug exposure: Maternal hormone mediation. *Neurobehav. Toxicol. Teratol.* **1985**, *7*, 511–517.
7. Hinde, K.; Skibiel, A.L.; Foster, A.B.; Rosso, L.D.; Mendoza, S.P.; Capitanio, J.P. Cortisol in mother's milk across lactation reflects maternal life history and predicts infant temperament. *Behav. Ecol.* **2015**, *26*, 269–281. [CrossRef]
8. Hahn-Holbrook, J.; Le, T.B.; Chung, A.; Davis, E.P.; Glynn, L.M. Cortisol in human milk predicts child BMI. *Obesity (Silver Spring)* **2016**, *24*, 2471–2474. [CrossRef]
9. Van der Voorn, B.; de Waard, M.; van Goudoever, J.B.; Rotteveel, J.; Heijboer, A.C.; Finken, M.J. Breast-Milk Cortisol and Cortisone Concentrations Follow the Diurnal Rhythm of Maternal Hypothalamus-Pituitary-Adrenal Axis Activity. *J. Nutr.* **2016**, *146*, 2174–2179. [CrossRef]
10. Adam, E.K.; Quinn, M.E.; Tavernier, R.; McQuillan, M.T.; Dahlke, K.A.; Gilbert, K.E. Diurnal cortisol slopes and mental and physical health outcomes: A systematic review and meta-analysis. *Psychoneuroendocrinology* **2017**, *83*, 25–41. [CrossRef]
11. Ruttle, P.L.; Javaras, K.N.; Klein, M.H.; Armstrong, J.M.; Burk, L.R.; Essex, M.J. Concurrent and longitudinal associations between diurnal cortisol and body mass index across adolescence. *J. Adolesc. Health* **2013**, *52*, 731–737. [CrossRef] [PubMed]
12. Wirix, A.J.; Finken, M.J.; von Rosenstiel-Jadoul, I.A.; Heijboer, A.C.; Nauta, J.; Groothoff, J.W.; Chinapaw, M.J.; Kist-van Holthe, J.E. Is There an Association Between Cortisol and Hypertension in Overweight or Obese Children? *J. Clin. Res. Pediatr. Endocrinol.* **2017**, *9*, 344–349. [CrossRef] [PubMed]
13. Patacchioli, F.; Cigliana, G. Maternal plasma and milk free cortisol during the first 3 days of breast-feeding following spontaneous delivery or elective cesarean section. *Gynecolog. Obstet. Invest.* **1992**, *34*, 159–163. [CrossRef] [PubMed]
14. Zigmond, A.S.; Snaith, R.P. The hospital anxiety and depression scale. *Acta Psychiatr. Scand.* **1983**, *67*, 361–370. [CrossRef] [PubMed]
15. Ma, G.; Yao, M.; Liu, Y.; Lin, A.; Zou, H.; Urlando, A.; Wong, W.W.; Nommsen-Rivers, L.; Dewey, K.G. Validation of a new pediatric air-displacement plethysmograph for assessing body composition in infants. *Am. J. Clin. Nutr.* **2004**, *79*, 653–660. [CrossRef] [PubMed]
16. Van der Voorn, B.; Martens, F.; Peppelman, N.S.; Rotteveel, J.; Blankenstein, M.A.; Finken, M.J.; Heijboer, A.C. Determination of cortisol and cortisone in human mother's milk. *Clin. Chim. Acta* **2015**, *444*, 154–155. [CrossRef] [PubMed]
17. Pruessner, J.C.; Kirschbaum, C.; Meinlschmid, G.; Hellhammer, D.H. Two formulas for computation of the

area under the curve represent measures of total hormone concentration versus time-dependent change. *Psychoneuroendocrinology* **2003**, *28*, 916–931. [CrossRef]

18. Kyle, U.G.; Schutz, Y.; Dupertuis, Y.M.; Pichard, C. Body composition interpretation. Contributions of the fat-free mass index and the body fat mass index. *Nutrition* **2003**, *19*, 597–604. [CrossRef]
19. TNO. *De Vijfde Landelijke Groeistudie*; TNO: Hague, The Netherlands, 2010.
20. Schonbeck, Y.; Talma, H.; van Dommelen, P.; Bakker, B.; Buitendijk, S.E.; HiraSing, R.A.; van Buuren, S. The world's tallest nation has stopped growing taller: The height of Dutch children from 1955 to 2009. *Pediatr. Res.* **2013**, *73*, 371–377. [CrossRef]
21. Figueiras, A.; Domenech-Massons, J.M.; Cadarso, C. Regression models: Calculating the confidence interval of effects in the presence of interactions. *Stat. Med.* **1998**, *17*, 2099–2105. [CrossRef]
22. De Weerth, C.; Zijl, R.H.; Buitelaar, J.K. Development of cortisol circadian rhythm in infancy. *Early Hum. Dev.* **2003**, *73*, 39–52. [CrossRef]
23. Ackermans, M.T.; Endert, E. LC-MS/MS in endocrinology: What is the profit of the last 5 years? *Bioanalysis* **2014**, *6*, 43–57. [CrossRef] [PubMed]
24. Koontz, M.B.; Gunzler, D.D.; Presley, L.; Catalano, P.M. Longitudinal changes in infant body composition: Association with childhood obesity. *Pediatr. Obes.* **2014**, *9*, e141–e144. [CrossRef]
25. Blair, J.; Adaway, J.; Keevil, B.; Ross, R. Salivary cortisol and cortisone in the clinical setting. *Curr. Opin. Endocrinol. Diabetes Obes.* **2017**, *24*, 161–168. [CrossRef] [PubMed]
26. Savas, M.; Wester, V.L.; de Rijke, Y.B.; Rubinstein, G.; Zopp, S.; Dorst, K.; van den Berg, S.A.A.; Beuschlein, F.; Feelders, R.A.; Reincke, M.; et al. Hair glucocorticoids as biomarker for endogenous Cushing's syndrome: Validation in two independent cohorts. *Neuroendocrinology* **2019**, *109*, 171–178. [CrossRef]
27. Smith, R.E.; Maguire, J.A.; Stein-Oakley, A.N.; Sasano, H.; Takahashi, K.; Fukushima, K.; Krozowski, Z.S. Localization of 11 beta-hydroxysteroid dehydrogenase type II in human epithelial tissues. *J. Clin. Endocrinol. Metab.* **1996**, *81*, 3244–3248. [CrossRef]
28. Macfarlane, A.J.; Blondel, B.; Mohangoo, A.D.; Cuttini, M.; Nijhuis, J.; Novak, Z.; Olafsdottir, H.S.; Zeitlin, J.; Euro-Peristat Scientific Committee. Wide differences in mode of delivery within Europe: Risk-stratified analyses of aggregated routine data from the Euro-Peristat study. *BJOG* **2016**, *123*, 559–568. [CrossRef]

7

Nutrition of Preterm Infants and Raw Breast Milk-Acquired Cytomegalovirus Infection: French National Audit of Clinical Practices and Diagnostic Approach

Anne-Aurelie Lopes [1,*], Valerie Champion [2] and Delphine Mitanchez [2]

1 Pediatric Emergency Department, AP-HP, Robert Debre Hospital, 48 Boulevard Serurier, 75019 Paris, France
2 Neonatology Department, AP-HP, Armand Trousseau Hospital, 26 Avenue du Dr Arnold Netter, 75012 Paris, France; valerie.champion@aphp.fr (V.C.); delphine.mitanchez@aphp.fr (D.M.)
* Correspondence: anne-aurelie.lopes@aphp.fr

Abstract: Raw breast milk is the optimal nutrition for infants, but it is also the primary cause of acquired cytomegalovirus (CMV) infection. Thus, many countries have chosen to contraindicate to feed raw breast milk preterm infants from CMV-positive mothers before a corrected age of 32 weeks or under a weight of 1500 g. French national recommendations have not been updated since 2005. An audit of the French practices regarding the nutrition with raw breast milk in preterm infants was carried out using a questionnaire sent to all neonatal care units. Diagnosed postnatal milk-acquired CMV infections have been analysed using hospitalisation reports. Seventy-five percent of the neonatal units responded: 24% complied with the French recommendations, 20% contraindicated raw breast milk to all infants before 32 weeks regardless of the mothers' CMV-status, whereas 25% fed all preterm infants unconditionally with raw breast milk. Thirty-five cases of infants with milk-acquired CMV infections have been reported. The diagnosis was undeniable for five patients. In France, a high heterogeneity marks medical practices concerning the use of raw breast milk and the diagnostic approach for breast milk-acquired CMV infection is often incomplete. In this context, updated national recommendations and monitored CMV infections are urgently needed.

Keywords: raw breast milk; cytomegalovirus; milk-acquired infections; preterm infant

---

1. Introduction

In the last fifty years, the development of neonatology reversed the prognosis of preterm infants with a weight over 1500 g from a mortality rate of 85% to a survival rate without sequelae of 85% [1,2]. This drop in mortality was accompanied by a steady decrease in severe morbidities [2]. It was mainly related to significant advances in lung maturation, respiratory support, and optimal nutrition [3]. Breast milk is a crucial part in the management of preterm infants with widely documented immunological and nutritional benefits [4]. Its composition adapts to the gestational age at birth to better protect preterm infants and to regulate their immune response [5–8]. It reduces the risk of infection and inflammatory phenomena, leading to a significant decrease in the incidence of bronchopulmonary dysplasia [9], retinopathy of prematurity [10] and necrotising enterocolitis (NEC) [11]. Nutritional values of breast milk also have a beneficial role in both short and long-term neurological development [12–14], and exposure to breast milk antigens promotes the development of tolerance and significantly reduces the risk of allergy and atopic diseases [15,16]. However, the long-term benefits of breast milk on the prevention of leukaemia [17], obesity [18], type 2 diabetes [19], and others are not yet fully assessed.

The risk of transmitting infections remains a barrier to the use of raw breast milk. To limit this risk, methods have been developed. Freezing reduces the risk of infection (mainly viral risk) without eliminating it, and pasteurisation affects nutritional and antimicrobial properties of breast milk [20]. Whilst there are no differences in neurodevelopmental outcomes in preterm infant fed preterm formula compared with those fed breast milk there is a significantly higher risk of developing NEC with formula [21]. Thus, in light of the improvement of knowledge on the benefits of breast milk, the risk of transmission of the commonly feared infections has been carefully reassessed, and contraindications have been increasingly restricted. With the temporary contraindication of breastfeeding caused by Herpes simplex or Herpes zoster lesions on the breast [22], the only definite contraindication of raw breast milk in developed western countries is maternal HIV-positivity [23,24], and the most discussed one is the maternal cytomegalovirus (CMV)-positivity regarding preterm infants.

CMV (cytomegalovirus) is reactivated by lactation in the mammary gland with a prevalence greater than 95% and is then transmitted via macrophages, monocytes, and virions present in raw breast milk [25,26]. In the mother milk of full-term infants, CMV is excreted as early as colostrum and during the first three months of lactation. In the mother milk of preterm infants, CMV excretion begins with a lower viral load and the onset of excretion is more variable. It usually begins in the first ten days of life, but may be present from the colostrum [27,28]. The standard diagnostic method of CMV infection was viral isolation on fibroblasts culture from a urine sample, but current polymerase chain reaction (PCR) techniques have better sensitivity and specificity (98.8% and 99.9%, respectively) and can be performed on urine or blood samples [29]. To conclude to a milk-acquired infection, congenital CMV infections should be eliminated by a negative CMV research on a blood or urine sample taken within the 21st days of life or on a salivary sample taken within the 21st days of life and before nutrition by unpasteurised breast milk [29,30]. In the case of CMV infection diagnosed after the 21st day of life, the positivity of the PCR could no longer differentiate congenital and postnatal infections. Then, only a negative CMV PCR on a specimen collected before the 21st day of life (cord blood or dried blood spots collected on blotting paper for newborn screening program) can eliminate the diagnosis of congenital infection. The reactivation of the virus in breast milk can be confirmed the same way, by viral isolation or PCR done on milk sample [31]. In the 1990s to 2000s, studies demonstrated that, in children born before a corrected age of 32 weeks or below a weight of 1500 g, the CMV transmission rate was over 50% in the first three months of life [27]. Moreover, 50% of preterm infants had symptomatic infections, and 15% of these infections were severe [26]. The main symptoms were apnoea, bradycardia, pneumonia, hepatitis, gastrointestinal tract symptoms, and haematological signs (thrombocytopenia, neutropenia, and lymphocytosis). These infections appeared between four and eight weeks of life and were responsible for significant clinical degradations that could be life-threatening, whereas the level of C-reactive protein remained low (10 to 20 mg/L). This clinical situation was called "sepsis-like". Thus, the international guidelines agreed not to feed preterm infants from CMV-positive mothers with raw breast milk before a corrected age of 32 weeks or below a weight of 1500 g [32–34].

In the 2010s, retrospective studies and reviews of the literature reassessed the risk of milk-acquired severe CMV infections and the prognosis of affected infants. The risk associated with symptomatic infections and "sepsis-like" were estimated to be low [35]. In particular, the risk of neurological sequelae (cognitive and motor) was similar to that of preterm infants without a history of postnatal CMV infections [25]. Therefore, since 2012, the American Academic of Pediatrics recommends nutrition with raw breast milk for all preterm infants [36]. However, publications have rapidly reported cases with severe "sepsis-like" and severe enteropathies suggestive of atypical NEC [37–40]. Several fatal cases have been reported [41,42]. Moreover, since 2015, large cohorts have shown that the incidence of bronchopulmonary dysplasia was significantly higher in infants with postnatal CMV infection [43]. The absence of long-term consequences has also been questioned [28].

Since 2005, the French recommendations maintained to not feed preterm infants from CMV-positive mothers with raw breast milk before a corrected age of 32 weeks or below a weight of 1500 g. The breast milk must then be pasteurised before its administration [32]. This recommendation is problematic for several reasons. Routine CMV screening of pregnant women is not recommended in France [44], and not all neonatal units have access to pasteurisation. Furthermore, several cases of postnatal breast milk-acquired CMV infections in infants fed raw breast milk before a corrected age of 32 weeks or below a weight of 1500 g have been published by French neonatal units [42,45,46]. Thus, this study aimed to evaluate the French national current clinical practices about breast milk nutrition of preterm infants, to carry out a first national census of raw breast milk-acquired CMV infections and to check the validity of this diagnosis.

2. Methods

2.1. Study Design

An observational, transverse, prospective, multicentre, descriptive study was conducted via a questionnaire sent by e-mail to all NICU (neonatal intensive care unit) and neonatal non-ICU, in mainland France and French overseas territories.

2.2. Outcome Measures

The questionnaire was sent by email to at least one doctor or breastfeeding counsellor from each unit from June 2015 to June 2016. Reminders were sent out every four months for one year as long as there was no answer. The answers were collected by e-mail and by post. The questionnaire was written in French and translated into English for this publication (Figure S1).

The questionnaire consisted of four parts. In the first part, general data on the neonatal unit were collected. In the second part, the current clinical practices of each service were requested. The information was related to the use of breast milk (frozen, pasteurised, raw mother milk, or donation of breast milk), the promotion of breastfeeding, and the access to a human milk bank. The third part concerned the conditions of use of raw breast milk (maternal CMV status, infants' term or weight) and the barriers to its use (mainly infectious risks). Finally, the last part of the questionnaire identified diagnosed cases of postnatal CMV infections imputed to raw breast milk (clinical signs and course).

Subsequently, the neonatal units reporting cases of breast milk-acquired CMV infections were contacted again between June 2016 and June 2017 to obtain the hospitalisation reports of the concerned infants.

2.3. Data Management

CMV infections have been classified as "proven", "highly probable", "probable", or "unlikely" breast milk-acquired infections.

CMV infections have been classified as "proven" if the infection occurred in infants from CMV-positive mothers fed raw breast milk with documented CMV reactivation in breast milk and without any other mode of transmission possible. A congenital infection must have been rejected. Both viral isolation culture and PCR methods were accepted to reject the congenital infection and confirm the infection in the blood or the urine of the preterm infant and to confirm the CMV reactivation in breast milk. Other possible modes of transmission had to be eliminated (PCR on residual blood from transfusions), and no other cause of infection must be found.

CMV infections have been classified as "highly probable" if the infection occurred in infants from CMV-positive mothers fed raw breast milk, but one of the following items was not documented: reactivation of CMV in breast milk, elimination of all other possible modes of transmission, and evidence of absence of congenital infection except mothers' CMV-positivity prior to pregnancy.

CMV infections were classified as "probable" if the infection occurred in infants from CMV-positive mothers fed raw breast milk, but two of the following items were undocumented: reactivation of CMV in breast milk, elimination of all other possible modes of transmission, and evidence of absence of congenital infection except mothers' CMV-positivity prior to pregnancy.

CMV infections have been classified as "unlikely" for other cases.

2.4. Statistical Analysis

The results for the quantitative variables were expressed in median (minimum—maximum). The results for the qualitative variables were expressed in numbers and percentages.

3. Results

The questionnaire was completed by 105 neonatal units including 58 NICU (88%) and 47 non-ICU (64%), representing an overall response rate of 75% (Figure 1). The participation rate was evenly distributed across regions, ranging from the smallest to the largest unit (Table S1).

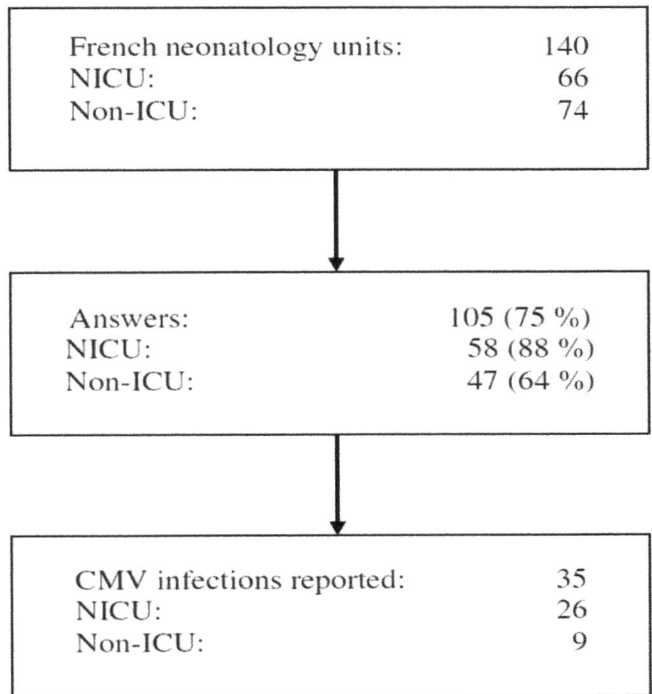

Figure 1. Flowchart. NICU: neonatal intensive care unit; ICU: intensive care unit; CMV: cytomegalovirus.

3.1. Current Clinical Practices

Ninety percent of NICU and 67% of non-ICU reported promoting breast milk nutrition with 70% of NICU and 63% of non-ICU having a breastfeeding counsellor, but only half of them with protocols to help initial breastfeeding. The storage methods of breast milk were freezing in 17 units, pasteurisation in 32 units, and both methods in 47 units.

The 36 neonatal units located in hospitals with a human milk bank responded to the questionnaire. Fifty-six other neonatal units (53%), including 35 NICU, had access to a human milk bank outside their hospital. Thirteen services (12%) reported not having access to a human milk bank. Among them, six neonatal units (5 NICU) were in overseas territories. The two NICU of the Reunion (overseas territory) were the only units to report the use of freeze-dried women's milk from the French human milk bank of Marmande.

Among the 92 neonatal units that had access to a human milk bank, if the infant's mother milk was unavailable, 87 (95%) routinely used pasteurised women's milk instead of formulas for preterm infants before a corrected age of 32 weeks. This corresponded to 51 NICU and 36 non-ICU. All NICU systematically used pasteurised women's milk before a corrected age of 30 weeks, except for a unit that used it systematically only for infants before 28 weeks. For infant over a corrected age of 32 weeks, 37 units (35%), including 19 NICU, used pasteurised women's milk for initial trophic nutrition, nutrition for infants with significant in utero growth retardation (birth weight <10th percentile and less than 1500 g) or for children with congenital digestive disorders, current digestive disorders, or renal failure.

3.2. Raw Breast Milk Use

Only two among 105 units declared never to use raw breast milk. Among the 103 units that used raw breast milk, 25% neonatal units fed all infants with raw milk, regardless of term, weight and the mother CMV status (Figure 2). Among them, seven units did not have access to a Human milk bank (including three overseas territories), and eight NICU decided to feed all preterm infants with raw breast milk, despite access to a Human milk bank.

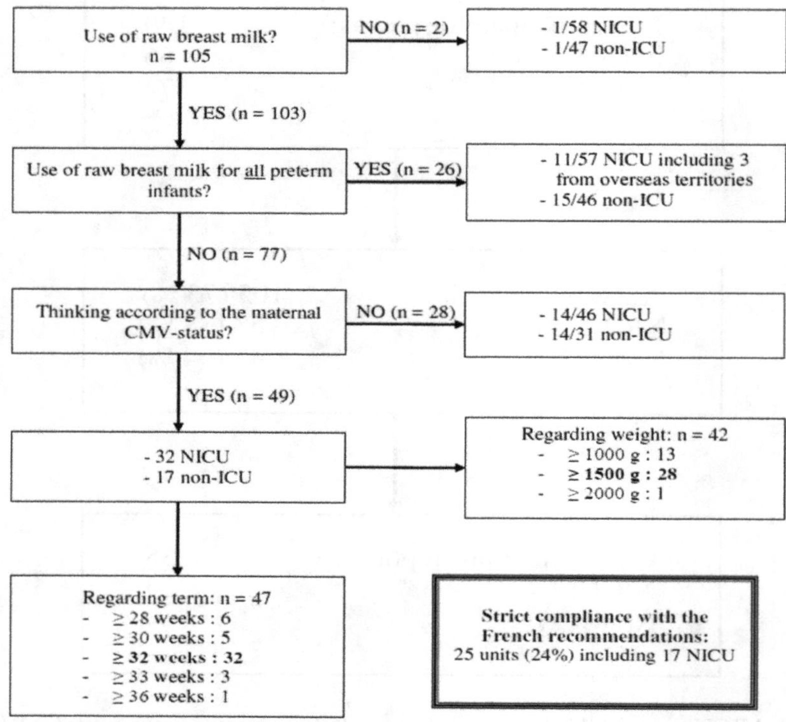

Figure 2. Summary of the current use of raw breast milk in France.

Seventy-three percent of the units used raw breast milk based on the infants' term or weight. Among them, 49 units gave raw milk according to the CMV maternal status. Thus, all infants born from CMV-negative mothers received raw breast milk from birth. On the other hand, in the case of maternal CMV-positivity, 32 units gave breast milk from a corrected age of 32 weeks, but some gave it either later or sooner (Figure 2). Although 1500 g was the most common weight limit used, 1000 g was also widely used, associated with a term limit of 28 weeks. Twenty-eight units gave raw breast milk based on infants' term, but not according to the maternal CMV status. Consequently, even infants born from CMV-negative mothers did not receive raw breast milk before a defined term or weight. The clear majority (21 including 11 NICU) gave raw breast milk from 32 weeks to all preterm infants. Other units gave it from terms ranging from 28 weeks to 35 weeks. Overall, 25 units (24%) complied with the French recommendations.

Among the 77 units that did not give unconditionally raw breast milk, 95% reported that the risk of transmission of infectious diseases was the main barrier. The most feared infections were caused by CMV (56 units including all NICU), HIV (43 units including 26 NICU), bacterial infections led by those caused by *Staphylococcus aureus* (33 units including 20 NICU) and HTLV-1 (10 NICU). Five units also reported that the current French recommendations were the principal barrier to the use of raw breast milk. Units that did not give raw breast milk before a corrected age of 32 weeks and below 1500 g, regardless of the maternal CMV-status, highlighted the contradiction of the French recommendations as the maternal CMV serology is not recommended during pregnancy. On the other hand, those who gave raw breast milk to all infants, regardless of their term, weight, and their mother's CMV-status, justified this approach by the numerous studies on the benefits of breast milk and the latest American recommendations. Other units pointed out that the absence of a human milk bank was of great importance in their decision and that it could have been otherwise. Moreover, some units changed their practices because of cases of severe postnatal infections.

3.3. Reported Postnatal CMV Infection Attributed to Raw Breast Milk Nutrition

Twenty-one units (20%) (17 NICU and 4 non-ICU) reported a total of 35 cases of postnatal CMV infections thought to be transmitted via raw breast milk between 2013 and 2016. Eight infants (23%) had asymptomatic infections, 11 (31%) had moderate signs (hepatic cytolysis, thrombocytopenia), and 16 (46%) had significant signs including 10 infants (29%) with "sepsis-like" infections. Two infants died in NICU during the infection, and another infant died a few months later from complications of this infection. Seventeen hospitalisation reports were obtained, including the reports of two of the three deceased infants and were classified as "proven", "highly probable", "probable", and "unlikely" (Table 1).

Table 1. Infection cases.

"Proven" Infections	Term at Birth	Weight at Birth	Age at Diagnosis (Day)	Symptoms	Missing Information	Source of Reference
1	27 weeks 4 days	550 g	50	"Sepsis-like", NEC, death	/	Lopes et al., 2016
2	27 weeks 4 days	1000 g	50	Asymptomatic	/	Lopes et al., 2016
3	26 weeks	810 g	70	"Sepsis-like", NEC,	/	This study
4	27 weeks	900 g	60	"Sepsis-like", NEC	/	This study
5	29 weeks	1200 g	53	Asymptomatic	/	Croly-Labourlette et al., 2006
"Highly probable" infections						
6	25 weeks 5 days	900 g	36	Thrombocytopenia, hyperleukocytosis	CMV PCR on residual blood from transfusions	This study
7	27 weeks	/	30	"Sepsis-like"	Elimination of congenital origin	This study
8	27 weeks 5 days	950 g	41	"Sepsis-lik", thrombocytopenia NEC, death	Elimination of congenital origin	This study
9	28 weeks	1125 g	60	Thrombocytopenia	CMV reactivation in breast milk (stopped before)	Boumahni et al., 2014
10	30 weeks	1500 g	15 and 40	Cholestasis "Sepsis-like"	CMV reactivation in breast milk	Radi et al., 2007
11	33 weeks	>2000 g	20	"Sepsis-like", NEC	Elimination of congenital origin	This study
12	33 weeks	>2000 g	20	Adenopathies	Elimination of congenital origin	This study
"Probable" infections						
13	25 weeks	570 g	90	Unconfirmed hearing loss	CMV reactivation in breast milk & Elimination of congenital origin	This study
14	32 weeks	>2000	35	"Sepsis-like"		This study
15	32 weeks	1950	60	Severe leukopenia		This study

CMV: cytomegalovirus; PCR: polymerase chain reaction; NEC: necrotising enterocolitis.

The five cases classified as "proven" infections were fed raw breast milk before their second week of life. The congenital origin of the infection was eliminated by a CMV PCR negative on the dried blood spots of the newborn screening program for all of them, excepted one infant with an intrauterine growth restriction who had negative research of CMV done on urine sample during his first week of life. The mean gestational age of birth of these children was 27 weeks (26–29 weeks). Two children had an asymptomatic infection diagnosed for one because of the symptomatic infection of his twin, and for the other during a pilot study. One infant received blood transfusions because of a win-to-twin transfusion syndrome with negative CMV PCR done on the residual blood (patient 1). His autopsy found typical CMV lesions in all organs including the entire digestive tract. Another infant who suffered from "sepsis-like" and NEC showed a CMV PCR positive on peritoneal liquid.

The seven cases classified as "highly probable" were all fed raw breast milk before their second week of life. When it was done, the congenital origin of the infection was eliminated by a CMV PCR negative on the dried blood spots of the newborn screening program. The children had a gestational age of birth between 25 and 33 weeks. Half of the infections were discovered on biological abnormalities. The mother of the twins born at 33 weeks with a weight over 2000 g was suffering from a CMV mastitis. Only two patients received treatment by ganciclovir: one died (patient 8), and the other showed numerous CMV reactivation (patient 10). The histological examination of the ileocaecal resection of patient 8 showed intense necrotic and pan-parietal inflammatory lesions with typical CMV lesions. This infant presented a persistent hepatocellular insufficiency associated with significant thrombocytopenia requiring numerous platelet transfusions. Four months later, during surgery for restoring the continuity of the gastrointestinal tract, his clinical condition deteriorated rapidly, and he died in the following hours.

The three cases classified as "probable" were all fed through raw breast milk from their first week of life. In these cases, even if the mothers were CMV-positive before pregnancy, the congenital origin was not eliminated, and the reactivation in the mother milk was not proven. The diagnostic was done after two months of life in the two cases.

Two reported cases considered as milk-acquired CMV infections were classified as "unlikely". Based on their history, they were probably congenital infections. One did not receive his mother milk but women pasteurised milk. For the second one, the CMV PCR done on the mother milk was negative.

4. Discussion

As a result of a high rate of participation, this work offers a global vision of clinical practices in France. All neonatal units recognised the fundamental issue of promoting breastfeeding and emphasised the importance of individual and adapted care, as shown by the higher importance given to the breastfeeding counsellor compared with the establishment of breastfeeding protocols. Regarding raw breast milk, 24% of units strictly complied with the French recommendations and 20% applied the same limits to all preterm infants, regardless of maternal CMV-status, whereas 25% of neonatal units fed all preterm infants unconditionally with raw breast milk. Most neonatal units believed that the French recommendations are outdated. Their current protocols were the result of reflections including French recommendations [32], recommendations from authorities of other countries [36] or by French experts [47], recent literature, possible access to a human milk bank, and their clinical experience. It resulted in a variety of protocols ranging from raw breast milk nutrition for all preterm infants to non-use of it before a corrected age of 36 weeks or below a weight of 2000 g.

These protocols were mainly based on the fear of severe breast milk-acquired CMV infections in preterm infants. However, this audit shows that the diagnostic approach to conclude such an infection was often incomplete. Out of the 17 hospitalisation reports obtained, the diagnosis was confirmed in only five cases. In the group of infections classified as "highly probable", the missing step was most often the elimination of congenital infection. In the case of infections classified as "probable", the two missing elements were both the elimination of congenital infection and the confirmation of the CMV reactivation in breast milk. The diagnosis was always made in the first months of life when the information can be retreived. Indeed, the retrospective way to eliminate a congenital infection is to perform a CMV PCR on a sample taken before the 21st day of life. In France, blotting papers for the newborn screening program are kept for 18 months. Viral DNA testing on the dried blood spots collected on this blotting paper could be done up to five years after birth [48] and the technique to perform a CMV PCR on it has evolved to improve the sensitivity and specificity to 99.9% [49,50]. Thus, the congenital origin of a CMV infection can be confirmed or denied. The second missing element was the proof of CMV reactivation in the mother milk. CMV excretion occurs from the first to the eighth week with a peak of viral load between the third and the fifth week. Freezing decreases the viral load while preserving the viral DNA. Thus, this research can be conducted afterwards, including that on frozen milk.

In the absence of an exhaustive diagnostic approach, it is impossible to know the exact number of postnatal breast milk-acquired CMV infections, as well as their risk factors and prognosis. A possible exhaustive diagnostic approach is presented in Figure 3. The only mode of transmission that is not eliminated by this approach is perinatal transmission when passing the birth canal. Few studies have investigated this mode of transmission, but they showed a near-zero risk in term infant as in preterm infants [26]. However, this approach investigates and eliminates all other sources of transmission. In the 2000s, prospective studies focused on eliminating congenital origin and confirming postnatal infection, without systematically eliminating the risk of transmission through blood products or through confirming the CMV reactivation in breast milk. This fact has been emphasised in the review of the literature by Kurath et al. in 2010 [25] and a meta-analysis conducted in 2017 by Lanzieri et al. [35]. The latter analysed all the studies carried out since 1980 in English, French, Spanish, and Portuguese. Its inclusion factors were known old maternal immunity, birth before a gestational age of 32 weeks or below a weight of 1500 g, elimination of congenital infection, confirmation of postnatal infection, and accuracy of the preservation mode of the breast milk received (pasteurised, frozen, or raw). Only 17 studies conducted between 2001 and 2011 could be included, and elimination of transmission via blood products was analysed, but was not an inclusion factor as few studies explicitly excluded it. These studies underlined the difficulty of analysing the results, considering the heterogeneity of the international recommendations and practices.

In our study, infants affected by CMV infections were born between 25 and 33 weeks and fed raw breast milk before their second week of life. Infections occurred between the 15th and 70th day of life. All reported cases of severe infections ("sepsis-like", ECUN, deaths) involved infants born before 30 weeks of age, except for one twin born at 33 weeks with a mother suffering from CMV mastitis. Eight cases involved infants born before 28 weeks with infections occurring until a corrected age of 36 weeks. Studies and reviews of the literature seem to agree that children born before a corrected age of 28 weeks or a weight below 1000 g are at higher risk of developing severe infections, and that 80% of "sepsis-like" concern infants born before 26 weeks [27,41]. One of the reasons is probably the reduced transplacental passage of protective maternal antibodies before the end of the 28th week [51]. The risk of severe infection appears to be increased if preterm infants receive raw breast milk during the first month of life and have comorbidities [52–54]. A group of French experts worked on the use of raw breast milk to harmonise practices and wrote the "First Recommendations for the Use of Raw Milk" [47]. The experts provided advice on all crucial steps in breastfeeding, from breastfeeding promotion to protein fortification and viral and bacteriological infectious contraindications. Regarding CMV, the contraindication only concerns infants born from CMV-positive mothers before a corrected age of 28 weeks or below a weight of 1000 g. For these infants, although raw colostrum can be administered within the first 2–3 days of life, milk must be pasteurised up to a corrected age of 31 weeks and 6 days to protect children for at least the first month of life. Six NICU followed these recommendations. However, this expert opinion, like the current French recommendations, raises the problem of CMV screening in pregnant women. The main argument for not recommending this non-targeted screening is the lack of effective treatment for congenital infections. However, this screening would promote hygiene measures to CMV-negative women [55] and facilitate compliance with the French recommendations concerning the nutrition of preterm infants with raw breast milk. Moreover, although no curative treatment exists, early treatment of infants born with congenital infection can reduce the rate of neurosensory sequelae [56].

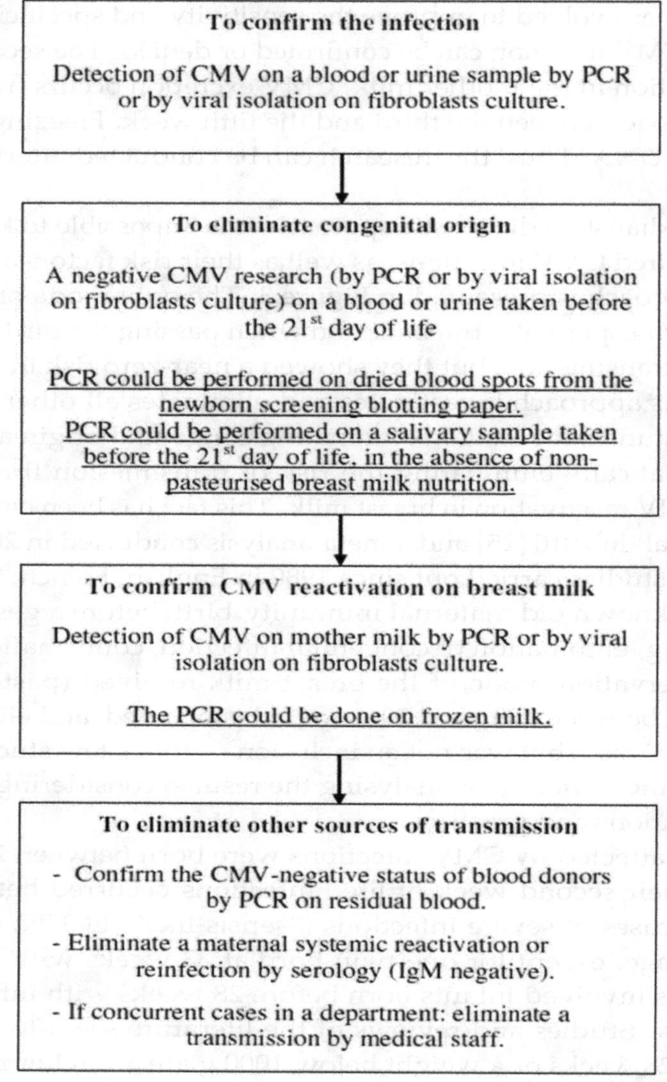

Figure 3. Possible exhaustive diagnostic approach of milk-acquired CMV infections. PCR: polymerase chain reaction.

Another issue raised by this study is the link between milk-acquired CMV infection and NEC. In our study, more than half of severe postnatal CMV infections were associated with NEC. The autopsy finding of one infant showed specific CMV lesions in the digestive tract [42], as the histological examination of the ileocaecal resection of a second infant, and a CMV PCR was positive on the peritoneal liquid of another infant. NEC is an acute inflammatory reaction with necrosis of the digestive tract and is the leading gastrointestinal cause of morbidity and mortality in preterm infants with, in very low birth weight, an incidence estimated at 11% [57]. Surgery is required for 50% of them and 35% die [57]. In CMV infection, the involvement of the digestive tract is mainly described in immunocompromised patients where the entire digestive tract can be affected and can lead to digestive perforation with a poor prognosis [58]. Studies have shown that raw breast milk nutrition significantly reduces the risk of NEC [58]. However, the link between NEC and postnatal CMV infection transmitted via breast milk (and thus via the digestive tract) is controversial. Although many case reports highlight this association [37,42], some prospective studies have shown no link between NEC and viral infections [59], while others have shown a significant incidence of CMV infections in acute digestive tract pathologies in preterm infants [57]. The digestive manifestations associated with a postnatal or congenital CMV infection appear to be diverse and include, in term or premature infants, NEC (including atypical) or digestive perforations as volvulus in low birth weight infants [60].

Our study has a major limitation. The questionnaire was essentially empirical and could be completed by a physician, a nurse, or a breastfeeding counsellor. The high level of participation and its even distribution across regions should provide an overview of French practices and enable an optimal census of diagnosed milk-acquired CMV infections. However, we faced a reporting bias and probably an underestimation of the cases. While many units have reported milk-acquired CMV infections, half have finally agreed to send us the hospitalisation reports. Moreover, some known cases have not been reported. The human milk bank of Ile-de-France is often consulted to determine the probability that CMV infections are milk-acquired infections. In 2015–2016, it confirmed four cases. These cases concern four neonatal units who responded to the audit, but none of them has reported the infections in our questionnaire. These cases, like most of the cases reported without an obtained hospitalisation report, occurred in neonatal units using raw breast milk before a corrected age of 32 weeks or below a weight of 1500 g. On the other hand, units that have turned back their practices because of the occurrence of milk-acquired CMV infections, or that continue voluntarily to not follow the French recommendations, have sent us the hospitalisation reports.

5. Conclusions

In the absence of an efficient technique to eliminate infectious risk while preserving the nutritional and immunological values of breast milk, consensus on the use of raw breast milk in preterm infants is needed. The French recommendations are indeed too restrictive but, given the heterogeneity of clinical practices and the likely underestimation of infectious risk, new recommendations seem challenging to formulate. The creation of a national registry of milk-acquired CMV infections with a structured diagnostic approach could be an effective way to assess the real infectious risk; identify a population at risk; and, in few years, write national recommendations. These recommendations will have, among others, to rule on the knowledge of maternal CMV status during pregnancy or in preterm births, as well as on the best screening methods for infants.

Author Contributions: Conceptualization, methodology, investigation, formal analysis and writing (original draft preparation) were done by A.-A.L. Writing (review and editing) and supervision were done by V.C. and D.M. All the authors critically reviewed the manuscript, approved the final manuscript as submitted and agree to be accountable for all aspects of the work.

References

1. Torchin, H.; Ancel, P.-Y.; Jarreau, P.-H.; Goffinet, F. Epidemiology of preterm birth: Prevalence, recent trends, short- and long-term outcomes. *J. Gynecol. Obstet. Biol. Reprod.* **2015**, *44*, 723–731. [CrossRef] [PubMed]
2. Ancel, P.-Y.; Goffinet, F.; EPIPAGE-2 Writing Group; Kuhn, P.; Langer, B.; Matis, J.; Hernandorena, X.; Chabanier, P.; Joly-Pedespan, L.; Lecomte, B.; et al. Survival and morbidity of preterm children born at 22 through 34 weeks' gestation in France in 2011: Results of the EPIPAGE-2 cohort study. *JAMA Pediatr.* **2015**, *169*, 230–238. [CrossRef] [PubMed]
3. Vidyasagar, D. Half a Century of Evolution of Neonatology: A Witness's Story. *Indian J. Pediatr.* **2015**, *82*, 1117–1125. [CrossRef] [PubMed]
4. Cleminson, J.S.; Zalewski, S.P.; Embleton, N.D. Nutrition in the preterm infant: What's new? *Curr. Opin. Clin. Nutr. Metab. Care* **2016**, *19*, 220–225. [CrossRef] [PubMed]

5. Lewis, E.D.; Richard, C.; Larsen, B.M.; Field, C.J. The Importance of Human Milk for Immunity in Preterm Infants. *Clin. Perinatol.* **2017**, *44*, 23–47. [CrossRef] [PubMed]
6. Araújo, E.D.; Gonçalves, A.K.; da Cornetta, M.C.; Cunha, H.; Cardoso, M.L.; Morais, S.S.; Giraldo, P.C. Evaluation of the secretory immunoglobulin A levels in the colostrum and milk of mothers of term and pre-term newborns. *Braz. J. Infect. Dis.* **2005**, *9*, 357–362. [CrossRef] [PubMed]
7. Mehta, R.; Petrova, A. Biologically active breast milk proteins in association with very preterm delivery and stage of lactation. *J. Perinatol.* **2011**, *31*, 58–62. [CrossRef] [PubMed]
8. Koenig, A.; de Albuquerque Diniz, E.M.; Barbosa, S.F.C.; Vaz, F.A.C. Immunologic factors in human milk: The effects of gestational age and pasteurization. *J. Hum. Lact.* **2005**, *21*, 439–443. [CrossRef] [PubMed]
9. Spiegler, J.; Preuß, M.; Gebauer, C.; Bendiks, M.; Herting, E.; Göpel, W.; German Neonatal Network (GNN). Does Breastmilk Influence the Development of Bronchopulmonary Dysplasia? *J. Pediatr.* **2016**, *169*, 76–80. [CrossRef] [PubMed]
10. Bharwani, S.K.; Green, B.F.; Pezzullo, J.C.; Bharwani, S.S.; Dhanireddy, R. Systematic review and meta-analysis of human milk intake and retinopathy of prematurity: A significant update. *J. Perinatol.* **2016**, *36*, 913–920. [CrossRef] [PubMed]
11. Donovan, S.M. The Role of Lactoferrin in Gastrointestinal and Immune Development and Function: A Preclinical Perspective. *J. Pediatr.* **2016**, *173*, S16–S28. [CrossRef] [PubMed]
12. Horta, B.L.; Loret de Mola, C.; Victora, C.G. Breastfeeding and intelligence: A systematic review and meta-analysis. *Acta Paediatr.* **2015**, *104*, 14–19. [CrossRef] [PubMed]
13. Belfort, M.B.; Rifas-Shiman, S.L.; Kleinman, K.P.; Guthrie, L.B.; Bellinger, D.C.; Taveras, E.M.; Gillman, M.W.; Oken, E. Infant feeding and childhood cognition at ages 3 and 7 years: Effects of breastfeeding duration and exclusivity. *JAMA Pediatr.* **2013**, *167*, 836–844. [CrossRef] [PubMed]
14. Victora, C.G.; Horta, B.L.; de Mola, C.L.; Quevedo, L.; Pinheiro, R.T.; Gigante, D.P.; Gonçalves, H.; Barros, F.C. Association between breastfeeding and intelligence, educational attainment, and income at 30 years of age: A prospective birth cohort study from Brazil. *Lancet Glob. Health* **2015**, *3*, e199–e205. [CrossRef]
15. Van Odijk, J.; Kull, I.; Borres, M.P.; Brandtzaeg, P.; Edberg, U.; Hanson, L.A.; Høst, A.; Kuitunen, M.; Olsen, S.F.; Skerfving, S.; et al. Breastfeeding and allergic disease: A multidisciplinary review of the literature (1966–2001) on the mode of early feeding in infancy and its impact on later atopic manifestations. *Allergy* **2003**, *58*, 833–843. [CrossRef] [PubMed]
16. Dogaru, C.M.; Nyffenegger, D.; Pescatore, A.M.; Spycher, B.D.; Kuehni, C.E. Breastfeeding and childhood asthma: Systematic review and meta-analysis. *Am. J. Epidemiol.* **2014**, *179*, 1153–1167. [CrossRef] [PubMed]
17. Amitay, E.L.; Keinan-Boker, L. Breastfeeding and Childhood Leukemia Incidence: A Meta-analysis and Systematic Review. *JAMA Pediatr.* **2015**, *169*, e151025. [CrossRef] [PubMed]
18. Pudla, K.J.; Gonzaléz-Chica, D.A.; Vasconcelos, F.D.A.G.D. Effect of breastfeeding on obesity of schoolchildren: Influence of maternal education. *Rev. Paul. Pediatr.* **2015**, *33*, 295–302. [CrossRef] [PubMed]
19. Horta, B.L.; Loret de Mola, C.; Victora, C.G. Long-term consequences of breastfeeding on cholesterol, obesity, systolic blood pressure and type 2 diabetes: A systematic review and meta-analysis. *Acta Paediatr.* **2015**, *104*, 30–37. [CrossRef] [PubMed]
20. Van Gysel, M.; Cossey, V.; Fieuws, S.; Schuermans, A. Impact of pasteurization on the antibacterial properties of human milk. *Eur. J. Pediatr.* **2012**, *171*, 1231–1237. [CrossRef] [PubMed]
21. Quigley, M.; Embleton, N.D.; McGuire, W. Formula versus donor breast milk for feeding preterm or low birth weight infants. *Cochrane Database Syst. Rev.* **2018**, *6*. [CrossRef] [PubMed]
22. Berens, P.; Eglash, A.; Malloy, M.; Steube, A.M. ABM Clinical Protocol #26: Persistent Pain with Breastfeeding. *Breastfeed. Med.* **2016**, *11*, 46–53. [CrossRef] [PubMed]
23. Little, K.M.; Hu, D.J.; Dominguez, K.L. HIV-1 and breastfeeding in the United States. *Adv. Exp. Med. Biol.* **2012**, *743*, 261–270. [CrossRef] [PubMed]
24. World Health Organization. *UNICEF Update on HIV and Infant Feeding*; World Health Organization: Geneva, Switzerland, 2016.
25. Kurath, S.; Halwachs-Baumann, G.; Müller, W.; Resch, B. Transmission of cytomegalovirus via breast milk to the prematurely born infant: A systematic review. *Clin. Microbiol. Infect.* **2010**, *16*, 1172–1178. [CrossRef] [PubMed]
26. Hamprecht, K.; Maschmann, J.; Vochem, M.; Dietz, K.; Speer, C.P.; Jahn, G. Epidemiology of transmission of cytomegalovirus from mother to preterm infant by breastfeeding. *Lancet* **2001**, *357*, 513–518. [CrossRef]

27. Vochem, M.; Hamprecht, K.; Jahn, G.; Speer, C.P. Transmission of cytomegalovirus to preterm infants through breast milk. *Pediatr. Infect. Dis. J.* **1998**, *17*, 53–58. [CrossRef] [PubMed]
28. Hamprecht, K.; Goelz, R. Postnatal Cytomegalovirus Infection through Human Milk in Preterm Infants: Transmission, Clinical Presentation, and Prevention. *Clin. Perinatol.* **2017**, *44*, 121–130. [CrossRef] [PubMed]
29. Ross, S.A.; Ahmed, A.; Palmer, A.L.; Michaels, M.G.; Sánchez, P.J.; Bernstein, D.I.; Tolan, R.W.; Novak, Z.; Chowdhury, N.; Fowler, K.B.; et al. Detection of congenital cytomegalovirus infection by real-time polymerase chain reaction analysis of saliva or urine specimens. *J. Infect. Dis.* **2014**, *210*, 1415–1418. [CrossRef] [PubMed]
30. Boppana, S.B.; Ross, S.A.; Shimamura, M.; Palmer, A.L.; Ahmed, A.; Michaels, M.G.; Sánchez, P.J.; Bernstein, D.I.; Tolan, R.W.; Novak, Z.; et al. Saliva polymerase-chain-reaction assay for cytomegalovirus screening in newborns. *N. Engl. J. Med.* **2011**, *364*, 2111–2118. [CrossRef] [PubMed]
31. Romero-Gómez, M.P.; Cabrera, M.; Montes-Bueno, M.T.; Cendejas-Bueno, E.; Segovia, C.; Pastrana, N.; Mingorance, J.; Omeñaca, F. Evaluation of cytomegalovirus infection in low-birth weight children by breast milk using a real-time polymerase chain reaction assay. *J. Med. Virol.* **2015**, *87*, 845–850. [CrossRef] [PubMed]
32. Agence française de sécurité sanitaire des aliments. Recommandations d'hygiène pour la préparation et la conservation des biberons. Available online: https://www.anses.fr/fr/system/files/MIC-Ra-BIB.pdf (accessed on 4 July 2015).
33. Gartner, L.M.; Morton, J.; Lawrence, R.A.; Naylor, A.J.; O'Hare, D.; Schanler, R.J.; Eidelman, A.I. Breastfeeding and the Use of Human Milk. *Pediatrics* **2005**, *115*, 496–506. [CrossRef] [PubMed]
34. Omarsdottir, S.; Casper, C.; Akerman, A.; Polberger, S.; Vanpée, M. Breastmilk handling routines for preterm infants in Sweden: A national cross-sectional study. *Breastfeed. Med.* **2008**, *3*, 165–170. [CrossRef] [PubMed]
35. Lanzieri, T.M.; Dollard, S.C.; Josephson, C.D.; Schmid, D.S.; Bialek, S.R. Breast milk-acquired cytomegalovirus infection and disease in VLBW and premature infants. *Pediatrics* **2013**, *131*, e1937–e1945. [CrossRef] [PubMed]
36. Eidelman, A.I.; Schanler, R.J.; Johnston, M.; Landers, S.; Noble, L.; Szucs, K.; Viehmann, L. Se Breastfeeding and the use of human milk. *Pediatrics* **2012**, *129*, e827–e841. [CrossRef]
37. Cheong, J.L.Y.; Cowan, F.M.; Modi, N. Gastrointestinal manifestations of postnatal cytomegalovirus infection in infants admitted to a neonatal intensive care unit over a five year period. *Arch. Dis. Child. Fetal Neonatal Ed.* **2004**, *89*, F367–F369. [CrossRef] [PubMed]
38. Okulu, E.; Akin, I.M.; Atasay, B.; Ciftçi, E.; Arsan, S.; Türmen, T. Severe postnatal cytomegalovirus infection with multisystem involvement in an extremely low birth weight infant. *J. Perinatol.* **2012**, *32*, 72–74. [CrossRef] [PubMed]
39. Takahashi, R.; Tagawa, M.; Sanjo, M.; Chiba, H.; Ito, T.; Yamada, M.; Nakae, S.; Suzuki, A.; Nishimura, H.; Naganuma, M.; et al. Severe postnatal cytomegalovirus infection in a very premature infant. *Neonatology* **2007**, *92*, 236–239. [CrossRef] [PubMed]
40. Fischer, C.; Meylan, P.; Bickle Graz, M.; Gudinchet, F.; Vaudaux, B.; Berger, C.; Roth-Kleiner, M. Severe postnatally acquired cytomegalovirus infection presenting with colitis, pneumonitis and sepsis-like syndrome in an extremely low birthweight infant. *Neonatology* **2010**, *97*, 339–345. [CrossRef] [PubMed]
41. Hamele, M.; Flanagan, R.; Loomis, C.A.; Stevens, T.; Fairchok, M.P. Severe morbidity and mortality with breast milk associated cytomegalovirus infection. *Pediatr. Infect. Dis. J.* **2010**, *29*, 84–86. [CrossRef] [PubMed]
42. Lopes, A.-A.; Belhabri, S.; Karaoui, L. Erratum: Clinical Findings and Autopsy of a Preterm Infant with Breast Milk-Acquired Cytomegalovirus Infection. *AJP Rep.* **2016**, *6*, e367. [CrossRef] [PubMed]
43. Kelly, M.S.; Benjamin, D.K.; Puopolo, K.M.; Laughon, M.M.; Clark, R.H.; Mukhopadhyay, S.; Benjamin, D.K.; Smith, P.B.; Permar, S.R. Postnatal Cytomegalovirus Infection and the Risk for Bronchopulmonary Dysplasia. *JAMA Pediatr.* **2015**, *169*, e153785. [CrossRef] [PubMed]
44. Collège National des Gynécologues et Obstétriciens Français. Cytomégalovirus et grossesse. Available online: http://www.cngof.fr/actualites/403-cytomegalovirus-et-grossesse (accessed on 2 March 2016).
45. Boumahni, B.; Robillard, P.-Y. Infection post-natale à cytomégalovirus chez l'enfant prématuré: Rôle du lait de mère. *Arch. Pédiatr.* **2014**, *21*, 1060–1061. [CrossRef] [PubMed]
46. Croly-Labourdette, S.; Vallet, S.; Gagneur, A.; Gremmo-Feger, G.; Legrand-Quillien, M.-C.; Ansquer, H.; Jacquemot, L.; Narbonne, V.; Lintanf, J.; Collet, N.; et al. Transmission du cytomégalovirus par le lait maternel cru aux enfants prématurés: Étude épidémiologique pilote. *Arch. Pédiatr.* **2006**, *13*, 1015–1021. [CrossRef] [PubMed]

47. Picaud, J.C.; Buffin, R.; Gremmo-Feger, G.; Rigo, J.; Putet, G.; Casper, C.; Working group of the French Neonatal Society on fresh human milk use in preterm infants. Review concludes that specific recommendations are needed to harmonise the provision of fresh mother's milk to their preterm infants. *Acta Paediatr.* **2018**, *107*, 1145–1155. [CrossRef] [PubMed]
48. Barbi, M.; Binda, S.; Primache, V.; Caroppo, S.; Didò, P.; Guidotti, P.; Corbetta, C.; Melotti, D. Cytomegalovirus DNA detection in Guthrie cards: A powerful tool for diagnosing congenital infection. *J. Clin. Virol.* **2000**, *17*, 159–165. [CrossRef]
49. Binda, S.; Caroppo, S.; Didò, P.; Primache, V.; Veronesi, L.; Calvario, A.; Piana, A.; Barbi, M. Modification of CMV DNA detection from dried blood spots for diagnosing congenital CMV infection. *J. Clin. Virol.* **2004**, *30*, 276–279. [CrossRef] [PubMed]
50. Göhring, K.; Dietz, K.; Hartleif, S.; Jahn, G.; Hamprecht, K. Influence of different extraction methods and PCR techniques on the sensitivity of HCMV-DNA detection in dried blood spot (DBS) filter cards. *J. Clin. Virol.* **2010**, *48*, 278–281. [CrossRef] [PubMed]
51. Mussi-Pinhata, M.M.; Pinto, P.C.G.; Yamamoto, A.Y.; Berencsi, K.; de Souza, C.B.S.; Andrea, M.; Duarte, G.; Jorge, S.M. Placental transfer of naturally acquired, maternal cytomegalovirus antibodies in term and preterm neonates. *J. Med. Virol.* **2003**, *69*, 232–239. [CrossRef] [PubMed]
52. Mussi-Pinhata, M.M.; Yamamoto, A.Y.; do Carmo Rego, M.A.; Pinto, P.C.G.; da Motta, M.S.F.; Calixto, C. Perinatal or early-postnatal cytomegalovirus infection in preterm infants under 34 weeks gestation born to CMV-seropositive mothers within a high-seroprevalence population. *J. Pediatr.* **2004**, *145*, 685–688. [CrossRef] [PubMed]
53. Mehler, K.; Oberthuer, A.; Lang-Roth, R.; Kribs, A. High rate of symptomatic cytomegalovirus infection in extremely low gestational age preterm infants of 22–24 weeks' gestation after transmission via breast milk. *Neonatology* **2014**, *105*, 27–32. [CrossRef] [PubMed]
54. Remington, J.; Klein, J.; Wilson, C.; Nizet, V.; Maldonado, Y. *Infectious Diseases of the Fetus and Newborn*, 7th ed.; Elsevier Saunders: Philadelphia, PA, USA, 2011.
55. Vauloup-Fellous, C.; Picone, O.; Cordier, A.-G.; Parent-du-Châtelet, I.; Senat, M.-V.; Frydman, R.; Grangeot-Keros, L. Does hygiene counseling have an impact on the rate of CMV primary infection during pregnancy? Results of a 3-year prospective study in a French hospital. *J. Clin. Virol.* **2009**, *46*, S49–S53. [CrossRef] [PubMed]
56. Kimberlin, D.W.; Jester, P.M.; Sánchez, P.J.; Ahmed, A.; Arav-Boger, R.; Michaels, M.G.; Ashouri, N.; Englund, J.A.; Estrada, B.; Jacobs, R.F.; et al. National Institute of Allergy and Infectious Diseases Collaborative Antiviral Study Group Valganciclovir for symptomatic congenital cytomegalovirus disease. *N. Engl. J. Med.* **2015**, *372*, 933–943. [CrossRef] [PubMed]
57. Omarsdottir, S.; Agnarsdottir, M.; Casper, C.; Orrego, A.; Vanpée, M.; Rahbar, A.; Söderberg-Nauclér, C. High prevalence of cytomegalovirus infection in surgical intestinal specimens from infants with necrotizing enterocolitis and spontaneous intestinal perforation: A retrospective observational study. *J. Clin. Virol.* **2017**, *93*, 57–64. [CrossRef] [PubMed]
58. You, D.M.; Johnson, M.D. Cytomegalovirus infection and the gastrointestinal tract. *Curr. Gastroenterol. Rep.* **2012**, *14*, 334–342. [CrossRef] [PubMed]
59. Skeath, T.; Stewart, C.; Waugh, S.; Embleton, N.; Cummings, S.; Berrington, J. Cytomegalovirus and other common enteric viruses are not commonly associated with NEC. *Acta Paediatr.* **2016**, *105*, 50–52. [CrossRef] [PubMed]
60. Goelz, R.; Hamprecht, K.; Klingel, K.; Poets, C.F. Intestinal manifestations of postnatal and congenital cytomegalovirus infection in term and preterm infants. *J. Clin. Virol. Off. Publ. Pan Am. Soc. Clin. Virol.* **2016**, *83*, 29–36. [CrossRef] [PubMed]

8

Variation and Interdependencies of Human Milk Macronutrients, Fatty Acids, Adiponectin, Insulin and IGF-II in the European PreventCD Cohort

Maria Grunewald [1], Christian Hellmuth [1], Franca F. Kirchberg [1], Maria Luisa Mearin [2], Renata Auricchio [3], Gemma Castillejo [4], Ilma R. Korponay-Szabo [5], Isabel Polanco [6], Maria Roca [7], Sabine L. Vriezinga [2], Katharina Werkstetter [1], Berthold Koletzko [1,*] and Hans Demmelmair [1,*]

1 Ludwig-Maximilians-Universität, Division of Metabolic and Nutritional Medicine, Dr. von Hauner Children's Hospital, University of Munich Medical Center, 80337 Munich, Germany
2 Department of Paediatrics, Leiden University Medical Center, 2300 Leiden, The Netherlands
3 Department of Medical Translational Sciences and European Laboratory for the Investigation of Food-Induced Diseases, University Federico II, 80131 Naples, Italy
4 Department of Pediatric Gastroenterology Unit, Hospital Universitari Sant Joan de Reus, URV, IIPV, 43201 Reus, Spain
5 Celiac Disease Center, Heim Pál Children's Hospital, 1089 Budapest, Hungary
6 Department of Pediatric Gastroenterology and Nutrition, La Paz University Hospital, 28033 Madrid, Spain
7 U. Enfermedad Celiaca e Inmunopatología Digestiva, Instituto de Investigación Sanitaria La Fe, 46026 Valencia, Spain
* Correspondence: office.koletzko@med.uni-muenchen.de (B.K.); hans.demmelmair@med.uni-muenchen.de (H.D.)

Abstract: Human milk composition is variable. The identification of influencing factors and interdependencies of components may help to understand the physiology of lactation. In this study, we analyzed linear trends in human milk composition over time, the variation across different European countries and the influence of maternal celiac disease. Within a multicenter European study exploring potential prevention of celiac disease in a high-risk population (PreventCD), 569 human milk samples were donated by women from five European countries between 16 and 163 days postpartum. Some 202 mothers provided two samples at different time points. Protein, carbohydrates, fat and fatty acids, insulin, adiponectin, and insulin-like growth factor II (IGF-II) were analyzed. Milk protein and n-6 long chain polyunsaturated fatty acids decreased during the first three months of lactation. Fatty acid composition was significantly influenced by the country of residence. IGF-II and adiponectin concentrations correlated with protein content ($r = 0.24$ and $r = 0.35$), and IGF-II also correlated with fat content ($r = 0.36$), suggesting a possible regulatory role of IGF in milk macronutrient synthesis. Regarding the impact of celiac disease, only the level in palmitic acid was influenced by this disease, suggesting that breastfeeding by celiac disease mothers should not be discouraged.

Keywords: human milk; celiac disease; hormones; fatty acids; duration of lactation; country; carbohydrate; fat

---

1. Introduction

Breastfeeding supports physiological infant growth and development [1]. The importance of early life nutrition has been stimulated in studies investigating human milk composition and influencing factors [2–5]. A recent meta-analysis found that the average energy content in human milk of mothers with term born babies hardly changes from lactation week 2 to weeks 10–12 [6]. However, at both time points, the energy content shows large inter-individual variation. This primarily reflects a high variation of milk fat content, but also protein and to a lesser extent lactose are variable [7]. Colostrum and transitional milk are clearly different from mature milk. After the second week of lactation, changes associated with the duration of lactation, like the decrease in protein content, only partially explain the variation in milk composition and other influencing factors, for example, maternal diet, have to be considered [7].

The fatty acid (FA) composition of human milk fat is dependent on maternal diet. This has been demonstrated for essential FA and their long chain polyunsaturated derivatives (LC-PUFA) [8], as well as for medium chain FA (MCFA, C8.0 to C14.0) contents in milk, which are influenced by the ratio of dietary carbohydrates to fat [9]. Milk protein is composed of casein and whey, which is mainly comprised by α-lactalbumin and lactoferrin, but also includes a variety of lower concentrated proteins and peptides [10]. Insulin, insulin-like growth factors, and adipokines are metabolic regulators that might modulate infantile metabolism after milk feeding [11,12]. The hormones in milk may be derived from the maternal circulation, as suggested for insulin [13], or they could be synthesized in the mammary gland [11]; and their concentrations may be related to other human milk components. Co-variation of peptide hormone and macronutrient concentrations in human milk might complicate the identification of growth promoting or growth attenuating effects to individual compounds. This could also in part explain why studies observing the relationship between human milk composition and infant growth often yield ambiguous results [14–17].

Celiac disease (CD) is an intolerance of gluten, a protein present in various cereals. The disease is associated with atrophy of the intestinal villi, inflammation of the jejunal mucosa, and intestinal malabsorption [18]. A lifelong gluten free diet (GFD) is required to improve the histopathology and symptoms of CD, such as steatorrhea, diarrhea, and abdominal distension [18]. However, there is a risk that adherence to a GFD induces nutritional deficiencies, as GFDs have been found to be low in iron, calcium, B-vitamins, and some fatty acids [19]. There are ambiguous findings in relation to the effect of a GFD on fatty acid status biomarkers [20,21]. It is currently not known whether human milk fatty acid composition is affected by maternal CD. So far, it has only been shown that CD affects cytokines in milk [22]. Significant effects of CD or GFD on macronutrient contents or fatty acid composition could be of importance for the nutrition of breast fed infants of CD mothers and might require specific dietary recommendations.

In this study, we determined protein, fat, carbohydrate, individual FA, insulin, adiponectin, and insulin-like growth factor II (IGF-II) in milk samples collected in the large European PreventCD prospective cohort study. We aimed to compare milk composition between mothers with CD and healthy mothers, to investigate any effects by country of residence and duration of lactation on milk composition and to analyze the variation and interdependencies of the measured milk components.

2. Materials and Methods

Human milk samples were collected from 2007 to 2010 within the PreventCD study [23]. Details on the study population are reported in Vriezinga et al. [24]. Briefly, healthy newborns were enrolled if they had at least one first-degree family member with biopsy-confirmed celiac disease and were tested positive for the risk alleles *HLA-DQ2* and/or *HLA-DQ8*. Infants born preterm or with any congenital disorder were excluded. Infants were randomized to the introduction of either small amounts of gluten or to placebo at the age of 16 weeks.

The PreventCD study was approved by the medical ethics committee of each participating center and complied with Good Clinical Practice guidelines (ICH-GCP) regulations. The study was conducted according to the Declaration of Helsinki. The PreventCD Current Controlled Trials number is ICTRP CTRP NTR890.

Milk samples for this study were donated by mothers in five European countries between 16 days and 163 days postpartum. The included milk samples were collected in the Netherlands (Leiden, $n = 116$), Italy (Naples, $n = 68$), Spain (Madrid, Valencia, and Barcelona, $n = 138$), Hungary (Budapest, $n = 120$), and Germany (Munich, $n = 127$).

Mothers were asked to express milk manually or by pump once a month during the first six months after birth without further specification for fore- or hind-milk sampling and time of day. Milk samples were first frozen at −20 °C in home freezers, transferred to the hospital on ice, and then stored at −80 °C. Samples for the reported analyses were aliquoted (1–2 mL) and randomly selected, aiming for two samples from each mother, with one sample collected until 3 months postpartum (early samples), and one sample collected during months 4 or 5 (late samples).

2.1. Measurements

Analytical procedures were previously described in a publication observing the association between milk components and the infant metabolome [25]. Measurement of total fat and total carbohydrates was performed via mid-infrared spectroscopy with a Human Milk Analyzer (MIRIS AB, Uppsala, Sweden) [26]. Owing to limited available sample volumes, the samples were diluted 1:3 with water. Samples were sonicated and heated to 40 °C prior to analysis. Tests with a diluted reference milk sample revealed intra- and inter-assay coefficients of variation (CVs) (7 and 13 determinations) for fat (5.3% and 6.6%) and carbohydrates (4.8% and 4.5%), comparable to the inter-assay CVs of undiluted milk samples (fat: 5.6% and carbohydrates: 4.3%). The calibration curve of eight different diluted samples versus the same eight undiluted samples showed high correlations with R^2 of 0.99 for fat and 0.90 for carbohydrates, respectively.

As the protein measurement by infrared spectroscopy (MIRIS) led to unsatisfactory CVs, the protein content was measured with an adapted Bradford method [27]. The intra batch—and inter batch—assay CVs of 4 and 16 determinations were calculated with 4.3% and 9.7%, respectively, using samples with 1.3 g/dL protein. Spiking recovery was determined to be 99.1% ± 27.6% in eight low (+0.27 g/dL) and 105.8% ± 16.5% in eight high (+0.44 g/dL) spiked samples.

Analysis of the FA composition of milk lipids was performed as previously described using 20 µL of milk [28]. The lipid bound FAs were converted in situ with acidic catalysis into FA methyl esters, which were subsequently extracted into hexane and analyzed by gas chromatography. The method enabled quantification of FA with 8 to 24 carbon atoms, including the major LC-PUFA. The weight percentages of 35 FA were determined with a mean CV of 4.9%, as estimated from 31 analyses of control milk aliquots measured along with study samples.

For the analysis of hormones, milk aliquots were thawed overnight at 4 °C and skimmed by centrifugation at 4000× *g* and 4 °C for 30 min. Total adiponectin concentration was measured with a commercially available ELISA kit (Biovendor RD191023100 High Sensitivity Adiponectin, Brno, Czech Republic) in 50 µL skimmed milk with a 1:3 dilution following the protocol of the manufacturer. The intra-batch and inter-batch CVs of 4 and 8 determinations were 4.5% and 4.8%, respectively. Spiking recovery was found to be 105.1% ± 14.0% in eight low (+2 ng/mL) and 91.6% ± 4.0% in eight high (+10 ng/mL) spiked determinations.

Insulin was measured with the Mercodia Insulin ELISA kit 10-1113-01 (Mercodia, Uppsala, Sweden) from 25 µL of undiluted, skimmed human milk, according to the protocol of the manufacturer. The intra-batch and inter-batch CVs of 4 and 8 determinations were 3.4% and 11.0%, respectively. Spiking recovery was determined to be 92.3% ± 14.8% in seven low (+21 mU/L) and 85.9% ± 7.2% in seven high (+42 mU/L) spiked samples.

IGF-II was determined with a radioimmunoassay from 30 µL of full fat milk by Mediagnost (Reutlingen, Germany) using the R-30 IGF-II RIA kit, according to the protocol of the manufacturer. The kit had already successfully been applied for the analysis of IGF-II in human milk [29].

2.2. Data Analysis

In order to evaluate the effects of duration of lactation and country of residence, data were divided into subsets of early (day 16–100) and late (day 101–163) lactation. Statistical analyses were performed independently on both subsets, that is, separately on the early and late samples. We identified outliers by calculating the numeric distance to its nearest neighbor. If this distance (gap) was bigger than one standard deviation of the corresponding parameter, the observations more distant from the mean were excluded from further analyses.

Using univariate linear regression, we tested for effects of individual factors (mode of delivery, maternal age at delivery, duration of gestation, infants' gender, birth weight, maternal pre-pregnancy weight, maternal pre-pregnancy body mass index (BMI), maternal CD status, day of lactation, or country of residence) on measured milk analytes. As potentially significant predictors for the multiple regression analysis, we selected the variates that showed Bonferroni corrected p-values below 0.2 in both data sets [30].

Potentially significant factors were included in the multiple linear regression analysis to test for effects of these factors on the standardized analyte concentrations. Standardization, the transformation of the analytes to have a mean of 0 and standard deviation of 1, was done in order to obtain comparable model estimates. We used weighted effects coding for the categorical variable "country of residence" (each variable is coded such that the estimated effects for each category are to be interpreted as deviations from the weighted mean of the whole data set) to test whether milk components from individual countries differed significantly from the global mean. Subsequently, we utilized analysis of variance (ANOVA) to test for significant differences in the means of the measured analytes across countries.

For the determination of the relationships among selected analytes, correlation coefficients according to Pearson were calculated for the early and late dataset, respectively.

For the exploration of intra-individual stability of concentrations and percentages, we related data points in the early data set to the corresponding data points in the late data set for the 202 mothers who donated two samples. Intra-individual comparisons were done with paired t-tests and correlation coefficients were calculated according to Pearson.

All statistical analyses were performed with the software R (version 3.0.2., the R foundation for statistical computing). We adjusted the confidence intervals and p-values that we report here for multiple testing (41 milk compounds) using Bonferroni's method.

3. Results

A total of 569 samples from 367 mothers were available. After outlier removal, the early dataset (lactation days 16 to 100) contained results from 319 milk samples with a minimum of 307 values for each analyte. The late dataset (lactation days 101 to 163) with 250 milk samples provided a minimum of 233 values for individual analytes. Early samples were collected on lactation days 42 ± 21 (mean ± SD) and late samples were collected 120 ± 8 days postpartum. A total of 202 of the late samples had an earlier sampled counterpart in the first subset from the same mother. The characteristics of the mothers and their children are summarized in Table 1.

Table 1. Characteristics of participating mothers and their infants.

Variable	M	SD	N *
Age mother, years	33.4	±3.9	357
Gestational age, weeks	39.3	±1.4	366
Pre-pregnancy BMI mother, kg/m^2	22.4	±3.4	175
Birth weight, g	3373	±455	364
	n	**%**	**N ***
Mothers with celiac disease	184	50.1	367
Exclusive breastfeeding at 4 months	264	77.9	339
Infant gender female	182	49.6	367

* N corresponds to the number of participants with available information, BMI, body mass index.

Day of lactation, country of residence, and CD status were identified as potentially relevant variables for milk composition. Pre-pregnancy BMI showed a positive correlation with human milk insulin (Figure 1), but was not considered in other analyses as we have this information only from a small subset of mothers.

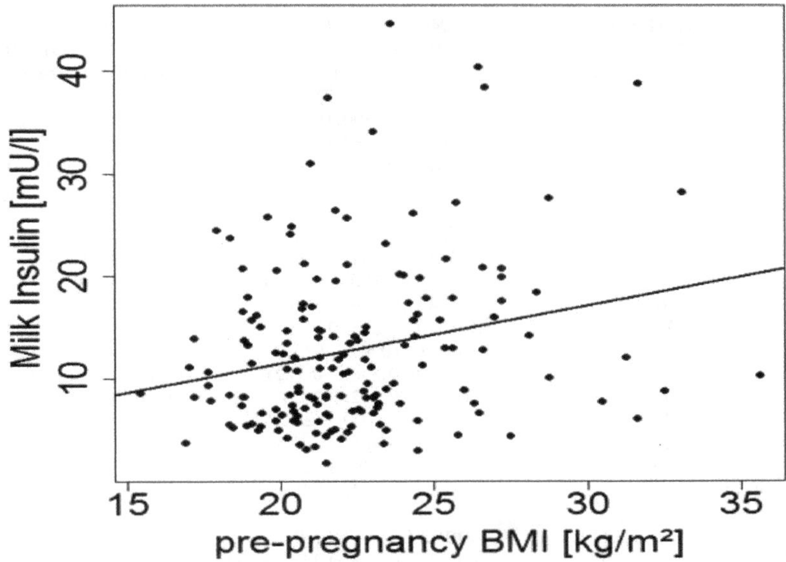

Figure 1. Milk insulin levels in early milk samples versus maternal pre-pregnancy body mass index (BMI) ($r = 0.24$, $p = 0.002$, $n = 175$).

3.1. *Influence of Maternal CD Status, Day of Lactation, and Country of Residence*

About half of the participating mothers were CD patients (Table 1). Five out of 184 mothers with CD did not follow a GFD. The early and late dataset showed that the milk of CD negative and positive women was not significantly different regarding the hormone and macronutrient concentrations. Among the FA percentages, only palmitic acid (C16:0) showed significantly decreased percentages in milk of mothers with CD compared with non-CD mothers. Taking all available data into account, palmitic acid contributed 22.3% ± 3.1% to total milk fatty acids in the healthy mothers and 22.0% ± 2.8% in mothers with CD.

Within the first three months of lactation, levels of protein, n-6 LC-PUFA percentages, n-3 eicosatrienoic acid (20:3n-3), capric acid (10:0), lauric acid (12:0), and the monounsaturated fatty acids (MUFA) C20:1n-9 and C24:1n-9 decreased significantly over time (Table 2). Day of lactation did not show significant effects on milk FA composition during months 4 and 5 postpartum (Table 3). During the first three months of lactation, most FA percentages differed significantly across the tested countries (Table 4, docosahexaenoic acid (DHA) in Figure 2A), and long-chain FA also differed by country in late samples (Table 5, DHA in Figure 2A). Comparisons of the individual FA between countries identified a huge number of differences, which were mostly similar in the early and the late data set (Tables 4 and 5). In the case of DHA, the mean value found in the early samples from Hungary was significantly lower than in the sample from all other countries, and in the late samples, values for Italy and Hungary were similarly low. This is also reflected in 57% and 73%, respectively, of Hungarian samples with DHA below 0.2%, while in the whole sample set, only 29% of the early and 51% of the late samples were below 0.2%. The highest DHA percentages were found in the samples from Spain and the Netherlands, where only 15% and 23%, respectively, of the early samples and 37% and 36%, respectively, of the late samples were below 0.2% DHA.

Table 2. Mean analyte concentrations (±SD) of early samples collected until day 100 of lactation.

	Mean ± SD	CD Mother	Day of Lactation	Country p
		β (CI: 0.06%; 99.94%)	β (CI: 0.06%; 99.94%)	
Hormones				
IGF-II, ng/mL	17.41 ± 6.09	−0.048 (−0.423; 0.326)	−0.005 (−0.014; 0.003)	**<0.001**
Insulin, mU/L	12.46 ± 8.19	−0.090 (−0.480; 0.300)	0.003 (−0.006; 0.012)	1
Adiponectin, ng/mL	19.28 ± 6.63	0.134 (−0.267; 0.534)	−0.005 (−0.014; 0.004)	1
macronutrients, g/dL				
Fat	2.2 ± 1.2	−0.202 (−0.600; 0.196)	−0.002 (−0.011; 0.007)	**0.031**
Carbohydrates	6.5 ± 0.4	−0.102 (−0.482; 0.278)	−0.002 (−0.010; 0.007)	0.701
Protein	1.16 ± 0.22	0.081 (−0.276; 0.439)	**−0.015 (−0.023; −0.007)**	**0.049**
Fatty Acids, wt %				
SFA				
C8:0	0.26 ± 0.10	0.129 (−0.258; 0.516)	−0.007 (−0.016; 0.001)	**0.002**
C10:0	1.36 ± 0.32	0.224 (−0.161; 0.609)	**−0.013 (−0.022; −0.004)**	0.122
C12:0	5.37 ± 1.69	0.244 (−0.150; 0.639)	**−0.01 (−0.019; −0.001)**	1
C13:0	0.04 ± 0.01	0.134 (−0.258; 0.526)	−0.002 (−0.011; 0.007)	**0.005**
C14:0	5.76 ± 1.62	0.131 (−0.268; 0.530)	−0.006 (−0.015; 0.003)	**0.031**
C15:0	0.32 ± 0.12	−0.068 (−0.404; 0.269)	0.001 (−0.007; 0.008)	**<0.001**
C16:0	22.16 ± 2.92	**−0.446 (−0.770; −0.122)**	0.002 (−0.005; 0.009)	**<0.001**
C17:0	0.31 ± 0.06	0.020 (−0.342; 0.382)	0.005 (−0.003; 0.013)	**<0.001**
C18:0	7.37 ± 1.33	−0.108 (−0.500; 0.284)	0.007 (−0.002; 0.015)	**<0.001**
C20:0	0.27 ± 0.10	−0.006 (−0.421; 0.409)	0.003 (−0.006; 0.013)	0.821
C22:0	0.10 ± 0.03	0.143 (−0.239; 0.525)	0.004 (−0.004; 0.013)	**<0.001**
C24:0	0.09 ± 0.04	0.181 (−0.184; 0.545)	−0.004 (−0.012; 0.004)	**<0.001**
MUFA				
C14:1	0.23 ± 0.11	−0.102 (−0.442; 0.237)	−0.004 (−0.011; 0.004)	**<0.001**
C15:1	0.07 ± 0.03	0.005 (−0.338; 0.348)	0.001 (−0.007; 0.008)	**<0.001**
C16:1 n-7	2.23 ± 0.69	−0.103 (−0.480; 0.274)	−0.006 (−0.015; 0.002)	**<0.001**
C18:1 n-9	35.33 ± 4.35	0.216 (−0.119; 0.550)	0.005 (−0.003; 0.012)	**<0.001**
C18:1 n-7	1.62 ± 0.25	0.185 (−0.223; 0.593)	−0.007 (−0.016; 0.002)	1
C20:1 n-9	0.46 ± 0.08	0.235 (−0.140; 0.610)	**−0.011 (−0.019; −0.003)**	0.272
C24:1 n-9	0.07 ± 0.02	0.306 (−0.042; 0.653)	**−0.015 (−0.022; −0.007)**	**<0.001**
PUFA				
n6				
C18:2 n-6	13.27 ± 4.16	−0.028 (−0.380; 0.323)	0.002 (−0.005; 0.010)	**<0.001**
C18:3 n-6	0.16 ± 0.05	−0.205 (−0.603; 0.193)	0.000 (−0.009; 0.009)	0.619
C20:2 n-6	0.30 ± 0.09	0.098 (−0.239; 0.435)	**−0.014 (−0.022; −0.007)**	**<0.001**
C20:3 n-6	0.44 ± 0.11	−0.010 (−0.374; 0.354)	**−0.019 (−0.027; −0.011)**	**<0.001**
C20:4 n-6	0.49 ± 0.11	0.066 (−0.294; 0.426)	**−0.013 (−0.021; −0.005)**	**<0.001**
C22:4 n-6	0.11 ± 0.03	0.137 (−0.191; 0.466)	**−0.014 (−0.021; −0.007)**	**<0.001**
C22:5 n-6	0.05 ± 0.02	0.167 (−0.171; 0.506)	**−0.013 (−0.021; −0.006)**	**<0.001**
n3				
C18:3 n-3	0.77 ± 0.39	−0.065 (−0.429; 0.298)	−0.001 (−0.009; 0.007)	**<0.001**
C20:3 n-3	0.05 ± 0.02	0.106 (−0.245; 0.458)	**−0.010 (−0.018; −0.002)**	**<0.001**
C20:5 n-3	0.07 ± 0.05	0.012 (−0.383; 0.408)	−0.005 (−0.014; 0.004)	**<0.001**
C22:5 n-3	0.15 ± 0.05	0.016 (−0.363; 0.396)	−0.007 (−0.016; 0.001)	**<0.001**
C22:6 n-3	0.29 ± 0.16	0.117 (−0.274; 0.508)	−0.009 (−0.017; 0.000)	**<0.001**
n9				
C20:3 n-9	0.02 ± 0.01	0.021 (−0.380; 0.423)	−0.003 (−0.012; 0.006)	**0.018**
Trans FA				
C16:1 trans	0.06 ± 0.02	−0.049 (−0.412; 0.314)	0.005 (−0.003; 0.013)	**<0.001**
C18:1 trans	0.31 ± 0.20	−0.296 (−0.672; 0.080)	0.004 (−0.005; 0.012)	**0.001**
C18:2 trans	0.10 ± 0.04	−0.010 (−0.359; 0.339)	0.002 (−0.005; 0.010)	**<0.001**

Influence of maternal celiac disease (CD) status and day of lactation are indicated by β estimates, and influence of country is indicated by the p-values from analysis of variance (ANOVA). Weighted effects coding was used to code the country. p-values and 95% confidence intervals were Bonferroni corrected (n = 41), resulting in an adjusted 99.88% confidence interval. Significant p-values and β estimates are printed in bold. SFA, saturated fatty acids, MUFA, monounsaturated fatty acids; PUFA, polyunsaturated fatty acid; IGF, insulin-like growth factor.

Table 3. Mean analyte concentrations (±SD) of late samples collected between days 101 to 163 of lactation.

	Global Mean ± SD	CD Mother	Day of Lactation	Country *p*
		β (CI: 0.06%; 99.94%)	β (CI: 0.06%; 99.94%)	
Hormones				
IGF-II, ng/mL	12.61 ± 3.25	0.055 (−0.393; 0.502)	−0.007 (−0.034; 0.021)	1
Insulin, mU/L	13.67 ± 9.15	−0.207 (−0.600; 0.186)	0.003 (−0.021; 0.027)	1
Adiponectin, ng/mL	17.56 ± 6.26	0.268 (−0.154; 0.689)	−0.008 (−0.034; 0.018)	1
macronutrients, g/dL				
Fat	2.4 ± 1.5	−0.035 (−0.482; 0.413)	0.000 (−0.027; 0.028)	1
Carbohydrates	6.6 ± 0.4	0.123 (−0.258; 0.504)	0.001 (−0.023; 0.024)	1
Protein	0.84 ± 0.18	0.094 (−0.339; 0.527)	−0.014 (−0.041; 0.012)	0.753
Fatty Acids, wt %				
SFA				
C8:0	0.21 ± 0.06	0.142 (−0.297; 0.580)	−0.004 (−0.031; 0.024)	1
C10:0	1.42 ± 0.33	0.317 (−0.119; 0.752)	−0.012 (−0.038; 0.015)	1
C12:0	5.76 ± 1.66	0.181 (−0.261; 0.623)	−0.007 (−0.034; 0.020)	1
C13:0	0.04 ± 0.01	0.031 (−0.386; 0.449)	0.004 (−0.022; 0.030)	**<0.001**
C14:0	6.24 ± 1.71	0.196 (−0.264; 0.656)	0.003 (−0.026; 0.031)	1
C15:0	0.33 ± 0.12	−0.097 (−0.469; 0.276)	0.010 (−0.013; 0.033)	**<0.001**
C16:0	22.33 ± 2.66	**−0.404 (−0.795; −0.012)**	−0.005 (−0.030; 0.019)	**<0.001**
C17:0	0.32 ± 0.06	−0.146 (−0.562; 0.270)	0.005 (−0.021; 0.031)	**<0.001**
C18:0	7.66 ± 1.34	−0.328 (−0.756; 0.100)	−0.002 (−0.029; 0.025)	**<0.001**
C20:0	0.24 ± 0.06	−0.197 (−0.637; 0.243)	−0.005 (−0.032; 0.022)	**0.012**
C22:0	0.09 ± 0.03	0.139 (−0.310; 0.588)	−0.002 (−0.030; 0.026)	**0.004**
C24:0	0.07 ± 0.03	0.212 (−0.240; 0.664)	−0.003 (−0.031; 0.025)	**0.024**
MUFA				
C14:1	0.23 ± 0.11	−0.114 (−0.487; 0.260)	0.005 (−0.018; 0.028)	**<0.001**
C15:1	0.08 ± 0.03	−0.010 (−0.391; 0.370)	0.009 (−0.015; 0.033)	**<0.001**
C16:1 n-7	2.14 ± 0.68	−0.033 (−0.465; 0.398)	0.003 (−0.024; 0.030)	**<0.001**
C18:1 n-9	34.87 ± 4.50	0.271 (−0.114; 0.656)	0.001 (−0.023; 0.025)	**<0.001**
C18:1 n-7	1.54 ± 0.25	0.089 (−0.365; 0.542)	−0.003 (−0.031; 0.025)	1
C20:1 n-9	0.42 ± 0.09	0.259 (−0.188; 0.706)	−0.008 (−0.036; 0.019)	1
C24:1	0.05 ± 0.02	0.304 (−0.147; 0.755)	−0.006 (−0.034; 0.022)	0.223
PUFA				
n6				
C18:2 n-6	12.93 ± 3.72	−0.106 (−0.497; 0.284)	0.005 (−0.019; 0.029)	**<0.001**
C18:3 n-6	0.15 ± 0.04	−0.243 (−0.685; 0.198)	−0.015 (−0.042; 0.012)	0.073
C20:2 n-6	0.25 ± 0.07	−0.068 (−0.456; 0.319)	−0.008 (−0.032; 0.016)	**<0.001**
C20:3 n-6	0.34 ± 0.07	−0.116 (−0.540; 0.308)	−0.025 (−0.052; 0.001)	**<0.001**
C20:4 n-6	0.43 ± 0.09	0.042 (−0.381; 0.466)	−0.016 (−0.043; 0.010)	**<0.001**
C22:4 n-6	0.09 ± 0.03	−0.015 (−0.397; 0.367)	−0.013 (−0.037; 0.011)	**<0.001**
C22:5 n-6	0.04 ± 0.02	0.064 (−0.316; 0.444)	−0.002 (−0.026; 0.022)	**<0.001**
n3				
C18:3 n-3	0.75 ± 0.39	−0.109 (−0.509; 0.291)	0.012 (−0.013; 0.037)	**<0.001**
C20:3 n-3	0.04 ± 0.01	−0.124 (−0.565; 0.317)	0.004 (−0.024; 0.031)	0.111
C20:5 n-3	0.06 ± 0.05	0.089 (−0.368; 0.546)	0.002 (−0.026; 0.031)	**0.027**
C22:5 n-3	0.14 ± 0.05	0.067 (−0.368; 0.502)	−0.001 (−0.028; 0.026)	**<0.001**
C22:6 n-3	0.24 ± 0.15	0.197 (−0.248; 0.641)	0.001 (−0.027; 0.029)	**<0.001**
n9				
C20:3 n-9	0.02 ± 0.01	−0.068 (−0.513; 0.378)	−0.012 (−0.039; 0.016)	**0.018**
Trans FA				
C16:1 trans	0.06 ± 0.02	−0.037 (−0.451; 0.378)	0.013 (−0.013; 0.038)	**<0.001**
C18:1 trans	0.30 ± 0.13	−0.229 (−0.672; 0.215)	−0.002 (−0.029; 0.026)	**0.004**
C18:2 trans	0.11 ± 0.04	−0.044 (−0.435; 0.348)	0.01 (−0.014; 0.035)	**<0.001**

Influence of maternal CD status and day of lactation are indicated by β estimates, and influence of country is indicated by the *p*-values from ANOVA. Weighted effects coding was used to code the country. *p*-values and 95% confidence intervals were Bonferroni corrected ($n = 41$), resulting in an adjusted 99.88% confidence interval. Significant *p*-values and β estimates are printed in bold.

Table 4. Human milk fatty acid composition found in the early samples according to the country of residence of the mothers.

	NL	It	ESP	HU	GER
SFA					
C8:0	0.29 ± 0.12 ab	0.22 ± 0.07 a	0.26 ± 0.09 c	0.25 ± 0.12	0.21 ± 0.06 bc
C10:0	1.38 ± 0.35	1.50 ± 0.34	1.37 ± 0.29	1.27 ± 0.33	1.31 ± 0.32
C12:0	5.46 ± 1.84	6.03 ± 1.73	5.23 ± 1.52	5.46 ± 1.96	5.05 ± 1.46
C13:0	0.04 ± 0.01	0.04 ± 0.01	0.04 ± 0.02 a	0.04 ± 0.01 b	0.04 ± 0.01 ab
C14:0	6.06 ± 1.92 a	6.44 ± 1.76 b	5.03 ± 1.42 abc	5.74 ± 1.73	6.33 ± 1.55 c
C15:0	0.31 ± 0.08 ab	0.35 ± 0.09 cd	0.25 ± 0.09 a cef	0.30 ± 0.11 eg	0.45 ± 0.12 bdfg
C16:0	21.54 ± 2.50 abc	24.09 ± 2.37 abd	19.79 ± 2.32 def	22.64 ± 2.50 eg	24.25 ± 2.38 cfg
C17:0	0.29 ± 0.05 a	0.33 ± 0.05	0.30 ± 0.10 b	0.30 ± 0.05 c	0.36 ± 0.06 abc
C18:0	7.38 ± 1.59 a	7.03 ± 1.03 b	6.97 ± 1.15 c	7.40 ± 1.15 d	8.13 ± 1.31 abcd
C20:0	0.30 ± 0.12 a	0.23 ± 0.04 a	0.29 ± 0.13	0.27 ± 0.12	0.27 ± 0.08
C22:0	0.12 ± 0.04 abc	0.08 ± 0.01	0.11 ± 0.08 a	0.09 ± 0.03 b	0.09 ± 0.03 c
C24:0	0.12 ± 0.05 abc	0.07 ± 0.02 a	0.09 ± 0.08	0.08 ± 0.03 b	0.07 ± 0.03 c
MUF A					
C14:1	0.25 ± 0.09 abc	0.24 ± 0.07 de	0.15 ± 0.07 adfg	0.20 ± 0.08 bfh	0.33 ± 0.12 cegh
C15:1	0.07 ± 0.02 a	0.09 ± 0.03 bc	0.06 ± 0.04 bd	0.07 ± 0.03 ce	0.10 ± 0.03 ade
C16:1n-7	2.44 ± 0.78 a	2.20 ± 0.42 b	1.77 ± 0.42 abcc	2.17 ± 0.55 ce	2.58 ± 0.82 ce
C18:1n-9	35.18 ± 3.54 ab	35.58 ± 3.83 cd	38.91 ± 4.33 acef	31.54 ± 3.07 bdeg	34.44 ± 3.35 fg
C18:1n-7	1.64 ± 0.27	1.56 ± 0.19	1.64 ± 0.21	1.59 ± 0.27	1.63 ± 0.28
C20:1n-9	0.47 ± 0.07	0.43 ± 0.06	0.47 ± 0.10	0.43 ± 0.07	0.48 ± 0.12
C24:1	0.08 ± 0.03 abc	0.06 ± 0.02 a	0.07 ± 0.04 d	0.06 ± 0.02 b	0.06 ± 0.02 cd
n-6 PUF A					
C18:2n-6	12.81 ± 3.21 abc	10.46 ± 2.71 ade	13.95 ± 3.94 dfg	16.50 ± 4.27 befh	10.51 ± 2.71 cgh
C18:3n-6	0.15 ± 0.06	0.16 ± 0.05	0.17 ± 0.09	0.17 ± 0.06	0.15 ± 0.04
C20:2n-6	0.29 ± 0.07 a	0.24 ± 0.07 bc	0.33 ± 0.10 bd	0.37 ± 0.08 a ce	0.25 ± 0.06 de
C20:3n-6	0.45 ± 0.09 a	0.44 ± 0.13	0.44 ± 0.12 b	0.47 ± 0.14 c	0.38 ± 0.10 abc
C20:4n-6	0.51 ± 0.12 a	0.45 ± 0.09 b	0.47 ± 0.10 c	0.56 ± 0.12 bcd	0.43 ± 0.09 ad
C22:4n-6	0.11 ± 0.03 a	0.10 ± 0.02 b	0.11 ± 0.08 c	0.14 ± 0.04 abcd	0.09 ± 0.02 d
C22:5n-6	0.05 ± 0.02 a	0.05 ± 0.02	0.05 ± 0.05 b	0.07 ± 0.02 abc	0.04 ± 0.01 c
n-3 PUF A					
C18:3n-3	1.11 ± 0.43 abcd	0.56 ± 0.28 ae	0.60 ± 0.28 bf	0.76 ± 0.34 c	0.80 ± 0.35 def
C20:3n-3	0.06 ± 0.02 a	0.03 ± 0.01 a	0.05 ± 0.06	0.05 ± 0.01	0.05 ± 0.02
C20:5n-3	0.09 ± 0.05 ab	0.05 ± 0.03 a	0.08 ± 0.09 c	0.05 ± 0.04 bcd	0.08 ± 0.05 d
C22:5n-3	0.18 ± 0.05 abc	0.11 ± 0.04 ad	0.14 ± 0.07 b	0.13 ± 0.04 ce	0.16 ± 0.06 de
C22:6n-3	0.31 ± 0.17 a	0.23 ± 0.10 b	0.35 ± 0.20 bc	0.21 ± 0.10 a cd	0.30 ± 0.19 d
n-9 PUF A					
C20:3n-9	0.03 ± 0.01 a	0.03 ± 0.01	0.02 ± 0.01 ab	0.02 ± 0.01	0.03 ± 0.01 b
Tr a ns F A					
C16:1t	0.06 ± 0.02 a	0.06 ± 0.02	0.06 ± 0.07 b	0.06 ± 0.02 c	0.08 ± 0.03 abc
C18:1t	0.25 ± 0.12 a	0.34 ± 0.36	0.29 ± 0.21 b	0.46 ± 0.43 abc	0.31 ± 0.15 c
C18:2tt	0.10 ± 0.03 a	0.10 ± 0.04 b	0.09 ± 0.10 c	0.09 ± 0.04 d	0.15 ± 0.05 abcd

a–h pairs with common superscripts indicate significant country differences ($p < 0.05$ after Bonferroni adjustment.

Country effects were less pronounced for hormones (e.g., adiponectin, Figure 2B) and carbohydrates. IGF-II, protein, and total fat concentrations varied by country during the first three months, but not in the later samples (data not shown in detail).

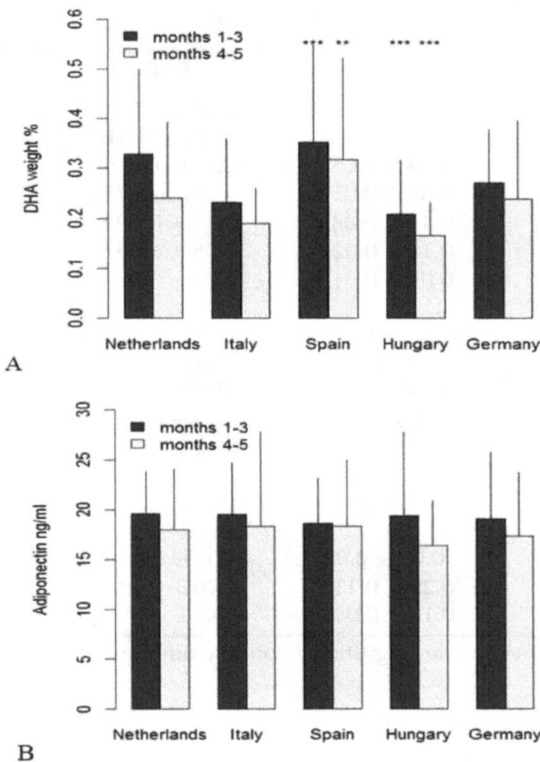

Figure 2. Mean values (+SD) of docosahexaenoic acid (DHA) weight% (**A**) and adiponectin concentration (**B**) per country in early and late milk samples; significant differences from the global means for DHA (months 1–3: 0.29%, months 4–5: 0.24%) and adiponectin (months 1–3: 19.3 ng/mL, months 4–5: 17.6 ng/mL) are indicated as ** for $p < 0.01$ and *** for $p < 0.001$.

Table 5. Human milk fatty acid composition found in the late samples according to the country of residence of the mothers.

	NL	It	ESP	HU	GER
SFA					
C8:0	0.21 ± 0.08	0.27 ± 0.17	0.21 ± 0.06	0.22 ± 0.07	0.21 ± 0.06
C10:0	1.34 ± 0.33	1.56 ± 0.34	1.40 ± 0.36	1.40 ± 0.33	1.44 ± 0.38
C12:0	5.46 ± 1.92	6.20 ± 1.77	5.79 ± 1.91	6.00 ± 1.70	5.44 ± 1.54
C13:0	0.04 ± 0.01 ^{ab}	0.05 ± 0.02 ^{ac}	0.03 ± 0.01 ^{cd}	0.04 ± 0.01 ^{e}	0.05 ± 0.01 ^{bde}
C14:0	6.17 ± 2.23	6.49 ± 1.50	5.77 ± 2.02	5.98 ± 1.78	6.74 ± 1.53
C15:0	0.31 ± 0.08 ^{ab}	0.35 ± 0.09 ^{cd}	0.25 ± 0.09 ^{ace}	0.29 ± 0.11 ^{f}	0.45 ± 0.12 ^{bdef}
C16:0	21.62 ± 2.39 ^{ab}	23.55 ± 2.51 ^{c}	19.79 ± 3.58 ^{acde}	22.33 ± 2.52 ^{df}	24.10 ± 2.19 ^{bef}
C17:0	0.31 ± 0.05 ^{a}	0.33 ± 0.06 ^{b}	0.28 ± 0.07 ^{bc}	0.31 ± 0.05 ^{d}	0.36 ± 0.06 ^{acd}
C18:0	7.63 ± 1.26	7.26 ± 0.97 ^{a}	6.87 ± 1.37 ^{bc}	7.72 ± 1.25 ^{b}	8.35 ± 1.46 ^{ac}
C20:0	0.29 ± 0.15 ^{ab}	0.33 ± 0.29 ^{cde}	0.22 ± 0.06 ^{ac}	0.22 ± 0.05 ^{bd}	0.24 ± 0.06 ^{e}
C22:0	0.11 ± 0.06 ^{abc}	0.09 ± 0.02	0.08 ± 0.03 ^{a}	0.08 ± 0.03 ^{b}	0.09 ± 0.03 ^{c}
C24:0	0.09 ± 0.06 ^{abc}	0.08 ± 0.03	0.07 ± 0.03 ^{a}	0.06 ± 0.02 ^{b}	0.06 ± 0.03 ^{c}
MUFA					
C14:1	0.24 ± 0.07 ^{ab}	0.22 ± 0.08	0.15 ± 0.07 ^{ac}	0.20 ± 0.09 ^{d}	0.33 ± 0.11 ^{bcd}
C15:1	0.07 ± 0.02 ^{a}	0.08 ± 0.03 ^{b}	0.05 ± 0.02 ^{bc}	0.07 ± 0.03 ^{d}	0.11 ± 0.03 ^{acd}
C16:1n-7	2.25 ± 0.72 ^{a}	1.87 ± 0.59 ^{b}	1.75 ± 0.51 ^{ac}	2.10 ± 0.53 ^{d}	2.49 ± 0.75 ^{bcd}
C18:1n-9	35.59 ± 3.57 ^{ab}	34.92 ± 4.21 ^{c}	39.58 ± 9.48 ^{acde}	31.31 ± 3.41 ^{bdf}	34.07 ± 3.19 ^{ef}
C18:1n-7	1.58 ± 0.26	1.45 ± 0.22	1.61 ± 0.45	1.59 ± 0.28	1.50 ± 0.25
C20:1n-9	0.48 ± 0.23	0.38 ± 0.07	0.41 ± 0.10	0.40 ± 0.09	0.44 ± 0.12
C24:1	0.06 ± 0.03	0.06 ± 0.02	0.05 ± 0.02	0.05 ± 0.01	0.05 ± 0.02
n-6 PUFA					

Table 5. *Cont.*

	NL	It	ESP	HU	GER
C18:2n-6	12.72 ± 2.66 [ab]	11.75 ± 3.54 [c]	12.82 ± 3.51 [de]	16.42 ± 4.38 [acdf]	10.35 ± 2.64 [bef]
C18:3n-6	0.15 ± 0.04	0.16 ± 0.04	0.15 ± 0.04	0.17 ± 0.05	0.14 ± 0.03
C20:2n-6	0.24 ± 0.05 [ab]	0.24 ± 0.05 [c]	0.26 ± 0.07 [de]	0.31 ± 0.07 [acdf]	0.20 ± 0.05 [bef]
C20:3n-6	0.33 ± 0.07	0.36 ± 0.05 [a]	0.34 ± 0.09	0.37 ± 0.10 [b]	0.30 ± 0.05 [ab]
C20:4n-6	0.42 ± 0.07 [a]	0.44 ± 0.08 [b]	0.40 ± 0.10 [c]	0.50 ± 0.11 [abcd]	0.40 ± 0.08 [d]
C22:4n-6	0.09 ± 0.03 [a]	0.10 ± 0.02 [b]	0.08 ± 0.03 [c]	0.12 ± 0.03 [abcd]	0.08 ± 0.02 [d]
C22:5n-6	0.04 ± 0.02 [a]	0.04 ± 0.01 [b]	0.04 ± 0.02 [c]	0.06 ± 0.02 [abcd]	0.04 ± 0.01 [d]
n-3 PUFA					
C18:3n-3	1.09 ± 0.43 [abc]	0.50 ± 0.28 [ad]	0.55 ± 0.23 [be]	0.72 ± 0.28 [c]	0.90 ± 0.48 [de]
C20:3n-3	0.05 ± 0.02	0.04 ± 0.02	0.04 ± 0.02	0.04 ± 0.01	0.04 ± 0.02
C20:5n-3	0.09 ± 0.11 [a]	0.05 ± 0.02	0.07 ± 0.05	0.04 ± 0.04 [ab]	0.08 ± 0.05 [b]
C22:5n-3	0.18 ± 0.09 [abc]	0.11 ± 0.03 [ad]	0.13 ± 0.06 [b]	0.12 ± 0.03 [ce]	0.16 ± 0.05 [de]
C22:6n-3	0.29 ± 0.35	0.19 ± 0.07	0.32 ± 0.20 [a]	0.18 ± 0.12 [a]	0.24 ± 0.14
n-9 PUFA					
C20:3n-9	0.02 ± 0.01 [a]	0.02 ± 0.01	0.02 ± 0.01 [ab]	0.02 ± 0.01	0.03 ± 0.01 [b]
Trans FA					
C16:1t	0.06 ± 0.02 [a]	0.07 ± 0.02	0.05 ± 0.02 [b]	0.06 ± 0.02 [c]	0.08 ± 0.02 [abc]
C18:1t	0.27 ± 0.12 [a]	0.28 ± 0.11 [b]	0.26 ± 0.13 [c]	0.42 ± 0.29 [abcd]	0.32 ± 0.12 [d]
C18:2tt	0.12 ± 0.04 [abc]	0.10 ± 0.04 [d]	0.08 ± 0.04 [ae]	0.09 ± 0.03 [bf]	0.14 ± 0.04 [cdef]

[a–h] pairs with common superscripts indicate significant country differences ($p < 0.05$ after Bonferroni adjustment).

3.2. *Correlations among Human Milk Components*

We focused on correlations that were consistently significant in both the early and late datasets (Table 6). Protein in milk was positively correlated with adiponectin and IGF-II levels. Milk fat content was not significantly related to adiponectin or insulin, but correlated positively with IGF-II and protein.

Table 6. Pearson correlations between the concentrations of macronutrients, hormones, and FA groups (weight%) stratified according to sample collection period.

	IGF-II	Insulin	Adip	Fat	CH	Protein	MUFA	PUFA
Collection during the First Three Months of Lactation (n = 319)								
Insulin	0.02							
Adip	0.15	−0.05						
Fat	**0.36 *****	0.09	0.06					
CH	−0.14	−0.06	−0.12	−0.16				
Protein	**0.24 *****	−0.03	**0.35 *****	**0.23 ****	−0.01			
MUFA	−0.12	**−0.20 ***	−0.1	−0.12	0.12	0.04		
PUFA	0.15	−0.04	0.02	−0.13	0.05	−0.05	**−0.33 *****	
SFA	−0.03	**0.21 ***	0.06	**0.21 ****	−0.15	0	**−0.56 *****	**−0.59 *****
Collection during Months 4 and 5 of Lactation (n = 250)								
	IGF-II	Insulin	Adip	Fat	CH	Protein	MUFA	PUFA
Insulin	**0.21 ***							
Adip	**0.30 *****	0.02						
Fat	**0.51 *****	0.17	0.12					
CH	−0.11	0	−0.05	−0.13				
Protein	**0.38 *****	0.07	**0.30 *****	**0.23 ***	0.03			
MUFA	−0.1	−0.2	−0.05	−0.09	−0.04	0.02		
PUFA	0.05	−0.07	−0.05	0.12	−0.04	−0.1	**−0.34 ****	
SFA	0.06	0.25	0.09	0	0.07	0.06	**−0.68 *****	**−0.46 *****

Note: * $p < 0.05$, ** $p < 0.01$, *** $p < 0.001$ after Bonferroni correction. Significant results are given in bold. Adip = Adiponectin, CH = carbohydrates.

3.3. *Intrainividual Relationships between Early and Late Milk Samples*

The relationships of the milk components in early and late samples from mothers who donated two samples are summarized in Table 7. The mean difference between the days of collection was 76 days (range 11 to 109 days). Most analytes showed significant correlations ($p < 0.05$, Table 7) with the exception of carbohydrates, protein, as well as caprylic (8:0), arachidic (20:0), and nervonic acid (24:1n9). Adiponectin and IGF-II concentrations showed closer relationships between both time points than insulin. LC-PUFA and odd-chain FA showed the strongest correlations between the two sampling points (e.g., arachidonic acid (AA) and DHA in Figure 3). Significantly lower values in the 4–5 months period than in the early period for protein and most FA agree with the decreases indicated by multiple linear regression analyses during the first three months (Table 7, *t*-test). The exception is capric acid, which decreased during the early period, but was found to be higher in the later period (Table 7). Additionally, DHA showed a significant decrease from the early sample compared with the later sample.

Table 7. Comparison of the concentrations measured in the early (from lactation day 16–100) and late samples (from lactation day 101–163) from the mothers who donated two samples ($n = 202$).

	Early (M ± SD)	**Late (M ± SD)**	***t*-Test *p***	**Correlation *r* (*p*)**
	Hormones and macronutrients			
IGF-II, ng/mL	17.16 ± 5.42	12.62 ± 3.30	**<0.001**	0.303 **(0.001)**
Insulin, mU/L	12.28 ± 8.06	13.72 ± 8.74	0.531	0.480 **(<0.001)**
Adiponectin, ng/mL	19.19 ± 6.06	17.61 ± 6.45	**0.013**	0.466 **(<0.001)**
Fat, g/dL	2.22 ± 1.20	2.54 ± 1.53	0.205	0.346 (<0.001)
Carbohydrates, g/dL	6.54 ± 0.43	6.63 ± 0.38	0.259	0.175 (0.543)
Protein, g/dL	1.15 ± 0.22	0.85 ± 0.18	**<0.001**	0.209 (0.128)
Fatty Acids, wt %				
C8:0	0.25 ± 0.10	0.21 ± 0.06	**<0.001**	0.208 (0.123)
C10:0	1.35 ± 0.32	1.42 ± 0.34	0.305	0.508 **(<0.001)**
C12:0	5.37 ± 1.67	5.74 ± 1.66	**0.032**	0.471 **(<0.001)**
C13:0	0.04 ± 0.01	0.04 ± 0.01	1	0.460 **(<0.001)**
C14:0	5.87 ± 1.66	6.23 ± 1.78	**0.013**	0.596 **(<0.001)**
C15:0	0.34 ± 0.12	0.33 ± 0.12	1	0.676 **(<0.001)**
C16:0	22.34 ± 2.85	22.24 ± 2.72	1	0.591 **(<0.001)**
C17:0	0.32 ± 0.06	0.32 ± 0.06	1	0.504 **(<0.001)**
C18:0	7.35 ± 1.33	7.63 ± 1.35	0.97	0.410 **(<0.001)**
C20:0	0.27 ± 0.09	0.23 ± 0.06	**<0.001**	0.167 (0.995)
C22:0	0.10 ± 0.03	0.09 ± 0.03	**0.002**	0.356 **(<0.001)**
C24:0	0.09 ± 0.03	0.07 ± 0.03	**<0.001**	0.355 **(<0.001)**
C14:1	0.24 ± 0.10	0.23 ± 0.11	1	0.651 **(<0.001)**
C15:1	0.08 ± 0.03	0.08 ± 0.03	1	0.651 **(<0.001)**
C16:1 n-7	2.25 ± 0.69	2.15 ± 0.70	1	0.594 **(<0.001)**
C18:1 n-9	35.25 ± 4.53	35.23 ± 4.54	1	0.605 **(<0.001)**
C18:1 n-7	1.62 ± 0.26	1.54 ± 0.25	**0.004**	0.488 **(<0.001)**
C20:1 n-9	0.46 ± 0.07	0.42 ± 0.09	**<0.001**	0.353 **(<0.001)**
C24:1	0.06 ± 0.02	0.05 ± 0.01	**<0.001**	0.217 (0.129)
C18:2 n-6	13.02 ± 4.19	12.76 ± 3.69	1	0.628 **(<0.001)**
C18:3 n-6	0.16 ± 0.05	0.15 ± 0.04	0.393	0.660 **(<0.001)**
C20:2 n-6	0.30 ± 0.09	0.24 ± 0.06	**<0.001**	0.569 **(<0.001)**
C20:3 n-6	0.44 ± 0.11	0.33 ± 0.07	**<0.001**	0.448 **(<0.001)**
C20:4 n-6	0.49 ± 0.11	0.43 ± 0.08	**<0.001**	0.575 **(<0.001)**
C22:4 n-6	0.11 ± 0.03	0.09 ± 0.03	**<0.001**	0.557 **(<0.001)**
C22:5 n-6	0.05 ± 0.02	0.04 ± 0.02	**<0.001**	0.525 **(<0.001)**
C18:3 n-3	0.77 ± 0.38	0.75 ± 0.40	1	0.514 **(<0.001)**
C20:3 n-3	0.05 ± 0.02	0.04 ± 0.01	**<0.001**	0.388 **(<0.001)**
C20:5 n-3	0.07 ± 0.05	0.06 ± 0.04	1	0.553 **(<0.001)**
C22:5 n-3	0.15 ± 0.05	0.13 ± 0.05	0.48	0.591 **(<0.001)**
C22:6 n-3	0.28 ± 0.16	0.23 ± 0.15	**<0.001**	0.632 **(<0.001)**
C20:3 n-9	0.02 ± 0.01	0.02 ± 0.01	1	0.534 **(<0.001)**
C16:1 trans	0.07 ± 0.03	0.06 ± 0.02	1	0.417 **(<0.001)**
C18:1 trans	0.31 ± 0.20	0.30 ± 0.13	1	0.386 **(<0.001)**
C18:2 trans	0.11 ± 0.04	0.11 ± 0.04	1	0.610 **(<0.001)**

Note: Means between the two samples were compared by paired *t*-test. Correlations between the concentrations of early and late samples were calculated according to Pearson. Significant *p*-values (<0.05 after Bonferroni correction) are given in bold.

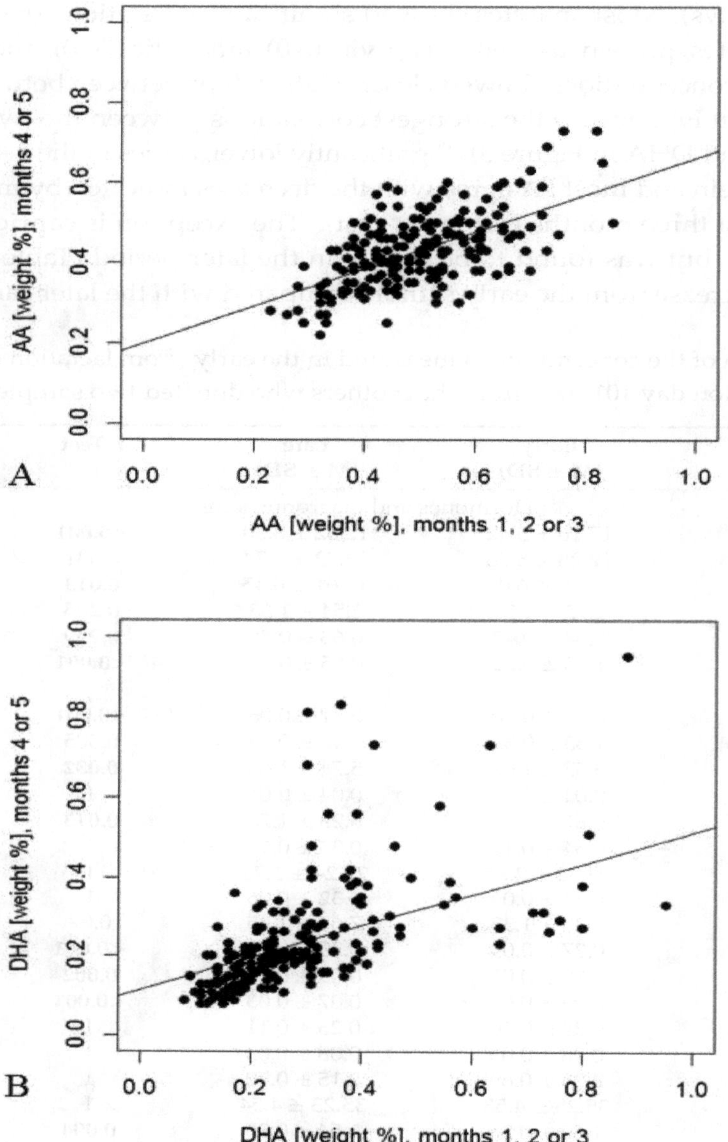

Figure 3. Weight percentages of arachidonic acid (AA) ((**A**), $r = 0.58$, $p < 0.001$) and docosahexaenoic acid (DHA) (**B**), $r = 0.63$, $p < 0.001$) measured in both early and late milk samples. Percentages were calculated for 202 mothers, who had provided samples during the first three months or during the fourth or fifth month of lactation, respectively.

4. Discussion

We observed a significant decrease of both milk protein and n-6 LC-PUFA during the first three months of lactation. Variations in the milk FA composition among the different countries were detected. Among the studied compounds, maternal CD only significantly influenced palmitic acid percentage, leading to lower values in the milk of mothers with CD.

In agreement with previous observations [31], milk carbohydrate contents remained stable over time. Human milk protein levels were higher in earlier lactation and continued to decrease beyond month 3 of lactation, similar to previous observations [7,32,33]. IGF-II and adiponectin showed a trend to decrease with time, which concurs with the assumption that IGFs and protein share common determinants or are directly associated [34]. Percentages of most saturated fatty acids SFA and MUFA (except C20:1n-9 and C24:1n-9) did not change with the duration of lactation. In contrast, LC-PUFA levels decreased. Maternal LC-PUFA stores are depleted due to the high requirements during pregnancy [35] and are further consumed during lactation, which leads to delayed recovery of DHA status after birth in breastfeeding women as compared with non-lactating women [36,37]. Diet and endogenous LC-PUFA synthesis from essential FA did not seem to compensate for the high demands. In our study population, milk fat content did not significantly increase with the day of lactation. Therefore, our results do not support the conclusion of Marangoni et al. [38], that lower LC-PUFA percentages with advancing lactation are compensated by an increase of total fat. The discrepant findings could be linked to the heterogeneity in the collection of our milk samples, while Marangoni et al. applied a defined sample collection procedure only allowing hind milk [38].

Correlations between early and late samples were low for macronutrients and only significant for milk fat, which may partially be the result of variation in conditions of sample collection. The considerable inter-individual differences of the time span between sample collections may have masked a significant intra individual correlation of protein levels. High PUFA and LC-PUFA correlation coefficients indicate a constancy of dietary habits, which define the individual PUFA and LC-PUFA levels, although levels generally decrease with time. For linoleic acid in human milk, it has been shown that about 30% is directly derived from diet and 70% is contributed by fat storage pools [39]. This also seems to apply to DHA [40] and could explain the high correlation coefficient observed for DHA. Nevertheless, single fish meals can markedly increase DHA in subsequent human milk feeds [3], although day-to-day variation is buffered by the contribution of FA from adipose tissue to milk fat [41,42]. Such single fish meals might have caused some of the observed high DHA-% and this could explain that the correlation between early and late DHA-% was not significant, as only those concentration pairs with at least one value above 0.45% were considered. A corresponding phenomenon was not seen for AA, which is assumed to be mainly contributed by endogenous synthesis from linoleic acid [43].

Our study showed that maternal CD and adherence to a GFD did not have any appreciable effect on milk macronutrients, hormones, and FA, with the exception of a lower palmitic acid percentage in the milk of CD mothers. Endogenous palmitic acid synthesis is stimulated by carbohydrate intake [44]. It is tempting to speculate that avoidance of gluten-containing grain-based foods could lead to a lower contribution of carbohydrates to energy intake, and hence lower palmitic acid synthesis. Comparisons of the diet of CD patients and healthy controls report lower carbohydrate or higher fat intake, respectively, with a GFD than in control groups in some studies, but not in all [45–47]. Previous studies have also reported lower n-6 LC-PUFA and higher or lower n-3 LC-PUFA in adult CD patients than in controls [20,21,48]. In this study population from five different countries, we could not find such differences in human milk. Patients with active CD showed higher plasma adiponectin values than healthy controls [49], but this seems not to apply for milk of mothers in remission with CD following a GFD. Olivares et al. had reported lower concentrations of protective immune mediators in milk of women with CD compared with milk from women without CD [22], but we did not identify further nutritionally important effects of CD on human milk. Therefore, breastfeeding can and should be encouraged also in women with CD and a GFD.

Total fat content was only different in the early samples between countries, whereas differences in FA composition were consistently found in both data sets. Potential differences in the lactation day at sample collection were considered in this analysis and do not explain country differences. Total lipid content in human milk is higher in hind-milk than in fore-milk [50]. As fore- or hind-milk collection was not specified in our study, differences of fat content could well be related to differences in sample collection and not reflect different dietary habits. The mode of sample collection does not affect FA composition (weight%), which remains stable during one feeding [51]. The significant variations across countries confirm previous studies that revealed that average human milk FA composition depends on the country and corresponding dietary habits [7,52,53]. While DHA levels were low in milk from Hungarian mothers, Spanish mothers showed the highest DHA levels, which corresponds with previous reports [54,55]. A contribution of at least 0.2% by DHA to total fatty acids in human milk and infant formulas has been considered important for the infant development [56,57], and even

0.3% has been recommended [58]. About 30% of the early samples and 51% of the late samples did not reach the 0.2% level, indicating that sea fish consumption or n-3 LC-PUFA supplement intake should be further encouraged in all included countries, but specifically in Hungary, increased efforts seem required.

Brenna et al. included 65 studies in their meta-analysis of human milk DHA and AA contents and found, on average, 0.32% ± 0.22% for DHA and 0.47% ± 0.13% for ARA [43]. In our study, DHA values were found to be somewhat lower (early samples 0.29% ± 0.16%, late samples 0.24% ± 015%), but AA values were very close to the reported worldwide average (0.49% ± 0.11%, 0.43% ± 0.09%, respectively). In the whole study population, and stratified according to country, the observed variation was smaller for AA than for DHA, which agrees with the findings in the meta-analysis [43] and the concept that DHA levels in milk depend mainly on dietary intake, while AA is mostly endogenously produced from linoleic acid and levels are related to the desaturase genotype [40]. Although linoleic acid status is usually not found to limit the endogenous AA synthesis [59], the finding that Hungarian samples were highest in linoleic acid and AA could suggest that a very high availability of linoleic acid supports high AA. Comparing α-linolenic and DHA percentages between the countries did not indicate associations between levels, confirming the importance of dietary DHA for appropriate milk levels.

The odd chain tridecanoic and pentadecanoic acids differed between countries and could indicate differences in dairy fat intake, as previously shown for plasma FA [60] or differences in fiber intake [61]. Protein and carbohydrate content did not show consistent differences between countries in the early and late data set. Observational studies in affluent populations and in developing countries have failed to identify dietary factors that influence milk protein or carbohydrates [62–65].

There was a significant positive correlation between human milk fat and protein. This correlation has been previously described for milk from mothers of very low birth weight infants [66] and in African mothers [67]. A joint regulation of milk protein and milk fat synthesis has been suggested based on in vitro studies [34,68]. The positive correlation of IGF-II with both protein and fat could be of interest, although regulatory effects of IGF-II in the mammary gland were proposed to be much smaller than IGF-I effects [69]. Adiponectin is significantly related to protein, but not to fat content, but models of the actions of adiponectin in the mammary gland have not been developed so far. We found no correlations between insulin and macronutrients in milk. Human milk insulin levels are related to plasma insulin levels and show comparable diurnal variations [13]. Maternal insulin levels were not available, but pre-pregnancy BMI is positively associated with human milk insulin in the present study, comparable to the results of other studies [70–72].

Strengths and Limitations

The combined analysis of macronutrients, FA, and selected hormones in our study enabled the parallel examination of day of lactation, country of residence, and CD status, which have not been studied before in large numbers of human milk samples. Some of the results have to be interpreted with caution as spot milk samples without full standardization of sampling have been studied, while 24 h collections of human milk and volume determinations would be more representative, enabling a meaningful consideration of potential effects of mixed feeding. Furthermore, interpretation is limited by partially missing information on maternal anthropometry and the ethnicity of the mothers.

5. Conclusions

Milk FA patterns depend on country of residence, which suggests significant dietary influences. In contrast, protein, fat, IGF-II, and adiponectin seem to depend on the individual metabolism. The observed relationships between protein, fat, and IGF-II could agree with an IGF involvement in the regulation of milk synthesis. As no major effects of CD on the studied human milk components were found, breastfeeding should be encouraged in women with CD and a GFD as in the general population.

Author Contributions: Conceptualization, M.L.M. and B.K.; Formal analysis, M.G. and F.F.K.; Funding acquisition, M.L.M. and B.K.; Investigation, M.G., R.A., G.C., I.R.K.-S., I.P., M.R., S.L.V., K.W., and H.D.; Methodology, H.D.; Supervision, M.L.M. and B.K.; Writing—original draft, M.G.; Writing—review & editing, C.H., F.F.K., M.L.M., R.A., G.C., I.R.K.-S., I.P., M.R., S.L.V., K.W., B.K., and H.D.

Acknowledgments: We thank Stefan Stromer (Ludwig-Maximilians-Universität München), who analysed the milk fatty acids; Yvonne Wijkhuisen, project manager of PreventCD, for support; Els Stoopman, who helped with the data management; and all the children and families who participated in this project.

References

1. Prell, C.; Koletzko, B. Breastfeeding and Complementary Feeding. *Dtsch. Arztebl. Int.* **2016**, *113*, 435–444. [CrossRef] [PubMed]
2. Van Beusekom, C.; Martini, I.A.; Rutgers, H.M.; Boersma, E.R.; Muskiet, F.A. A carbohydrate-rich diet not only leads to incorporation of medium-chain fatty acids (6:0-14:0) in milk triglycerides but also in each milk-phospholipid subclass. *Am. J. Clin. Nutr.* **1990**, *52*, 326–334. [CrossRef] [PubMed]
3. Lauritzen, L.; Jorgensen, M.H.; Hansen, H.S.; Michaelsen, K.F. Fluctuations in human milk long-chain PUFA levels in relation to dietary fish intake. *Lipids* **2002**, *37*, 237–244. [CrossRef] [PubMed]
4. Grote, V.; Verduci, E.; Scaglioni, S.; Vecchi, F.; Contarini, G.; Giovannini, M.; Koletzko, B.; Agostoni, C. Breast milk composition and infant nutrient intakes during the first 12 months of life. *Eur. J. Clin. Nutr.* **2015**, *70*, 250–256. [CrossRef] [PubMed]
5. Armand, M.; Bernard, J.Y.; Forhan, A.; Heude, B.; Charles, M.A.; EDEN Mother-Child Cohort Study Group. Maternal nutritional determinants of colostrum fatty acids in the EDEN mother-child cohort. *Clin. Nutr.* **2018**, *37*, 2127–2136. [CrossRef] [PubMed]
6. Gidrewicz, D.A.; Fenton, T.R. A systematic review and meta-analysis of the nutrient content of preterm and term breast milk. *BMC Pediatrics* **2014**, *14*, 216. [CrossRef] [PubMed]
7. Jensen, R.G. *Handbook of Milk Composition*; Academic Press: NewYork, NY, USA, 1995.
8. Bravi, F.; Wiens, F.; Decarli, A.; Dal Pont, A.; Agostoni, C.; Ferraroni, M. Impact of maternal nutrition oh breast-milk composition: A systematic review. *Am. J. Clin. Nutr.* **2016**, *104*, 646–662. [CrossRef]
9. Nasser, R.; Stephen, A.M.; Goh, Y.K.; Clandinin, M.T. The effect of a controlled manipulation of maternal dietary fat intake on medium and long chain fatty acids in human breast milk in Saskatoon, Canada. *Int. Breastfeed. J.* **2010**, *5*, 3. [CrossRef]
10. Ballard, O.; Morrow, A.L. Human Milk Composition. *Pediatric Clin. N. Am.* **2013**, *60*, 49–74. [CrossRef]
11. Grosvenor, C.E.; Picciano, M.F.; Baumrucker, C.R. Hormones and growth factors in milk. *Endocr. Rev.* **1993**, *14*, 710–728. [CrossRef]
12. Newburg, D.S.; Woo, J.G.; Morrow, A.L. Characteristics and Potential Functions of Human Milk Adiponectin. *J. Pediatr.* **2010**, *11*, S41–S46. [CrossRef] [PubMed]
13. Cevreska, S.; Kovacev, V.P.; Stankovski, M.; Kalamaras, E. The presence of immunologically reactive insulin in milk of women, during the first week of lactation and its relation to changes in plasma insulin concentration. *God. Zb. Med. Fak. Skopje* **1975**, *21*, 35–41. [PubMed]
14. Woo, J.G.; Guerrero, M.L.; Altaye, M.; Ruiz-Palacios, G.M.; Martin, L.J.; Dubert-Ferrandon, A.; Newburg, D.S.; Morrow, A.L. Human milk adiponectin is associated with infant growth in two independent cohorts. *Breastfeed. Med.* **2009**, *4*, 101–109. [CrossRef] [PubMed]
15. Prentice, P.; Ong, K.K.; Schoemaker, M.H.; van Tol, E.A.; Vervoort, J.; Hughes, I.A.; Acerini, C.L.; Dunger, D.B. Breast milk nutrient content and infancy growth. *Acta Paediatr.* **2016**, *105*, 641–647. [CrossRef] [PubMed]
16. Heinig, M.J.; Nommsen, L.A.; Peerson, J.M.; Lonnerdal, B.; Dewey, K.G. Energy and protein intakes of breast-fed and formula-fed infants during the first year of life and their associationwith growth velocity: The DARLING Study. *Am. J. Clin. Nutr.* **1993**, *58*, 152–161. [CrossRef] [PubMed]
17. Eriksen, K.G.; Christensen, S.H.; Lind, M.V.; Michaelsen, K.F. Human milk composition and infant growth. *Curr. Opin. Clin. Nutr. Metab. Care* **2018**, *21*, 200–206. [CrossRef] [PubMed]
18. Green, P.H.R.; Cellier, C. Medical progress: Celiac disease. *N. Engl. J. Med.* **2007**, *357*, 1731–1743. [CrossRef]
19. Thompson, T.; Dennis, M.; Higgins, L.A.; Lee, A.R.; Sharrett, M.K. Gluten-free diet survey: Are Americans with coeliac disease consuming recommended amounts of fibre, iron, calcium and grain foods? *J. Hum. Nutr. Diet.* **2005**, *18*, 163–169. [CrossRef]

20. Van Hees, N.J.M.; Giltay, E.J.; Geleijnse, J.M.; Janssen, N.; van der Does, W. DHA Serum Levels Were Significantly Higher in Celiac Disease Patients Compared to Healthy Controls and Were Unrelated to Depression. *PLoS ONE* **2014**, *9*, e97778. [CrossRef]
21. Russo, F.; Chimienti, G.; Clemente, C.; Ferreri, C.; Orlando, A.; Riezzo, G. A possible role for ghrelin, leptin, brain-derived neurotrophic factor and docosahexaenoic acid in reducing the quality of life of coeliac disease patients following a gluten-free diet. *Eur. J. Nutr.* **2017**, *56*, 807–818. [CrossRef]
22. Olivares, M.; Albrecht, S.; De Palma, G.; Ferrer, M.D.; Castillejo, G.; Schols, H.A.; Sanz, Y. Human milk composition differs in healthy mothers and mothers with celiac disease. *Eur. J. Nutr.* **2015**, *54*, 119–128. [CrossRef] [PubMed]
23. Hogen Esch, C.E.; Rosen, A.; Auricchio, R.; Romanos, J.; Chmielewska, A.; Putter, H.; Ivarsson, A.; Szajewska, H.; Koning, F.; Wijmenga, C.; et al. The PreventCD Study design: towards new strategies for the prevention of coeliac disease. *Eur. J. Gastroenterol. Hepatol.* **2010**, *22*, 1424–1430. [CrossRef] [PubMed]
24. Vriezinga, S.L.; Auricchio, R.; Bravi, E.; Castillejo, G.; Chmielewska, A.; Crespo Escobar, P.; Kolacek, S.; Koletzko, S.; Korponay-Szabo, I.R.; Mummert, E.; et al. Randomized feeding intervention in infants at high risk for celiac disease. *N. Engl. J. Med.* **2014**, *371*, 1304–1315. [CrossRef] [PubMed]
25. Hellmuth, C.; Uhl, O.; Demmelmair, H.; Grunewald, M.; Auricchio, R.; Castillejo, G.; Korponay-Szabo, I.R.; Polanco, I.; Roca, M.; Vriezinga, S.L.; et al. The impact of human breast milk components on the infant metabolism. *PLoS ONE* **2018**, *13*, e0197713. [CrossRef] [PubMed]
26. Casadio, Y.S.; Williams, T.M.; Lai, C.T.; Olsson, S.E.; Hepworth, A.R.; Hartmann, P.E. Evaluation of a mid-infrared analyzer for the determination of the macronutrient composition of human milk. *J. Hum. Lact.* **2010**, *26*, 376–383. [CrossRef] [PubMed]
27. Polberger, S.; Lönnerdal, B. Simple and Rapid Macronutrient Analysis of Human Milk for Individualized Fortification: Basis for Improved Nutritional Management of Very-Low-Birth-Weight Infants? *J. Pediatr. Gastr. Nutr.* **1993**, *17*, 283–290. [CrossRef] [PubMed]
28. Stimming, M.; Mesch, C.M.; Kersting, M.; Kalhoff, H.; Demmelmair, H.; Koletzko, B.; Schmidt, A.; Bohm, V.; Libuda, L. Vitamin E content and estimated need in German infant and follow-on formulas with and without long-chain polyunsaturated fatty acids (LC-PUFA) enrichment. *J. Agric. Food Chem.* **2014**, *62*, 10153–10161. [CrossRef]
29. Goelz, R.; Hihn, E.; Hamprecht, K.; Dietz, K.; Jahn, G.; Poets, C.; ElmLinger, M. Effects of Different CMV-Heat-Inactivation-Methods on Growth Factors in Human Breast Milk. *Pediatr. Res.* **2009**, *65*, 458–461. [CrossRef]
30. Vittinghoff, E.; Glidden, D.; Shiboski, S.; McCulloch, C. *Regression Methods in Biostatistics: Linear, Logistic, Survival, and Repeated Measures Models*; Springer: New York, NY, USA, 2005.
31. Mitoulas, L.R.; Kent, J.C.; Cox, D.B.; Owens, R.A.; Sherriff, J.L.; Hartmann, P.E. Variation in fat, lactose and protein in human milk over 24h and throughout the first year of lactation. *Br. J. Nutr.* **2002**, *88*, 29–37. [CrossRef]
32. Shehadeh, N.; Aslih, N.; Shihab, S.; Werman, M.J.; Sheinman, R.; Shamir, R. Human milk beyond one year post-partum: Lower content of protein, calcium, and saturated very long-chain fatty acids. *J. Pediatrics* **2006**, *148*, 122–124. [CrossRef]
33. Lonnerdal, B.; Erdmann, P.; Thakkar, S.K.; Sauser, J.; Destaillats, F. Longitudinal evolution of true protein, amino acids and bioactive proteins in breast milk: A developmental perspective. *J. Nutr. Biochem.* **2017**, *41*, 1–11. [CrossRef] [PubMed]
34. Anderson, S.M.; Rudolph, M.C.; McManaman, J.L.; Neville, M.C. Secretory activation in the mammary gland: It's not just about milk protein synthesis. *Breast Cancer Res.* **2007**, *9*, 204–217. [CrossRef] [PubMed]
35. Herrera, E.; Amusquivar, E.; López-Soldado, I.; Ortega, H. Maternal lipid metabolism and placental lipid transfer. *Horm. Res. Paediatr.* **2006**, *65*, 59–64. [CrossRef] [PubMed]
36. Hornstra, G. Essential fatty acids in mothers and their neonates. *Am. J. Clin. Nutr.* **2000**, *71*, 1262s–1269s. [CrossRef] [PubMed]
37. Jorgensen, M.H.; Nielsen, P.K.; Michaelsen, K.F.; Lund, P.; Lauritzen, L. The composition of polyunsaturated fatty acids in erythrocytes of lactating mothers and their infants. *Matern. Child Nutr.* **2006**, *2*, 29–39. [CrossRef]
38. Marangoni, F.; Agostoni, C.; Lammardo, A.M.; Giovannini, M.; Galli, C.; Riva, E. Polyunsaturated fatty acid

concentrations in human hindmilk are stable throughout 12-months of lactation and provide a sustained intake to the infant during exclusive breastfeeding: An Italian study. *Br. J. Nutr.* **2000**, *84*, 103–109. [PubMed]

39. Demmelmair, H.; Baumheuer, M.; Koletzko, B.; Dokoupil, K.; Kratl, G. Metabolism of U13C-labeled linoleic acid in lactating women. *J. Lipid Res.* **1998**, *39*, 1389–1396.
40. Demmelmair, H.; Koletzko, B. Lipids in human milk. *Best Pract. Res. Clin. Endocrinol. Metab.* **2018**, *32*, 57–68. [CrossRef]
41. Innis, S.M. Fatty acids and early human development. *Early Hum. Dev.* **2007**, *83*, 761–766. [CrossRef]
42. Demmelmair, H.; Sauerwald, T.; Fidler, N.; Baumheuer, M.; Koletzko, B. Polyunsaturated fatty acid metabolism during lactation. *World Rev. Nutr. Diet.* **2001**, *88*, 184–189.
43. Brenna, J.T.; Varamini, B.; Jensen, R.G.; Diersen-Schade, D.A.; Boettcher, J.A.; Arterburn, L.M. Docosahexaenoic and arachidonic acid concentrations in human breast milk worldwide. *Am. J. Clin. Nutr.* **2007**, *85*, 1457–1464. [CrossRef]
44. Hudgins, L.C.; Hellerstein, M.; Seidman, C.; Neese, R.; Diakun, J.; Hirsch, J. Human fatty acid synthesis is stimulated by a eucaloric low fat, high carbohydrate diet. *J. Clin. Investig.* **1996**, *97*, 2081–2091. [CrossRef] [PubMed]
45. Kinsey, L.; Burden, S.T.; Bannerman, E. A dietary survey to determine if patients with coeliac disease are meeting current healthy eating guidelines and how their diet compares to that of the British general population. *Eur. J. Clin. Nutr.* **2008**, *62*, 1333–1342. [CrossRef] [PubMed]
46. Melini, V.; Melini, F. Gluten-Free Diet: Gaps and Needs for a Healthier Diet. *Nutrients* **2019**, *11*, 170. [CrossRef]
47. Capristo, E.; Addolorato, G.; Mingrone, G.; De Gaetano, A.; Greco, A.V.; Tataranni, P.A.; Gasbarrini, G. Changes in body composition, substrate oxidation, and resting metabolic rate in adult celiac disease patients after a 1-y gluten-free diet treatment. *Am. J. Clin. Nutr.* **2000**, *72*, 76–81. [CrossRef] [PubMed]
48. Solakivi, T.; Kaukinen, K.; Kunnas, T.; Lehtimaki, T.; Maki, M.; Nikkari, S.T. Serum fatty acid profile in celiac disease patients before and after a gluten-free diet. *Scand. J. Gastroenterol.* **2009**, *44*, 826–830. [CrossRef] [PubMed]
49. Russo, F.; Chimienti, G.; Clemente, C.; D'Attoma, B.; Linsalata, M.; Orlando, A.; De Carne, M.; Cariola, F.; Semeraro, F.P.; Pepe, G.; et al. Adipokine profile in celiac patients: Differences in comparison with patients suffering from diarrhea-predominant IBS and healthy subjects. *Scand. J. Gastroenterol.* **2013**, *48*, 1377–1385. [CrossRef] [PubMed]
50. Mizuno, K.; Nishida, Y.; Taki, M.; Murase, M.; Mukai, Y.; Itabashi, K.; Debari, K.; Iiyama, A. Is increased fat content of hindmilk due to the size or the number of milk fat globules? *Int. Breastfeed. J.* **2009**, *4*, 7. [CrossRef] [PubMed]
51. Emery, W.B., 3rd; Canolty, N.L.; Aitchison, J.M.; Dunkley, W.L. Influence of sampling on fatty acid composition of human milk. *Am. J. Clin. Nutr.* **1978**, *31*, 1127–1130. [CrossRef]
52. Yuhas, R.; Pramuk, K.; Lien, E.L. Human milk fatty acid composition from nine countries varies most in DHA. *Lipids* **2006**, *41*, 851–858. [CrossRef]
53. Keikha, M.; Bahreynian, M.; Saleki, M.; Kelishadi, R. Macro- and Micronutrients of Human Milk Composition: Are They Related to Maternal Diet? A Comprehensive Systematic Review. *Breastfeed. Med.* **2017**, *12*, 517–527. [CrossRef] [PubMed]
54. Barreiro, R.; Diaz-Bao, M.; Cepeda, A.; Regal, P.; Fente, C.A. Fatty acid composition of breast milk in Galicia (NW Spain): A cross-country comparison. *Prostaglandins Leukot. Essent. Fatty Acids* **2018**, *135*, 102–114. [CrossRef] [PubMed]
55. Decsi, T.; Olah, S.; Molnar, S.; Burus, I. Low contribution of docosahexaenoic acid to the fatty acid composition of mature human milk in Hungary. *Adv. Exp. Med. Biol.* **2000**, *478*, 413–414. [CrossRef] [PubMed]
56. Koletzko, B.; Lien, E.; Agostoni, C.; Bohles, H.; Campoy, C.; Cetin, I.; Decsi, T.; Dudenhausen, J.W.; Dupont, C.; Forsyth, S.; et al. The roles of long-chain polyunsaturated fatty acids in pregnancy, lactation and infancy: Review of current knowledge and consensus recommendations. *J. Perinat. Med.* **2008**, *36*, 5–14. [CrossRef] [PubMed]
57. FAO. *Fats and Fatty Acids in Human Nutrition—Report of an Expert Consultation*; FAO: Rome, Italy, 2010.

58. Koletzko, B.; Boey, C.C.; Campoy, C.; Carlson, S.E.; Chang, N.; Guillermo-Tuazon, M.A.; Joshi, S.; Prell, C.; Quak, S.H.; Sjarif, D.R.; et al. Current information and Asian perspectives on long-chain polyunsaturated fatty acids in pregnancy, lactation, and infancy: Systematic review and practice recommendations from an early nutrition academy workshop. *Ann. Nutr. Metab.* **2014**, *65*, 49–80. [CrossRef] [PubMed]
59. Demmelmair, H.; MacDonald, A.; Kotzaeridou, U.; Burgard, P.; Gonzalez-Lamuno, D.; Verduci, E.; Ersoy, M.; Gokcay, G.; Alyanak, B.; Reischl, E.; et al. Determinants of Plasma Docosahexaenoic Acid Levels and Their Relationship to Neurological and Cognitive Functions in PKU Patients: A Double Blind Randomized Supplementation Study. *Nutrients* **2018**, *10*, 1944. [CrossRef] [PubMed]
60. Brevik, A.; Veierod, M.B.; Drevon, C.A.; Andersen, L.F. Evaluation of the odd fatty acids 15:0 and 17:0 in serum and adipose tissue as markers of intake of milk and dairy fat. *Eur. J. Clin. Nutr.* **2005**, *59*, 1417–1422. [CrossRef] [PubMed]
61. Weitkunat, K.; Schumann, S.; Nickel, D.; Hornemann, S.; Petzke, K.J.; Schulze, M.B.; Pfeiffer, A.F.H.; Klaus, S. Odd-chain fatty acids as a biomarker for dietary fiber intake: A novel pathway for endogenous production from propionate. *Am. J. Clin. Nutr.* **2017**, *105*, 1544–1551. [CrossRef] [PubMed]
62. Nommsen, L.A.; Lovelady, C.A.; Heinig, M.J.; Lonnerdal, B.; Dewey, K.G. Determinants of energy, protein, lipid, and lactose concentrations in human milk during the first 12 mo of lactation: The DARLING Study. *Am. J. Clin. Nutr.* **1991**, *53*, 457–465. [CrossRef]
63. Yang, T.; Zhang, Y.; Ning, Y.; You, L.; Ma, D.; Zheng, Y.; Yang, X.; Li, W.; Wang, J.; Wang, P. Breast milk macronutrient composition and the associated factors in urban Chinese mothers. *Chin. Med. J.* **2014**, *127*, 1721–1725.
64. Quinn, E.A.; Largado, F.; Power, M.; Kuzawa, C.W. Predictors of breast milk macronutrient composition in Filipino mothers. *Am. J. Hum. Biol.* **2012**, *24*, 533–540. [CrossRef] [PubMed]
65. Bzikowska-Jura, A.; Czerwonogrodzka-Senczyna, A.; Oledzka, G.; Szostak-Wegierek, D.; Weker, H.; Wesolowska, A. Maternal Nutrition and Body Composition During Breastfeeding: Association with Human Milk Composition. *Nutrients* **2018**, *10*, 1379. [CrossRef] [PubMed]
66. Weber, A.; Loui, A.; Jochum, F.; Buhrer, C.; Obladen, M. Breast milk from mothers of very low birthweight infants: Variability in fat and protein content. *Acta Paediatr.* **2001**, *90*, 772–775. [CrossRef] [PubMed]
67. Roels, O.A. Correlation between the fat and the protein content of human milk. *Nature* **1958**, *182*, 673. [CrossRef] [PubMed]
68. Qi, L.; Yan, S.; Sheng, R.; Zhao, Y.; Guo, X. Effects of Saturated Long-chain Fatty Acid on mRNA Expression of Genes Associated with Milk Fat and Protein Biosynthesis in Bovine Mammary Epithelial Cells. *Asian Australas. J. Anim. Sci.* **2014**, *27*, 414–421. [CrossRef] [PubMed]
69. Prosser, C.G. Insulin-like growth factors in milk and mammary gland. *J. Mammary Gland Biol. Neoplasia* **1996**, *1*, 297–306. [CrossRef] [PubMed]
70. Ahuja, S.; Boylan, M.; Hart, S.L.; Román-Shriver, C.; Spallholz, J.E.; Pence, B.C.; Sawyer, B.G. Glucose and Insulin Levels are Increased in Obese and Overweight Mothers' Breast-Milk. *Food Nutr. Sci.* **2011**, *2*, 201–206. [CrossRef]
71. Ley, S.H.; Hanley, A.J.; Sermer, M.; Zinman, B.; O'Connor, D.L. Associations of prenatal metabolic abnormalities with insulin and adiponectin concentrations in human milk. *Am. J. Clin. Nutr.* **2012**, *95*, 867–874. [CrossRef] [PubMed]
72. Demmelmair, H.; Koletzko, B. Variation of Metabolite and Hormone Contents in Human Milk. *Clin. Perinatol.* **2017**, *44*, 151–164. [CrossRef]

9

Human Milk Omega-3 Fatty Acid Composition is Associated with Infant Temperament

Jennifer Hahn-Holbrook [1,*], Adi Fish [1] and Laura M. Glynn [2]

[1] Department of Psychology, University of California, Merced, 5200 North Lake Rd, Merced, CA 95343, Canada; afish@ucmerced.edu
[2] Department of Psychology, Chapman University, Orange, CA 92866, USA; lglynn@chapman.edu
* Correspondence: jhahn-holbrook@ucmerced.edu

Abstract: There is growing evidence that omega-3 (n-3) polyunsaturated fatty-acids (PUFAs) are important for the brain development in childhood and are necessary for an optimal health in adults. However, there have been no studies examining how the n-3 PUFA composition of human milk influences infant behavior or temperament. To fill this knowledge gap, 52 breastfeeding mothers provided milk samples at 3 months postpartum and completed the Infant Behavior Questionnaire (IBQ-R), a widely used parent-report measure of infant temperament. Milk was assessed for n-3 PUFAs and omega-6 (n-6) PUFAs using gas-liquid chromatography. The total fat and the ratio of n-6/n-3 fatty acids in milk were also examined. Linear regression models revealed that infants whose mothers' milk was richer in n-3 PUFAs had lower scores on the negative affectivity domain of the IBQ-R, a component of temperament associated with a risk for internalizing disorders later in life. These associations remained statistically significant after considering covariates, including maternal age, marital status, and infant birth weight. The n-6 PUFAs, n-6/n-3 ratio, and total fat of milk were not associated with infant temperament. These results suggest that mothers may have the ability to shape the behavior of their offspring by adjusting the n-3 PUFA composition of their milk.

Keywords: breastfeeding; breast milk; temperament; fatty acids; LC-PUFA; omega-3; omega-6; DHA; AA; children; early life nutrition

---

1. Introduction

Early life nutrition plays a foundational role in brain development [1–3]. In recent decades, research has shown that exposure to human milk and the variation in its composition contribute meaningfully to children's behavior, cognition, and disease risk [4–6]. The American Academy of Pediatrics recommends that human milk be the sole source of infant nutrition for the first 6 months of life [7], a sensitive period characterized by rapid brain development [2,3]. One key nutritional factor that is present in human milk and that is necessary for an optimal brain development during this period are omega-3 (n-3) polyunsaturated fatty-acids (PUFAs) [8,9].

Human milk contains relatively high levels of n-3 PUFAs, which are essential to visual, motor, and cognitive development [8,9]. Among the 11 n-3 PUFAs, the three most important and prevalent in human milk are alpha-linolenic acid (ALA), eicosapentaenoic acid (EPA), and docosahexaenoic acid (DHA) [5,10]. ALA is the most common n-3 PUFA in human milk [10] (and the adult diet) and can be converted into EPA and DHA [11]. DHA is the most abundant n-3 PUFA in the central nervous system in mammals and forms the structural matrix of grey matter and retinal membranes [9,12]. EPA is used to produce eicosanoids, signaling molecules that play numerous roles, including reducing inflammation in the body and the brain [13,14]. The U.S. Department of Health and Human Services 2015–2020 Dietary Guidelines for Americans recommend that all adults, particularly pregnant and breastfeeding women, consume 8 ounces of seafood per week, providing approximately 250 mg of

EPA and DHA per day [15]. Breast-fed infants have significantly higher levels of n-3 PUFAs in their plasma lipids at three months than do infants given formula lacking n-3 fortification [16]. An autopsy study showed that the rate of accumulation of DHA is approximately 5.0 mg a day in the brains of breast-fed infants versus 2.3 mg a day in infants fed non-DHA fortified formula [17].

Numerous studies have shown that deficiencies in n-3 PUFAs are related to mood and anxiety disorders [18,19]. In adults, n-3 supplementation has benefits for the prevention and treatment of major depression [20], bipolar disorder [21], and anxiety disorders [22]. Much less is known about how early variations in the exposure to n-3 PUFAs impact the mood and behavior of children. However, animal models suggest that early n-3 exposure can have a lasting impact on offspring temperament and behavioral phenotypes. For example, feeding pregnant rats diets deficient in n-3 PUFAs increases anxiety-like behavior in rat pups, and upregulates anxiogenic-related glucocorticoid receptors in the frontal cortex, hypothalamus, and hippocampus [23]. These pre-clinical studies are consistent with correlational studies in human children. For example, in a diverse study of 255 women, eating a diet higher in n-3 relative to n-6 fatty acids during pregnancy buffered Black infants against the detrimental effects of maternal stress on infant regulatory capacities [24]. Plasma DHA levels have also been found to negatively correlate with depressive symptoms in children and adolescents with bipolar disorder [25].

No studies, however, could be found examining whether the n-3 PUFA composition of milk influences the infant mood or anxiety in humans, although several studies have linked cortisol levels in milk to infant temperament [26–28]. For example, one study showed that higher levels of cortisol in milk predicted an enhanced performance on the autonomic stability cluster on the Neonatal Behavioral Assessment Scale in neonates [27]. Studies have also found that cortisol levels in mothers' milk are positively correlated with a negative affectivity and fear reactivity in humans [26,28]. Most of what we know about lactational programing comes from animal models, and findings are generally consistent with the notion that milk is an important early moderator of the infant phenotype [29–31]. For example, in a study of Rhesus Macaques, heavier mothers with more reproductive experience were able to supply more calories to their infant through milk [32]. Moreover, infants whose mothers supplied more calories through milk in the early postnatal period showed higher activity levels and a greater confidence in a stressful setting later in infancy [32]. In sum, research has neglected the question of whether the fatty acid composition of milk influences infant temperament in humans.

To fill this gap, the current study tests whether the n-3 PUFA composition of mothers' milk is associated with the temperament of their infants. To address this question, milk samples were collected from 52 mothers of 3-month old infants and assessed for n-3 PUFA levels using gas-liquid chromatography. Mothers also completed the Rothbart Revised Infant Behavior Questionnaire (IBQ-R) [33], a widely-used parental-report instrument that assesses three broad dimensions of infant temperament (negative affectivity, orienting/regulation, and surgency/extraversion). Given that n-3 PUFAs and higher n-3/n-6 ratios have been found to be protective against mood disorders and anxiety symptoms [20], we predicted that n-3 PUFAs and the n-3/n-6 ratio in milk would be inversely correlated with the negative affectivity dimension of the IBQ-R. n-3 PUFAs have also been linked to enhanced executive functioning in children [9]. Therefore, we predicted that milk n-3 PUFAs levels would be positively correlated with scores on the orienting/regulation temperament dimension. We had no predictions regarding the surgency/extraversion temperament dimension. Exploratory analyses are also presented; they test whether the levels of n-6 PUFAs, total PUFAs or total milk fat concentrations are associated with infant temperament.

2. Methods

2.1. Participants

Fifty-two breastfeeding mothers and their three-month-old infants were enrolled in a large longitudinal study of early development from a medical center in Southern California. To be eligible to participate in the study, participants had to be over the age of 18, English-speaking, with a singleton intrauterine pregnancy. Women were ineligible for this study if they used alcohol, tobacco, illicit drugs, had cervical or uterine abnormalities, used medications that impacted the endocrine function, had a diagnosis of a disease influencing the neuroendocrine function, or had an infant admittance to the Neonatal Intensive Care Unit at birth because of compromised health (e.g., intrauterine growth restriction and respiratory distress syndrome).

After mothers gave informed consent to participate in the study, they were asked to come into the laboratory at 3 months postpartum (M = 3.01 months, SD = 0.25) to provide milk samples and fill out a survey regarding their infants' temperament. This study was approved by the Institutional Review Board at the University of California, Irvine (ethics approval code HS# 2002–2441, first approved: January 31, 2003; renewed most recently: 25 February 2019).

2.2. Determination of Milk Fatty Acid Levels

Mothers were asked to empty the contents of one breast with an electric breast pump into a sterile plastic container (Medela, Inc., McHenry, IL, USA). In an effort to ensure that the mother's milk donation for the study would not adversely impact infant nutrition, providing milk samples was made an optional part of this larger longitudinal study, and mothers were only asked to empty the contents of one breast, leaving milk in the other breast for the infant. Before the collection, the mothers were asked to clean the breast and nipple area with an antibacterial wipe and wait until the area dried (to leave open the possibility to examine the microbial composition of the milk for later research). The milk samples were then immediately aliquoted into polypropylene tubes and stored at 70 °C until they were assessed for fatty acids. The time of day of the milk collection was recorded and modestly correlated with the n-3 fatty acid composition of the milk (Pearson's $r = -0.344$, $p = 0.015$). The time of day of the sample collection was not related to any of the other fatty acids' composite variables (Pearson's r ranged from −0.175 to −0.008; $ps > 0.153$).

The fatty acid composition of the breast milk was analyzed by gas-liquid chromatography in prepared fatty acid methyl esters. The total lipids were extracted from the milk by a method described previously [34], using tridecanoin as the internal standard [35]. The thawed milk samples were shaken vigorously and saponified in 6% ethanolic KOH for 1 h at 37 °C. The mixture was extracted twice with hexane (20 min on rotator), and spun to separate the phases. The hexane layers were then combined and evaporated under a gentle stream of nitrogen to reduce lipid peroxidation. The fatty acid methyl esters were prepared by heating the reconstituted samples in 12% boron trifluoride-methanol for 10 min at 100 °C in tightly sealed tubes. The derivatized samples were separated with a Hewlett-Packard gas chromatograph equipped with an Omegawax 250 capillary column and isothermal oven.

The total of the n-3 PUFAs was computed by summing the total fats from ALA, EPA, DHA, and a rare n-3 PUFA detected in milk, Eicosatrienoic acid (ETE). The total of the n-6 fatty acids was computed by summing the total fats from Linolelaidic acid, Arachidic acid, Linoleic acid, Linolenic acid, Dihomo-gamma-linolenic acid (DGLA), Arachidonic acid (AA), and Eicosadienoic Acid. The n-6/n-3 PUFA ratio was computed by dividing the total fats from n-6 PUFAs by the total fats from n-3 PUFAs. Higher ratios represent milk that has more n-6 fatty acids relative to n-3s. The total PUFA concentration in milk was determined by summing the levels of n-3 and n-6 PUFAs.

2.3. Infant Temperament

To assess the infant temperament, mothers were asked to fill out the Rothbart Revised Infant Behavior Questionnaire (IBQ-R) during their laboratory visit [33]. The IBQ-R includes 191 specific questions addressing concrete behaviors such as, "During a peek-a-boo game, how often did the baby smile?" and "How often during the last week did the baby startle to a sudden or loud noise?" To prevent errors in recall, the scale only asks mothers about recently occurring events, using a 7-point Likert scale (1-never to 7-always). The IBQ-R measures three broad dimensions of temperament: negative affectivity, surgency/extraversion, and orienting/regulation. The negative affectivity dimension is created by averaging the scores across four subscales assessing infant sadness, fear, falling reactivity, and distress to limitations. The orienting/regulation dimension is created by averaging across four subscales of mothers' ratings of infants' cuddliness/affiliation, low intensity pleasure, duration of orienting, and soothability. The surgency/extraversion dimension is a composite averaged from six subscales assessing infant approach, vocal reactivity, high intensity pleasure, smiling and laughter, activity level, and perceptual sensitivity. This widely used parental-report instrument has been shown to be reliable across parental reports [33] and to correlate well with behavioral observations of infants [36]. The IBQ-R has been validated for use for infants aged 3 to 12 months, scores are relatively stable over the first year of life [36], and the scale takes approximately 30 min to complete [33]. As part of the larger longitudinal study, mothers also completed the IBQ-R at 6 months. See Table S1 in the Supplemental Materials for exploratory analyses testing the association between the milk fatty acid composition at 3 months and the infant temperament at 6 months.

2.4. Demographic and Health Information

Various demographic and health measures were tested as potential covariates. Maternal reports of race/ethnicity, age, education level, income, parity, marital status, and breastfeeding exclusivity were collected during a structured interview. A medical record review was conducted to assess the birth outcomes, including the infant sex, gestational age at delivery, and birth weight and length. The early pregnancy BMI (at 15 weeks) and weight gain during pregnancy (weight in pounds at 37 weeks-15 weeks) were collected during laboratory visits as part of the larger longitudinal study. At 3 months, the infant weight was assessed using a digital scale (Midmark, Versailles, OH, USA), and the height was determined while the child lay in a supine position. The child BMI percentiles (BMIP) at birth and 3 months were calculated using an SPSS macro that fits the child's height and weight to standard WHO growth curves and generates a child's BMI z-score standardized for age and sex [37,38]. For ease of interpretation, these z-scores were converted to percentiles.

2.5. Statistical Analysis Strategy

First, preliminary analyses were performed to check that the variables were normally distributed. Outliers that were greater than 3 standard deviations above or below the mean were winsorized to bring them to within 2 standard deviations before the analysis. We planned to log-transform any skewed variables; however, after winsorization, all variables were normally distributed. Second, we sought to identify potential confounds by testing whether demographic or health characteristics were associated with fatty acid concentrations in milk. Linear regression models were run with various demographic (age, income, education, marital status, race/ethnicity and infant sex) and health (maternal BMI, weight gain in pregnancy, gestational age at birth, exclusive breastfeeding status, and infant BMIP at birth and at 3 months) covariates entered simultaneously to predict n-3, n-6, n-6/n-3 ratios, and the total milk fat. Demographic or health variables that were associated with any one of the milk fatty acid composite variables with a p-value < 0.10 were included as covariates in the subsequent analysis. For the primary analysis, a multivariate linear regression was used to test whether the n-3, n-6, n-6/n-3 ratios, total PUFAs, or total milk fat predicted the negative affectivity or orienting/regulation dimension of the IBQ-R, adjusting for potential confounds. We also ran an exploratory analysis to see whether the fatty acid composition of milk was associated with the surgency/extraversion factor. If there was a significant association, we then used a follow-up linear regression analysis to test: (i) which specific sub-scales that made up the IBQ-R temperament dimension were significantly related to the fatty acid composite, and (ii) which specific fatty acid type (e.g., DHA vs. ALA) predicted the IBQ-R temperament dimension. Finally, we tested whether infant sex or exclusive breastfeeding moderated any observed significant association between the fatty acid levels and IBQ-R dimension. A moderation analysis was carried out by creating cross products between the potential moderator (infant sex, exclusive breastfeeding) and fatty acid levels, and the cross-products were then included in a linear regression model with the constituent variables and covariates. All analyses were performed in SPSS version 21.0. The findings were considered statistically significant if the *p*-values were under 0.05. The effect sizes (Standardized Betas or β) are also provided for all analyses, regardless of the significance level.

3. Results

3.1. Preliminary and Descriptive Analyses

The demographic and health information of the samples is presented in Table 1. The fatty acids composition of the milk samples are presented in Table 2. Several milk samples were more than three standard deviations higher than the mean in terms of n-3 PUFA levels (n = 1), EPA levels (n = 2), ALA levels (n = 1), and ETE levels (n = 1) and were winsorized to within 2 standard deviations of the mean before the statistical analysis.

Table 1. Sample characteristics and their association with the fatty acid composition of the milk.

	Mean/%	Standard Deviation	Range	Omega-3	Omega-6	Omega-6/3 Ratio	Total Fat
				Stand. β	Stand. β	Stand. β	Stand. β
Maternal Characteristics							
Maternal age	29.67	4.86	19.2–39.9	**0.407** t	0.285	−0.066	0.254
Education	2.70	1.051	0–4	0.113	−0.014	−0.167	−0.060
Household Income	69,489	33,980	25k–105k	0.008	−0.186	−0.286	−0.181
Pre-Pregnancy BMI	24.17	5.98	16.4–47.4	−0.102	−0.086	−0.045	−0.026
Pregnancy Weight Gain (lbs)	35.60	13.27	9.00–71.00	0.103	0.221	0.168	0.243
Parity (% Primiparous)	48.1%		1–4	0.085	−0.053	−0.123	−0.076
Exclusive Breastfeeding	63.27%			0.133	0.168	0.027	0.260
% Married	75%			−0.223	0.341	**0.593** *	0.223
Race/Ethnicity							
% White	58.3%						
% Latina	18.8%			0.006	0.118	0.117	0.220
% Asian	10.4%			0.057	−0.006	−0.052	0.015
% Multi-Ethnic/Other	12.5%			−0.152	−0.011	0.170	−0.145
Infant Characteristics							
Birth Weight (grams)	3465.49	386.874	2470–4220	0.104	0.405	**0.449** t	0.215
Gestational Age at Birth (weeks)	39.6822	1.12	37.1–42.3	−0.093	−0.070	0.090	−0.147
BMIP at Birth	56.92%	0.30	0.34–98%	−0.114	−0.125	−0.175	−0.164
BMIP at 3 mos	46.25%	0.27	0.02–97%	0.164	0.101	−0.034	−0.013
% Female Infants	48%			0.117	0.181	0.035	0.120

Note: Race/ethnicity was dummy coded to create contrasts to compare Hispanic, Asian, and Multi-Ethnic/Other groups to whites. Married was coded as 1 = Married, 0 = Not married; Infant sex was coded as Female = 2, Male = 1. Bolded coefficients indicate those with *p*-values < 0.10 = t and *p*-values < 0.05 = *. BMIP = Body Mass Index Percentile.

See Table 1 for the results of the linear regression analysis testing for associations between sociodemographic and health factors and the milk fatty acid composition. Married mothers had significantly higher n-6/n-3 ratios in their milk than mothers who were not married (p = 0.010). Older mothers tended to have higher levels of n-3 PUFAs in their milk (p = 0.060). Babies with a higher birth weight also tended to have higher n-6/n-3 ratios in their milk (p = 0.086). Infant sex, gestational age at delivery, and infant BMIP at birth or 3 months were not associated with the milk fatty acid composition. Likewise, mothers' pre-pregnancy BMI, weight gain in pregnancy, income, education, exclusive breastfeeding status, parity and race/ethnicity did not predict fatty acid levels in milk. Therefore, only the maternal age, marital status, and infant birth weight were included as covariates in the subsequent linear regression models.

Table 2. Milk fatty acid concentrations.

	IUPAC Name	Mean	Standard Deviation	Range
		(ug/mL)	(ug/mL)	(ug/mL)
Omega-3 Fatty Acids				
Linolenic acid (ALA)	(9Z,12Z,15Z)-octadeca-9,12,15-trienoic acid	13.80	6.15	4.26–42.25
Eicosatrienoic acid (ETE)	(11Z,14Z,17Z)-icosa-11,14,17-trienoic acid	0.74	1.02	0.02–7.00
Eicosapentaenoic acid (EPA)	(5Z,8Z,11Z,14Z,17Z)-icosa-5,8,11,14,17-pentaenoic acid	1.09	1.16	0.06–7.00
Docosahexaenoic acid (DHA)	(4Z,7Z,10Z,13Z,16Z,19Z)-docosa-4,7,10,13,16,19-hexaenoic acid	2.72	1.91	0.77–10.71
Omega-6 Fatty Acids				
Linolelaidic acid	(9E,12E)-octadeca-9,12-dienoic acid	1.16	0.30	1.00–3.08
Arachidic acid	($1^{13}C$)icosanoic acid	194.60	72.78	65.12–398.72
Linoleic acid	(9Z,12Z)-octadeca-9,12-dienoic acid	0.54	.06	0.51–0.89
Linolenic acid	(9Z,12Z,15Z)-octadeca-9,12,15-trienoic acid	2.26	1.71	0.14–8.79
Dihomo-gamma-linolenic acid (DGLA)	(8Z,11Z,14Z)-icosa-8,11,14-trienoic acid	5.41	2.21	1.41–10.55
Arachidonic acid (AA)	(5Z,8Z,11Z,14Z)-icosa-5,8,11,14-tetraenoic acid	1.17	0.94	0.12–4.92
Eicosadienoic Acid	(11E,14E)-icosa-11,14-dienoic acid	3.72	1.78	1.04–9.01
Composite Fatty Acid Variables				
Total Omega-3		18.36	7.98	6.66–55.64
Total Omega-6		208.85	77.88	70.11–433.86
Omega-6/Omega-3 Ratio		12.12	4.36	4.86–27.14
Total Milk PUFAs		227.21	83.57	83.58–489.50
Total Milk Fat		942.51	346.76	398–2301

The average infant score on the surgency/extraversion factor was 3.92 (SD = 0.88), the negative affectivity factor was 2.99 (SD = 0.56), and the orienting regulation factor was 5.02 (SD = 0.62). These mean scores are similar to those reported in the original validation study that had a larger sample size [33].

3.2. Primary Analysis

See Table 3 for the results of the multivariate linear regression analyses testing the association between the fatty acid composite variables and the three primary temperament dimensions of the IBQ-R. These analyses revealed that only higher levels of n-3 PUFA levels predicted lower scores on the negative affectivity dimension (see Figure 1). This association remained statistically significant after adjustment for the total milk fat content ($\beta = -0.443$, $p = 0.023$) and when all covariates were removed from the model ($\beta = -0.335$, $p = 0.015$). In addition, controlling for the time of day of the milk collection did not change the significant association between n-3 fatty acids and negative affectivity.

Table 3. The association between the milk fatty acid composition and the infant temperament assessed with multivariate linear regression models.

	Negative Affectivity	Orienting/Regulation	Surgency/Extraversion
	Standardized β (*p*-Value)	Standardized β (*p*-Value)	Standardized β (*p*-Value)
Omega-3	−0.352 (0.020) *	−0.014 (0.927)	−0.108 (0.479)
Omega-6	−0.249 (0.106)	0.131 (0.394)	0.053 (0.727)
Omega-6/3 ratio	0.134 (0.387)	0.159 (0.297)	0.179 (0.236)
Total PUFAs	−0.266 (0.083)	0.127 (0.408)	0.042 (0.784)
Total Milk Fat	−0.124 (0.401)	−0.004 (0.981)	−0.039 (0.791)

Note: All coefficients are statistically adjusted for the maternal age, mother's marital status, and infant birth weight. * $p < 0.05$.

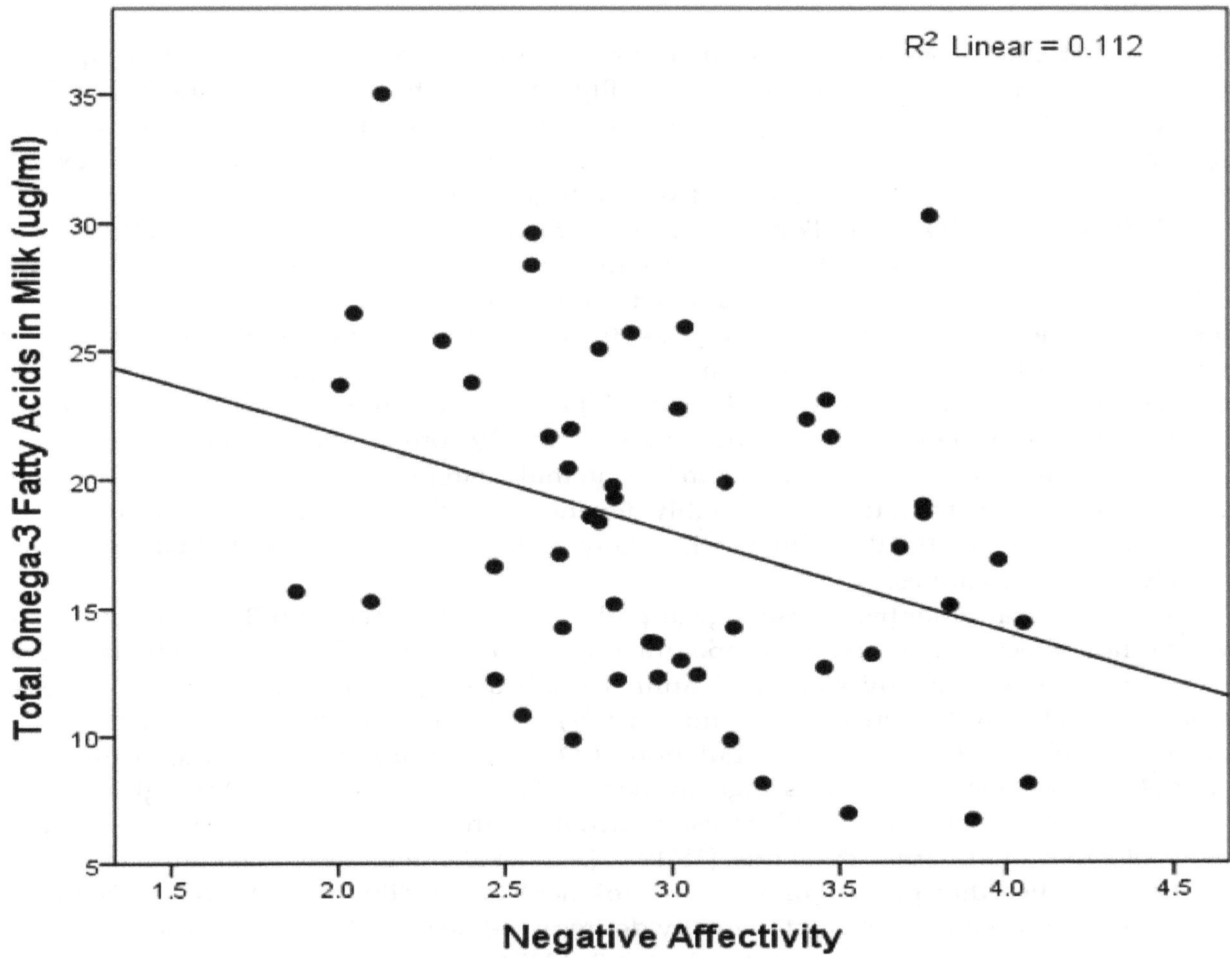

Figure 1. The scatterplot of the total omega-3 fatty acids in the milk and the infant negative affectivity.

Because the milk n-3 PUFA levels predicted a negative affectivity, we performed a follow-up analysis to test how the n-3 PUFAs predicted each of the four subscales that comprised this dimension of the IBQ-R. Higher n-3 PUFAs were associated with less sadness ($\beta = -0.349$, $p = 0.021$) and less distress to limitations ($\beta = -365$, $p = 0.017$). Milk n-3s were not significantly related to infant fear (β -0.187, $p = 0.219$) or falling reactivity ($\beta = -0.087$, $p = 0.584$), although these effects were in the same direction as those observed for sadness and limitations to distress.

In addition, given that n-3 PUFAs predicted negative affectivity, we tested whether specific subtypes of n-3 PUFAs (ALA, EPA, DHA, or ETE) were, independently, related to negative affectivity. Mothers with higher ALA in their milk reported that their infants had significantly less negative affectivity ($\beta = -0.368$, $p = 0.015$). Although they did not reach the criterion for statistical significance, the DHA, EPA, and ETE levels were all negatively associated with negative affectivity (DHA: β -0.178, $p = 0.229$; EPA: $\beta = -0.251$, $p = 0.095$; ETE: $\beta = -0.103$, $p = 0.472$).

3.3. Moderation Analysis

Neither the infant sex, nor the breastfeeding exclusivity, significantly moderated the association between the milk n-3 PUFA levels and negative affectivity (sex: $\beta = -0.170$, $p = 0.780$; breastfeeding exclusivity: $\beta = 0.975$, $p = 0.071$).

4. Discussion

The present study found evidence to support a link between the n-3 PUFA composition of human milk and infant temperament. Specifically, infants whose mothers had higher levels of n-3 PUFAs in their milk were reported to display lower levels of negative affectivity at 3 months than did infants whose mothers had lower levels of n-3 PUFAs in their milk. To the extent that negative affectivity in infancy is associated with a higher risk for internalizing disorders in later childhood [39,40], n-3 PUFAs in milk may represent a novel developmental origins pathway through which environmental exposures influence the risk for later mental health disorders. To our knowledge, this is the first study to report an association between the variation in the n-3 PUFAs levels in milk and the temperament in humans. One previous study did report that there was no difference in the temperaments of infants who were randomly assigned to receive formula supplemented with DHA (vs. non-DHA-supplemented formula) [41] (see [42] for similar null results with rhesus macaques). However, formula supplementation studies are not directly comparable to studies of human milk, since n-3 PUFAs are metabolized differently in human milk than they are in formula [43], and since the absorption of fatty acids from formula is highly dependent on the specific type of oil from which the n-3s were harvested [44]. Still, the results of this study should be considered preliminary until they can be replicated in larger studies.

There are several potential physiological pathways through which n-3 PUFAs in milk could influence infant affect regulation and temperament. Most directly, n-3 PUFAs and their derivatives help to regulate neurotransmission, and animal studies suggest that deficiencies increase the serotonin 2 (5-HT_2) and decrease dopamine 2 (D_2) receptor density in the frontal cortex [45]. The upregulation of 5-HT_2 and downregulation of D_2 in the brain have been implicated in mood disorders [46]. Less directly, n-3 PUFAs might influence infant negative affectivity through inflammatory pathways [18,19,47]. n-3 PUFAs, and EPA especially, have anti-inflammatory properties and reduce the levels of pro-inflammatory cytokines [18,19,47]. In adults, we know from animal and human experimental studies that pro-inflammatory cytokines can readily cross the blood–brain barrier and induce sickness behavior characterized by depressive-like symptoms such as low mood, social withdrawal, and anxiety [48]. The extent to which n-3s PUFAs regulate inflammatory processes in early development is unknown, but future research could investigate if n-3 PUFAs' levels in milk are related to inflammatory processes in infants and if, by doing so, they indirectly influence negative affectivity.

It was notable that, of the three primary types of n-3 PUFAs in milk, only higher levels of ALA were significantly associated with negative affectivity. The DHA and EPA levels were also inversely correlated with negative affectivity, but not to a statistically significant degree. It would be premature for readers to conclude, however, that only ALA (and not DHA or EPA) in milk influences infant temperament given that all three of the primary n-3 PUFAs were negatively correlated with negative affectivity, with effect sizes in the small-to-medium range. Future studies that combine the methods used here with direct assessments of infants' plasma levels of ALA, DHA, and EPA are necessary to address the question of whether it is n-3 PUFAs in general, or one subtype of n-3 PUFA in particular, that influences infant temperament.

In their strongest form, these results could have several potential policy implications. First, the maternal diet can influence the levels of n-3 PUFAs in milk and, by doing so, may influence infant temperament. For example, breast milk EPA and DHA concentrations are closely linked to maternal dietary EPA and DHA intake [49], and randomized control trials have shown that mothers given n-3 PUFA supplements show corresponding increases in the n-3 PUFA composition of their milk [50,51]. Unfortunately, this study did not include information on maternal diets, and only two mothers in our study reported taking omega-3 PUFA supplements, so we were not able to test this hypothesis. Future studies could examine whether increasing the dietary intake of n-3 PUFAs in breastfeeding women would lead to a reduced negative affectivity in infants. Second, considering that negative affectivity in infancy predicts internalizing disorders (i.e., anxiety/depression) in later childhood [39,40], perhaps supplementing breastfeeding mothers with n-3 PUFAs could help ameliorate the risk for later mental health problems. While this possibility is only hypothetical, maternal diets during pregnancy and lactation are modifiable and present promising targets for the prevention of adverse developmental outcomes in children [52,53].

Although this study had several strengths, including the direct assessment of the fatty acid composition of milk and the carefully characterized cohort, these results should be considered in the context of several limitations. First, we relied on maternal reports of infant temperament, which may be biased. Despite this, the IBQ-R has in previous studies been found to correlate highly with more objective measures of infant temperament (e.g., behavioral observations) [36]. Moreover, the association between the reports of mothers and other caregivers is generally high [33]. Still, future research would benefit from including additional object measures of infant temperament and behavior. Second, this study was correlational and cannot rule out the possibility that a confounding factor may explain the observed association between the n-3 PUFA levels in milk and infant temperament. To address this possibility, we tested whether a number of demographic (e.g., income, education) and health (e.g., maternal BMI, weight gain in pregnancy) factors predicted the fatty acid composition of milk. Only the marital status, maternal age, and infant birth weight predicted the fatty acid composition of milk, and statistically adjusting for these covariates did not negate the association between n-3 PUFA levels and negative affectivity in this study. Regardless, there are numerous bio-active factors in milk, such as cortisol, which have been shown to correlate with total milk fat [54] and negative affectivity in infants [26]. However, given that we found no association between the total fat or n-6 fatty acid content of milk and infant temperament, we believe that the n-3 composition of milk and cortisol levels in milk likely represent distinct lactational programming pathways. Furthermore, the association between n-3 PUFA levels in milk and negative affectivity remains statistically significant after adjusting for the total fat content of the milk, suggesting that it is n-3 PUFAs specifically, and not richer milk generally, that shapes infant temperament. Finally, this study did not include information on the last time mothers had breastfed or on the total milk volume that mothers expressed. We were unable to identify any studies that tested how the time since the last feeding or the volume of milk production impacts the omega-3 fatty acid composition of milk. Future research is needed to determine whether these factors are associated with LC PUFAs and could therefore have influenced these results.

Findings from this study add to the growing body of research demonstrating that the variation in the composition of mothers' milk plays an important role in shaping the development of offspring. Specifically, we found that milk that was richer in n-3 PUFAs was associated with reduced sadness and distress in infants. These new data are consistent with previous research linking n-3 PUFAs to an improved mood and mental health in adults [18–22]. We hope that the exciting research taking place in the field of lactational programming will open up new possibilities for preventing mood disturbances.

Author Contributions: Methodology, investigation, project administration, funding acqusition L.M.G., formal analysis, J.H.-H. and A.F., writing—original draft, J.H.-H., writing—review and editing, J.H.-H., A.F., L.M.G.

Acknowledgments: The authors thank the families who participated in this project and the staff at the UCI Women and Children's Health and Well-Being project for their excellent work.

References

1. Prado, E.L.; Dewey, K.G. Nutrition and brain development in early life. *Nutr. Rev.* **2014**, *72*, 267–284. [CrossRef] [PubMed]
2. Keunen, K.; Van Elburg, R.M.; Van Bel, F.; Benders, M.J. Impact of nutrition on brain development and its neuroprotective implications following preterm birth. *Pediatr. Res.* **2015**, *77*, 148. [CrossRef] [PubMed]
3. Cusick, S.E.; Georgieff, M.K. The role of nutrition in brain development: The golden opportunity of the "first 1000 days". *J. Pediatr.* **2016**, *175*, 16–21. [CrossRef] [PubMed]
4. Belfort, M.B.; Anderson, P.J.; Nowak, V.A.; Lee, K.J.; Molesworth, C.; Thompson, D.K.; Doyle, L.W.; Inder, T.E. Breast milk feeding, brain development, and neurocognitive outcomes: A 7-year longitudinal study in infants born at less than 30 weeks' gestation. *J. Pediatr.* **2016**, *177*, 133–139. [CrossRef]

5. Martin, C.; Ling, P.R.; Blackburn, G. Review of infant feeding: Key features of breast milk and infant formula. *Nutrients* **2016**, *8*, 279. [CrossRef]
6. Innis, S.M.; Gilley, J.; Werker, J. Are human milk long-chain polyunsaturated fatty acids related to visual and neural development in breast-fed term infants? *J. Pediatr.* **2001**, *139*, 532–538. [CrossRef]
7. Eidelman, A.I.; Schanler, R.J. Breastfeeding and the use of human milk. *Pediatrics* **2012**, *5*, 323–324.
8. Birch, D.G.; Birch, E.E.; Hoffman, D.R.; Uauy, R.D. Retinal development in very-low-birth-weight infants fed diets differing in omega-3 fatty acids. *Investig. Ophthalmol. Vis. Sci.* **1992**, *33*, 2365–2376.
9. Innis, S.M. Dietary omega 3 fatty acids and the developing brain. *Brain. Res.* **2008**, *1237*, 35–43. [CrossRef]
10. Jensen, R.G. Lipids in human milk. *Lipids* **1999**, *34*, 1243–1271. [CrossRef]
11. Brenna, J.T.; Salem, N., Jr.; Sinclair, A.J.; Cunnane, S.C. α-Linolenic acid supplementation and conversion to n-3 long-chain polyunsaturated fatty acids in humans. *Prostaglandins Leukot. Essent. Fat. Acids* **2009**, *80*, 85–91. [CrossRef] [PubMed]
12. Giusto, N.; Salvador, G.; Castagnet, P.; Pasquare, S.; de Boschero, M.I. Age-associated changes in central nervous system glycerolipid composition and metabolism. *Neurochem. Res.* **2002**, *27*, 1513–1523. [CrossRef] [PubMed]
13. Meydani, S.N. Effect of (n-3) polyunsaturated fatty acidson cytokine production and their biologic function. *Nutrition* **1996**, *12*, S8–S14. [CrossRef]
14. Endres, S.; Ghorbani, R.; Kelley, V.E.; Georgilis, K.; Lonnemann, G.; Van Der Meer, J.W.; Cannon, J.G.; Rogers, T.S.; Klempner, M.S.; Weber, P.C. The effect of dietary supplementation with n—3 polyunsaturated fatty acids on the synthesis of interleukin-1 and tumor necrosis factor by mononuclear cells. *N. Engl. J. Med.* **1989**, *320*, 265–271. [CrossRef] [PubMed]
15. U.S Department of Health and Human Services. *2015–2020 Dietary Guidelines for Americans*, 8th ed.; U.S Department of Health and Human Services: Washington, DC, USA, 2015.
16. Decsi, T.; Kelemen, B.; Minda, H.; Burus, I.; Kohn, G. Effect of type of early infant feeding on fatty acid composition of plasma lipid classes in full-term infants during the second 6 months of life. *J. Pediatr. Gastroenterol. Nutr.* **2000**, *30*, 547–551. [CrossRef] [PubMed]
17. Cunnane, S.C.; Francescutti, V.; Brenna, J.T.; Crawford, M.A. Breast-fed infants achieve a higher rate of brain and whole body docosahexaenoate accumulation than formula-fed infants not consuming dietary docosahexaenoate. *Lipids* **2000**, *35*, 105–111. [CrossRef] [PubMed]
18. Su, K.P.; Matsuoka, Y.; Pae, C.U. Omega-3 polyunsaturated fatty acids in prevention of mood and anxiety disorders. *Clin. Psychopharmacol. Neurosci.* **2015**, *13*, 129. [CrossRef]
19. Su, K.P. Biological Mechanism of Antidepressant Effect of Omega–3 Fatty Acids: How Does Fish Oil Act as a 'Mind-Body Interface'? *Neurosignals* **2009**, *17*, 144–152. [CrossRef]
20. Lin, P.Y.; Huang, S.Y.; Su, K.P. A meta-analytic review of polyunsaturated fatty acid compositions in patients with depression. *Biol. Psychiatry* **2010**, *68*, 140–147. [CrossRef]
21. Stoll, A.L.; Severus, W.E.; Freeman, M.P.; Rueter, S.; Zboyan, H.A.; Diamond, E.; Cress, K.K.; Marangell, L.B. Omega 3 fatty acids in bipolar disorder: A preliminary double-blind, placebo-controlled trial. *Arch. Gen. Psychiatry* **1999**, *56*, 407–412. [CrossRef]
22. Buydens-Branchey, L.; Branchey, M.; Hibbeln, J.R. Associations between increases in plasma n-3 polyunsaturated fatty acids following supplementation and decreases in anger and anxiety in substance abusers. *Prog. Neuro-Psychopharmacol. Biol. Psychiatry* **2008**, *32*, 568–575. [CrossRef] [PubMed]
23. Bhatia, H.S.; Agrawal, R.; Sharma, S.; Huo, Y.-X.; Ying, Z.; Gomez-Pinilla, F. Omega-3 fatty acid deficiency during brain maturation reduces neuronal and behavioral plasticity in adulthood. *PLoS ONE* **2011**, *6*, e28451. [CrossRef] [PubMed]
24. Brunst, K.J.; Enlow, M.B.; Kannan, S.; Carroll, K.N.; Coull, B.A.; Wright, R.J. Effects of prenatal social stress and maternal dietary fatty acid ratio on infant temperament: Does race matter? *Epidemiology* **2014**, *4*, 1000167. [PubMed]
25. Clayton, E.H.; Hanstock, T.L.; Hirneth, S.J.; Kable, C.J.; Garg, M.L.; Hazell, P.L. Long-chain omega-3 polyunsaturated fatty acids in the blood of children and adolescents with juvenile bipolar disorder. *Lipids* **2008**, *43*, 1031–1038. [CrossRef] [PubMed]

26. Grey, K.R.; Davis, E.P.; Sandman, C.A.; Glynn, L.M. Human milk cortisol is associated with infant temperament. *Psychoneuroendocrinology* **2013**, *38*, 1178–1185. [CrossRef]
27. Hart, S.; Boylan, L.M.; Border, B.; Carroll, S.R.; McGunegle, D.; Lampe, R.M. Breast milk levels of cortisol and Secretory Immunoglobulin A (SIgA) differ with maternal mood and infant neuro-behavioral functioning. *Infant Behav. Dev.* **2004**, *27*, 101–106. [CrossRef]
28. Nolvi, S.; Uusitupa, H.M.; Bridgett, D.J.; Pesonen, H.; Aatsinki, A.K.; Kataja, E.L.; Korja, R.; Karlsson, H.; Karlsson, L. Human milk cortisol concentration predicts experimentally induced infant fear reactivity: Moderation by infant sex. *Dev. Sci.* **2018**, *21*, e12625. [CrossRef]
29. Hinde, K. Lactational programming of infant behavioral phenotype. In *Building Babies*; Springer: Berlin/Heidelberg, Germany, 2013; pp. 187–207.
30. Dettmer, A.M.; Murphy, A.M.; Guitarra, D.; Slonecker, E.; Suomi, S.J.; Rosenberg, K.L.; Novak, M.A.; Meyer, J.S.; Hinde, K. Cortisol in neonatal mother's milk predicts later infant social and cognitive functioning in rhesus monkeys. *Child Dev.* **2018**, *89*, 525–538. [CrossRef]
31. Petrullo, L.; Hinde, K.; Lu, A. Steroid hormone concentrations in milk predict sex-specific offspring growth in a nonhuman primate. *Am. J. Hum. Biol.* **2019**, *31*, e23315. [CrossRef]
32. Hinde, K.; Capitanio, J.P. Lactational programming? Mother's milk energy predicts infant behavior and temperament in rhesus macaques (Macaca mulatta). *Am. J. Primatol. Off. J. Am. Soc. Primatol.* **2010**, *72*, 522–529. [CrossRef]
33. Gartstein, M.A.; Rothbart, M.K. Studying infant temperament via the revised infant behavior questionnaire. *Infant Behav. Dev.* **2003**, *26*, 64–86. [CrossRef]
34. Francois, C.A.; Connor, S.L.; Bolewicz, L.C.; Connor, W.E. Supplementing lactating women with flaxseed oil does not increase docosahexaenoic acid in their milk. *Am. J. Clin. Nutr.* **2003**, *77*, 226–233. [CrossRef] [PubMed]
35. Jacobson, J.L.; Jacobson, S.W.; Muckle, G.; Kaplan-Estrin, M.; Ayotte, P.; Dewailly, E. Beneficial effects of a polyunsaturated fatty acid on infant development: Evidence from the Inuit of Arctic Quebec. *J. Pediatr.* **2008**, *152*, 356–364. [CrossRef] [PubMed]
36. Worobey, J.; Blajda, V.M. Temperament ratings at 2 weeks, 2 months, and 1 year: Differential stablity of activity and emotionality. *Dev. Psychol.* **1989**, *25*, 257. [CrossRef]
37. World Health Organization. *WHO Child Growth Standards: Length/Height-for-Age, Weight-for-Age, Weight-for-Length, Weight-for-Height and Body Mass Index-for-Age: Methods and Development*; World Health Organization: Geneva, Switzerland, 2006.
38. Cole, T.J.; Green, P.J. Smoothing reference centile curves: The LMS method and penalized likelihood. *Stat. Med.* **1992**, *11*, 1305–1319. [CrossRef]
39. Gartstein, M.A.; Putnam, S.P.; Rothbart, M.K. Etiology of preschool behavior problems: Contributions of temperament attributes in early childhood. *Infant Ment. Health J.* **2012**, *33*, 197–211. [CrossRef]
40. Rende, R.D. Longitudinal relations between temperament traits and behavioral syndromes in middle childhood. *J. Am. Acad. Child Adolesc. Psychiatry* **1993**, *32*, 287–290. [CrossRef]
41. Auestad, N.; Halter, R.; Hall, R.T.; Blatter, M.; Bogle, M.L.; Burks, W.; Erickson, J.R.; Fitzgerald, K.M.; Dobson, V.; Innis, S.M. Growth and development in term infants fed long-chain polyunsaturated fatty acids: A double-masked, randomized, parallel, prospective, multivariate study. *Pediatrics* **2001**, *108*, 372–381. [CrossRef]
42. Champoux, M.; Hibbeln, J.R.; Shannon, C.; Majchrzak, S.; Suomi, S.J.; Salem Jr, N.; Higley, J.D. Fatty acid formula supplementation and neuromotor development in rhesus monkey neonates. *Pediatr. Res.* **2002**, *51*, 273. [CrossRef]
43. Carnielli, V.P.; Verlato, G.; Pederzini, F.; Luijendijk, I.; Boerlage, A.; Pedrotti, D.; Sauer, P. Intestinal absorption of long-chain polyunsaturated fatty acids in preterm infants fed breast milk or formula. *Am. J. Clin. Nutr.* **1998**, *67*, 97–103. [CrossRef]
44. de Souza, C.O.; Leite, M.E.Q.; Lasekan, J.; Baggs, G.; Pinho, L.S.; Druzian, J.I.; Ribeiro, T.C.M.; Mattos, Â.P.; Menezes-Filho, J.A.; Costa-Ribeiro, H. Milk protein-based formulas containing different oils affect fatty acids balance in term infants: A randomized blinded crossover clinical trial. *Lipids Health Dis.* **2017**, *16*, 78. [CrossRef] [PubMed]
45. Delion, S.; Chalon, S.; Hérault, J.; Guilloteau, D.; Besnard, J.C.; Durand, G. Chronic dietary α-linolenic acid

deficiency alters dopaminergic and serotoninergic neurotransmission in rats. *J. Nutr.* **1994**, *124*, 2466–2476. [CrossRef] [PubMed]

46. Meltzer, H. Serotonergic dysfunction in depression. *Br. J. Psychiatry* **1989**, *155*, 25–31. [CrossRef]
47. Stahl, L.A.; Begg, D.P.; Weisinger, R.S.; Sinclair, A.J. The role of omega-3 fatty acids in mood disorders. *Curr. Opin. Investig. Drugs* **2008**, *9*, 57–64.
48. Eisenberger, N.I.; Berkman, E.T.; Inagaki, T.K.; Rameson, L.T.; Mashal, N.M.; Irwin, M.R. Inflammation-induced anhedonia: Endotoxin reduces ventral striatum responses to reward. *Biol. Psychiatry* **2010**, *68*, 748–754. [CrossRef]
49. Francois, C.A.; Connor, S.L.; Wander, R.C.; Connor, W.E. Acute effects of dietary fatty acids on the fatty acids of human milk. *Am. J. Clin. Nutr.* **1998**, *67*, 301–308. [CrossRef]
50. Weseler, A.R.; Dirix, C.E.; Bruins, M.J.; Hornstra, G. Dietary arachidonic acid dose-dependently increases the arachidonic acid concentration in human milk. *J. Nutr.* **2008**, *138*, 2190–2197. [CrossRef]
51. Makrides, M.; Neumann, M.; Gibson, R.A. Effect of maternal docosahexaenoic acid (DHA) supplementation on breast milk composition. *Eur. J. Clin. Nutr.* **1996**, *50*, 352–357.
52. O'Neil, A.; Itsiopoulos, C.; Skouteris, H.; Opie, R.S.; McPhie, S.; Hill, B.; Jacka, F.N. Preventing mental health problems in offspring by targeting dietary intake of pregnant women. *BMC Med.* **2014**, *12*, 208. [CrossRef]
53. Greer, F.R.; Sicherer, S.H.; Burks, A.W. Effects of early nutritional interventions on the development of atopic disease in infants and children: The role of maternal dietary restriction, breastfeeding, timing of introduction of complementary foods, and hydrolyzed formulas. *Pediatrics* **2008**, *121*, 183–191. [CrossRef]
54. Hinde, K.; Skibiel, A.L.; Foster, A.B.; Del Rosso, L.; Mendoza, S.P.; Capitanio, J.P. Cortisol in mother's milk across lactation reflects maternal life history and predicts infant temperament. *Behav. Ecol.* **2014**, *26*, 269–281. [CrossRef] [PubMed]

10

Expression of Granulysin, Perforin and Granzymes in Human Milk over Lactation and in the Case of Maternal Infection

Alecia-Jane Twigger [1,*,†], Gwendoline K. Küffer [2,†], Donna T. Geddes [3] and Luis Filgueria [2]

1 Institute for Stem Cell Research, Helmholtz Center Munich, 85764 Munich, Germany
2 Faculty of Science and Medicine, University of Fribourg, 1700 Fribourg, Switzerland; gwendoline.kueffer@gmail.com (G.K.K.); luis.filgueira@unifr.ch (L.F.)
3 School of Molecular Sciences, Faculty of Science, The University of Western Australia, Perth 6009, Australia; donna.geddes@uwa.edu.au
* Correspondence: alecia-jane.twigger@helmholtz-muenchen.de
† These authors contributed equally to this work.

Abstract: Human milk has been previously found to contain various types of leukocytes however specific characteristics of these cells, such as whether they contain cytolytic antimicrobial proteins that may induce pathogen directed cell death, are unknown. This project aims to examine the presence and localization of immune proteins such as perforin, granulysin and granzymes in human milk cells at the protein and mRNA level. Genes encoding these proteins were confirmed in human milk cell samples, which were particularly enriched in early milk and in the case of maternal infection. Fluorescence activated cell sorting (FACS) was used to investigate the co-expression of these proteins with pan-immune cell marker CD45 and epithelial marker EPCAM. Co-expression of antimicrobial proteins was found predominantly in CD45 positive cells, also increasing in the case of maternal infection. Our study suggests that human milk contains cells that carry hallmarks of activated or memory T-cells which are enriched early in lactation and in the case of maternal infection. Presence and prevalence of these cells in human milk may indicate a role in the protection of the maternal breast or for delivery to the vulnerable infant.

Keywords: human milk; milk cells; immune cells; antimicrobial proteins

---

1. Introduction

Human milk contains all the necessary components required to satisfy the nutritional requirements of the infant, as well as immunological factors that support survival and thriving of the child. At birth, full term newborns are exposed to both vaginal bacteria and gut microbiota, some of which may be pathogenic [1]. Whilst infants have more or less a complete immune system, it is still highly immature [1–3] and requires contact with foreign antigens and stimulation such as from human milk to develop effective and specific defence mechanisms [2,3]. Human milk proteins, such as lactoferrin, certain caseins [4,5] and lysozyme, along with other bioactive molecules such as oligosaccharides, defensins, cytokines, chemokines, growth factors and anti-oxidants [1,3] support the development of the immune system at the same time as providing antimicrobial and antiviral effects [2]. Of note, secretory IgA (sIgA) antibodies found in human milk and produced by maternal plasma cells is an important antibody directed against microbes and food antigens that have challenged the maternal immune response [2]. The presence of immune cells, such as lymphocytes, has been shown in human milk [1–3,6,7], which increase in number when the infant has an infection even in an asymptomatic mother [8]. Moreover, the immune cell content of milk increases to a much greater degree during maternal infection, particularly during mastitis. It is therefore hypothesized that leukocytes entering human milk might play a role for the infant but may also result from protection of the breast tissue [3].

Generally, if a pathogenic or non-host cell (such as bacteria) is detected, the immune system is activated, leading primed leukocytes such as cytotoxic t-cells and natural killer cells to release cytolytic granules. These granules contain the bioactive molecules perforin [9] and granulysin (synthetic drugs include novobiocin [10]), which work together to form pores in the cell to allow the entry of a third component, granzymes into pathogenic cells, and trigger bacterial cell programmed death and possibly also apoptosis of the host cell [11–14]. Granzymes are serine proteases and of the twelve granzymes already described, five have been found in the human (A, B, H, K and M) and ten have been identified in rodents (A-G, K, M and N) [13]. Whilst immune cells are known to exist in human milk with their numbers and distribution changing in relation to the health status of either the mother or the child [3,7,8,15], the presence of associated cytotoxic immune proteins perforin, granzymes and granulysin have not yet been identified in human milk cells. Presence of these proteins in human milk leukocytes would indicate the existence of activated or memory t-cells which have recently or may be actively fighting pathogenic cells which may be of importance either for the protection of the maternal breast or infant. The aim of this study is to determine the presence of these antimicrobial proteins in human milk cells and determine whether they are normally expressed across different stages of lactation in healthy participants or in the case of breast inflammatory conditions such as mastitis.

2. Materials and Methods

2.1. Human Milk Collection

The study was approved by the Swissethics Committee (2016-00309, Switzerland), the Human Research Ethics Committee of The University of Western Australia (UWA, RA/4/1/4397) and the Australian Breastfeeding Association (ABA; 2014–5). All participants provided informed written consent to engage in the study and all methods were carried out according to the approved guidelines. Thirty-six mothers were recruited through the Hospital of Fribourg, ABA meetings and the website humanlactationresearchgroup.com. Mothers were on average 34.4 years of age (range from 27 to 45 years of age) (Table 1). All infants, with 53% being male, were born term with a median of 278 days of gestation (range from 249 to 301 days) with 60% delivered vaginally (Table 1). Milk samples were collected 4–142 days post-partum and a single pre-partum secretion was collected 5 days before birth (Table 1). After collection, milk samples were brought directly to the laboratory to be processed.

Table 1. Demographics of study participants engaged in the study.

	Median (Range)		
	All Participants	**PCR Participants**	**Flow Cytometry Participants**
Maternal characteristics	*n* = 36	*n* = 24	*n* = 13
Age (years)	34 (27–45)	33 (27–45)	35.5 (34–38)
Body Mass Index (BMI)	24 (19.8–31.9)	22.5 (19.8–27.9)	25.6 (22–31.9)
Parity	2 (1–4)	2 (1–4)	2 (1–3)
Infant characteristics	*n* = 36	*n* = 24	*n* = 13
Gestational age (days)	278 (249–301)	278 (249–301)	275 (252–281)
Infant age at collection (days)	47 (4–142)	45 (4–142)	57 (37–84)
Milk characteristics	*n* = 85	*n* = 70	*n* = 15
Volume of milk (mL)	50 (0.61–490)	50 (0.61–490)	62 (35–195)
Total cell count (cells/mL)	16.4 (1.9–214.5)	16.55 (1.9–214.5)	13.8 (4.9–63.8)
Viability (%)	97.4 (53.2–100)	98.1 (53.2–100)	93.6 (84.7–96.5)

2.2. Milk Cell Isolation

Each milk sample was diluted in equal volume of Phosphate Buffer Saline (PBS) (Gibco, Thermo Fisher Scientific, Wilmington, DE, USA) and centrifuged at 800 g for 20 min at 20 °C. The fat and skim layer of the milk was removed before washing the cell pellet twice in sterile PBS and the cells were resuspended in 5–10 mL of PBS. Cells were used fresh for flow cytometry or frozen and stored at −80 °C for RNA extraction and corresponding analysis.

2.3. RNA Extraction

Total RNA was extracted from frozen cell pellets, previously collected as part of a larger study. Mini RNeasy extraction kit (Qiagen, Valencia, CA, USA) was used according to the manufacturer's protocol. The concentration and purity of RNA was measured using NanoDrop 2000 (Thermo Fisher Scientific, Wilmington, DE, USA). All extracted RNA was of a high quality with a 260/280 ratio between 1.8 and 2.2. Pooled resting mammary tissue RNA taken from five donors aged 40–55 was purchased from Aligent Technologies (Catalogue number: 540045, lot number: 0006135096, Aligent Technologies, Santa Clara, CA, USA).

2.4. cDNA Generation

RNA was reverse transcribed into cDNA using the cDNA archive kit (Life Technologies, Carlsbad, CA, USA) following the manufacturer's instructions. 50 µL reactions were incubated in a Bio-Rad C1000 96-well gradient block thermal cycler and held at 25 °C for 10 min, followed by 37 °C for 120 min, 85 °C for 5 min and finally at 4 °C until collection.

2.5. Quantitative Real Time Polymerase Chain Reaction (qRT-PCR)

Gene expression was investigated through quantitative real time PCR using Taqman probes (Table S1, Life Technologies, Thermo fisher, CA, USA) with the 7500 Fast qRT-PCR system (Life Technologies). Each sample was measured in triplicate or where necessary, in duplicate. Cycle time (CT) values were obtained for each sample and subsequently, relative quantitation (RQ) was calculated using $2^{Ct(control)-Ct(sample)} \pm$ SD, where genes were normalized to resting breast tissue and GAPDH was used as a housekeeping control gene.

2.6. Sequencing Library Research

Genes coding for cytolytic immune proteins perforin (PRF1), granulysin (GNLY) and granzymes A, B, H and M (GZMA, GZMB, GZMH, GZMM) were searched in an RNA-sequencing dataset [16], which explored the transcriptome of prepartum secretions (PS) and human milk (HM) cells as well as resting mammary tissue (RMT). Previously, $1.1 \times 10^5 - 19.3 \times 10^5$ cells/mL were isolated from PS samples collected from four women at 38–40 weeks of pregnancy. All participants provided follow-up samples of $0.4 \times 10^6 - 43.5 \times 10^6$ cells/mL HM at 1, 3, 6 and 12 months of lactation [16]. mRNA was extracted from the isolated cells, the quantity was then standardized [17,18] and the samples were processed for library preparation. Moreover, RMT taken from five women aged 40–55 years (Catalogue number: 540045, Lot number: 0006135096, Agilent Technologies, Santa Clara, CA, USA) was pooled and mRNA was likewise processed for library preparation. Illumina HiSeq2500 version 3 was used to sequence all samples with a production of a minimum of 20 million 50 base paired single end reads. SOAP aligner 2 was used to align 865,913,217 clean reads to the human genome where only 2 mismatches were allowed, resulting in 414,203,980 clean transcripts. Gene expression levels were expressed as RPKM (Reads Per Kilobase per Million mapped reads) [19] and annotated with the algorithm Basic Local Alignment Search Tools (BLAST) (2.2.23). Plots of the genes of interest expression patterns were made, as described below.

2.7. Flow Cytometry

Flow cytometry was performed in cells isolated from fresh milk samples by either staining immediately (n = 11) or fixed in 1% paraformaldehyde 2/3% sucrose in PBS for subsequent staining the following day (n = 4). When immediately stained, 2 million cells were separated into Eppendorf tubes. Conjugated extracellular antibodies were added to cells (Table S2) in 100 µL of 2% foetal bovine serum (Fisher Biotec, Wembley, WA, Australia) PBS and incubated for 30 min at 4 °C shielded from light. When immediately fixed, the cells were stained the next day with antibodies against membrane proteins (Table S2), diluted in PBS for 30 min on ice and in the dark. All stained cells were then washed twice in PBS (10,000 g for 30 s) and fixed in 3% paraformaldehyde 2/3% sucrose in PBS for 20 min. Subsequently, cells were washed again twice in PBS. While optimizing the technique, it was observed that the antibody against granzyme A worked better when the permeabilization was conducted with 0.05% Tween, therefore antibodies for intracellular staining were diluted in 0.3% saponin or 0.05% Tween in PBS, were added for 30 min, at room temperature, in the dark. Cells were subsequently washed once with 0.1% saponin or 0.05% Tween in PBS (10000 g for 30 s) and then in PBS before resuspending the cells in PBS for subsequent data acquisition. Cells were either analyzed with a BD Accuri C6 plus flow cytometer or in case of triple stainings, cells were measured with a BD FACS Canto. FCS files were then analyzed with the version 10.2 of the software FlowJo™. To avoid doublets, single cells were gated using forward scatter area (FSC-A) versus forward scatter height (FSC-H) (Figure S1). Single cells were further separated in three populations (Figure S1) to examine the presence of granzyme A, granzyme B, granulysin and perforin in immune and epithelial cells.

2.8. Statistical Analysis

Statistical analyses were carried out using R 3.3.2. for Mac OSX, with additional packages ggplot2 [20], lattice [21], nlme [22], FactoMineR [23] and factoextra for longitudinal plots, box and whisker plots, mixed linear effects models, principal component analysis (PCA) and plots respectively. Longitudinal spaghetti plots of PS cells, HM cells and RMT gene expression obtained from the sequencing dataset of PRF1, GNLY, GZMA, GZMB, GZMH and GZMM were plotted. Linear mixed effects modeling was used to investigate correlation between qRT-PCR analyzed gene expression products and lactation stage, with participant being a fixed effect. Box and whisker plots were created for gene expression products of all genes resulting from qRT-PCR analysis of HM cells taken from healthy participants. Correlations between expression of the different genes in HM cells taken from healthy participants assessed with qRT-PCR was examined using pairs plots and PCA analysis. Differences in gene expression products assessed with qRT-PCR between healthy and mastitis participants were investigated using PCA and dot plots.

3. Results

3.1. Analysis of mRNA Encoding Antimicrobial Proteins in Human Milk Cells

3.1.1. Higher Expression of Immune Cell Genes in the Mammary Gland and Milk Cells Taken during Pregnancy and Early Lactation

Analysis of a prior human mammary transcriptome dataset (GEO Series accession number GSE85494) for immune related genes perforin (PRF1), granulysin (GNLY), granzyme A, B, H and M (GZMA, GZMB, GZMH, GZMM) found the highest expression in pre-partum secretions compared with purchased resting mammary tissue (RMT) mRNA (see Section 2, RNA extraction) and human milk (HM) cells (Figure 1). Overall, the average Reads Per Kilobase per Million mapped reads (RPKM) expression of HM cells for these genes were highest in the prepartum secretions, except for PRF1 which had a similar expression in RMT. Interestingly, whilst post-partum the levels of gene expression generally decreased over the course of 12 months, it appeared there was a slight increase in the expression of GZMA, GZMB, GZMH and PRF1 from 6 to 12 months in 1–2 samples.

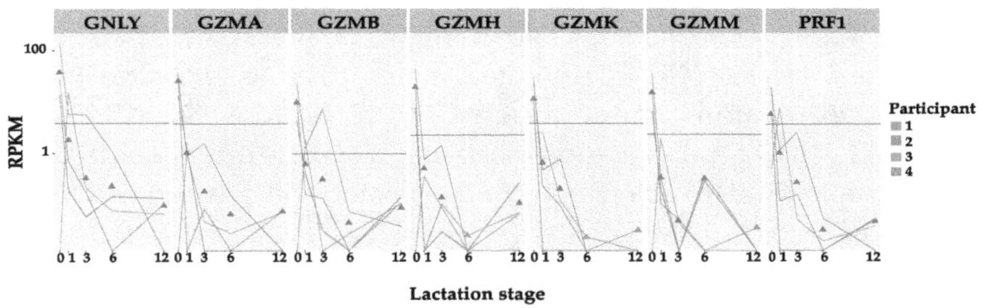

Figure 1. Expression of the genes encoding granzyme A (GZMA), granzyme B (GZMB), granzyme H (GZMH), granzyme M (GZMM), granulysin (GNLY) and perforin (PRF1) expressed in Reads Per Kilobase per Million mapped reads (RPKM) in longitudinal human milk cells (coloured lines) and pooled resting mammary tissue (RMT) (straight red line). Four lactating participants provided pre-partum secretion (PS) cells and four subsequent human milk cell samples at months 1, 3, 6 and 12 of lactation. Average expression at each time point is represented by grey triangles. In general, there is a decrease over lactation period with the highest expression in the pre-partum secretions. Moreover, PS cells show higher gene expression for all immune proteins in comparison with RMT.

3.1.2. Expression Level of Immune Protein Encoding Genes Shows Little Association with Time Post-Partum

Expression analysis of the immune cell gene products was expanded in a larger pool of participants (n = 24) who provided multiple (1–3) HM cell samples within the first six months of lactation for qRT-PCR analysis (Figure 2). A total of 65 HM cell samples from healthy participants were analysed for PRF1, GZMA, GZMB, GZMH, GZMM, GNLY, the gene encoding the immune cell marker CD45 (PTPRC) and epithelial cell adhesion marker (EPCAM). Many of the HM cell samples expressed all genes, where EPCAM was the most highly expressed gene and GZMM was the least expressed gene (Figure 2). The highest variation of gene expression between participants was found in GZMB (Figure 2, Table S3). Interestingly GZMB expression was found to be negatively associated with lactation stage (p-value 0.047, Table S4, Figure S2). GZMA, GZMH, GZMM, GNLY and PTPRC showed no association between expression levels and time post-partum (Table S4, Figure S2) whereas PRF1 had a borderline significant decrease (p-value 0.068) (Table S4). Analysis between expression of selected gene products with infant post-partum age revealed inter-individual differences, with participant as an influencing factor on the levels of gene expression.

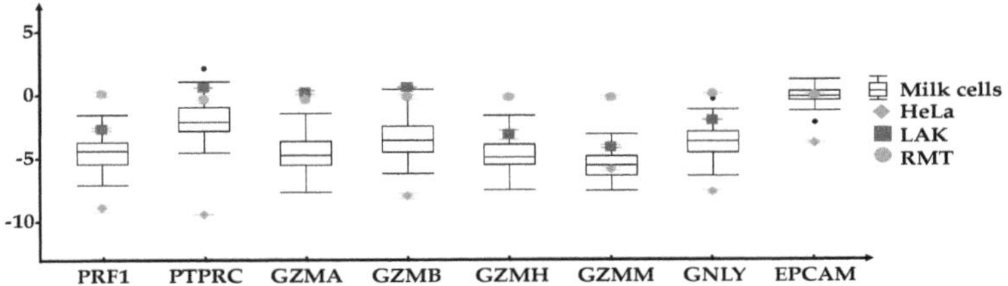

Figure 2. Box and whisker plots of the expression of the immune related genes PRF1, PTPRC, GZMA, GZMB, GZMH, GZMM, GNLY and the epithelial marker EPCAM in 65 HM cell samples (⊟). For each gene, the range of expression is shown by the whiskers of the plot and the interquartile ranges are displayed as the upper and lower sections of the boxes. The median expression in milk cells for each gene is represented by the horizontal line going through the box. In the case of milk cell outliers, these are represented by black circles. HeLa cells (◆) were used as a negative control whereas Lymphokine Activated Killer cells (LAK, ■) were a positive control for immune markers. All genes were normalized to resting mammary tissue (RMT, ●). The measured standard error of the mean for these reference samples are represented by error bars. All immune related genes were expressed in the HM cells, although in some cases having a lower expression compared to RMT and LAK.

3.1.3. Negative Association between EPCAM and Immune Markers

Principal component analysis (PCA) revealed a negative association between expression of EPCAM and the immune cell related gene products PTPRC, GZMA, GZMB, GZMH, GZMM, GNLY and PRF1 (Figure 3) with 51.3% of total variation explained by the differences in these genes (Figure 3a). Linear analysis of the markers (Figure 3b) showed an association between mRNA levels of PRF1 with GZMA (r^2 = 0.74), GZMH (r^2 = 0.72), GZMM (r^2 = 0.61), PTPRC (r^2 = 0.54) or GNLY (r^2 = 0.72). Furthermore, associations between expression of PTPRC and GZMA (r^2 = 0.58) as well as GNLY with GZMH (r^2 = 0.81) or GZMM (r^2 = 0.78) were found. There also appears to be a correlation between expression of GZMH with GZMM (r^2 = 0.71) or GZMB (r^2 = 0.51) (Figure 3b). In contrast, there is a negative association between expression of EPCAM and PTPRC (r^2 = 0.18), GNLY (r^2 = 0.19) and GZMA (r^2 = 0.22) (Figure 3b).

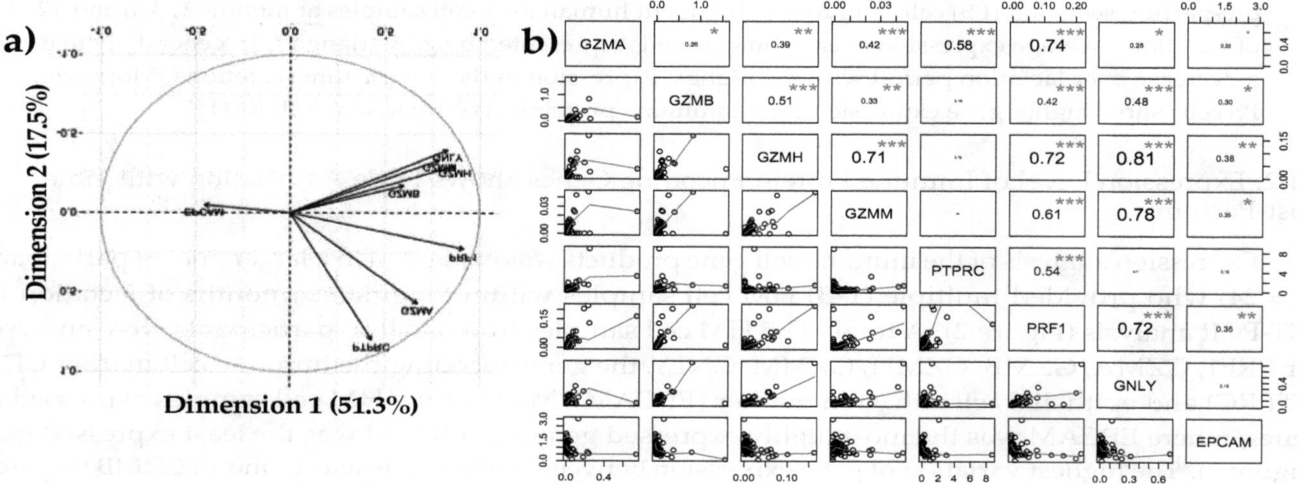

Figure 3. Associations between immune (GZMA, GZMB, GZMH, GZMM, GNLY, PRF1, PTPRC) and epithelial cell markers (EPCAM) analysed with (**a**) principal component analysis (PCA) and (**b**) Linear modelling. Half of the variation could be explained by difference between EPCAM and the immune markers. Moreover, 17.5% was due to the difference between expression of genes encoding granzyme B (GZMB), granzyme H (GZMH), granzyme M (GZMM) and granulysin (GNLY) compared to granzyme A (GZMA), perforin (PRF1) and immune cell marker PTPRC. Linear associations displayed a positive association of gene expression between PRF1 and GZMA, PRF1 and GZMB, PRF1 and PTPRC as well as between GZMA and GZMB. On the other hand a negative association exists between expression of EPCAM and GNLY. *** represents highly correlative genes (r^2 > 0.5), ** moderately correlative (0.5 > r^2 > 0.3) and * low correlation between genes (r^2 < 0.3).

3.1.4. Participants with Mastitis Show a Higher Expression of Immune Genes Compared to Healthy Participants

Three participants with mastitis (one with an abscess) provided HM cell samples from the affected breast. Moreover, two of the participants provided an additional sample from the adjacent healthy breast. Compared to the healthy breast, the two mastitis samples from the infected breast displayed a higher expression of immune cell related genes (Figure 4). There was much higher expression of PTPRC in the mastitis sample compared to the adjacent breast in both participants (Figure 4). In addition, the expression of GZMA, GZMB and PRF1 was increased in the mastitis sample of one participant when compared to the adjacent breast (Figure 4a(i)). Principal component analysis (PCA) of gene expression of all healthy and mastitic HM cell samples revealed great variation between healthy participants and the mastitis or breast abscess samples (Figure 4b).

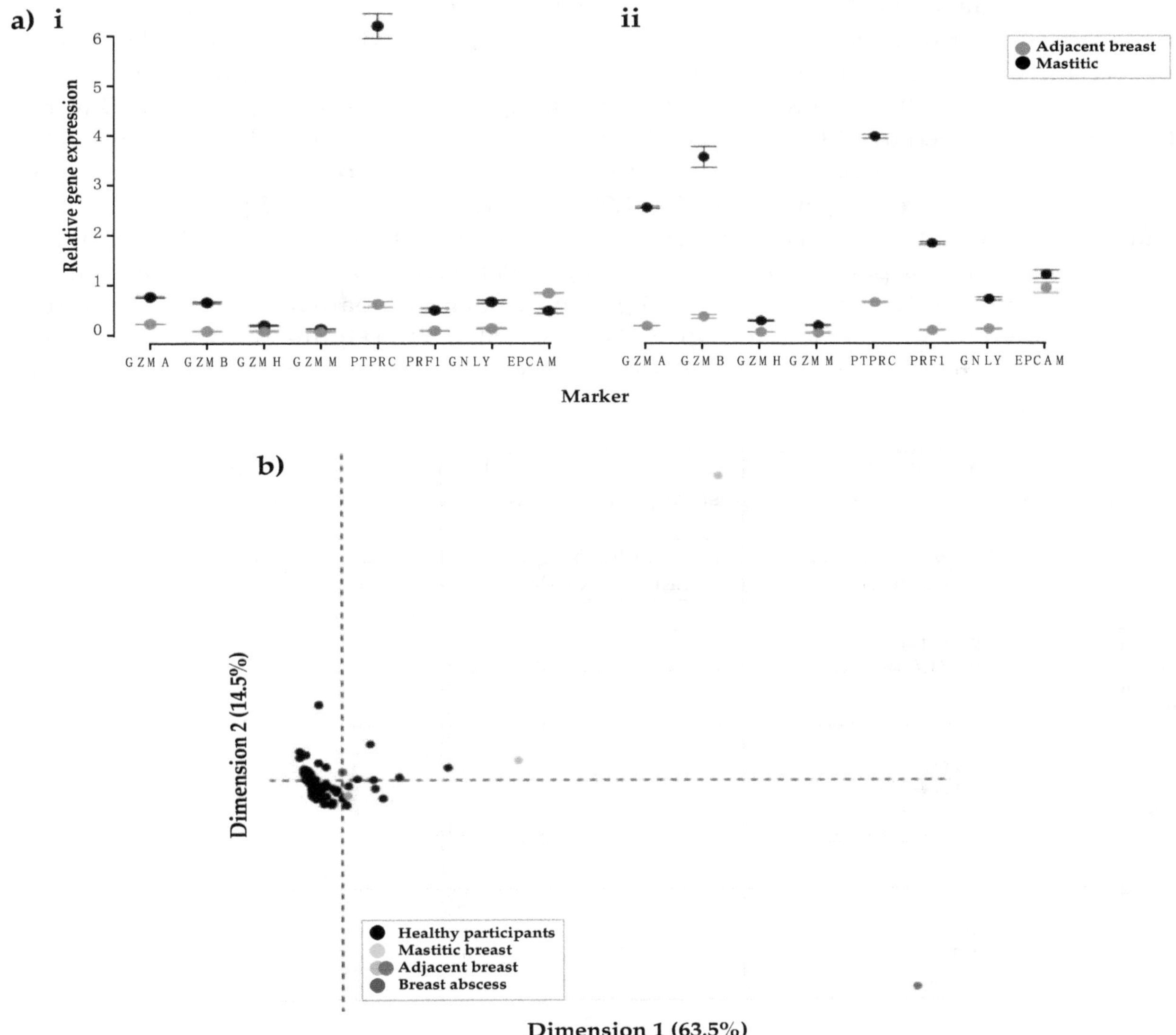

Figure 4. Comparisons of gene expression of immune genes in HM cells taken under different conditions. (**a**) Compares gene expression of HM cells taken from two participants (**i** and **ii**) with breasts affected by mastitis compared to the adjacent breast. PTPRC gene expression was upregulated in both participants (**i** and **ii**), whereas GZMA, GZMB and PRF1 was higher only in the second participant. Error bars represent the calculated standard error of the mean. (**b**) Principal component analysis (PCA) of the variance found between immune related gene expression in human milk cells taken from healthy participants compared to those from participants with mastitis or a breast abscess.

3.2. Analysis of Antimicrobial Proteins in Human Milk Cells

3.2.1. Expression at the Protein Level of All Immune Proteins in Healthy Participants

Flow cytometry was conducted to investigate the presence of the immune proteins in a healthy lactating population with infants under three months post-partum. Single cells were gated in each sample before separation into three cell populations (Figure S1). Both epithelial (EPCAM) and immune cell (CD45) markers were expressed in all samples with a median of 4.5% and 7.8% respectively, in the total cell population (Table 2). The presence of granulysin and perforin was also confirmed in all samples with a median of 1.6% and 1.4% of cells (Table 2), respectively. Granzyme A was not found in one out of eight samples, whereas granzyme B was not found in two out of twelve samples.

The median percentage of cells of healthy participants expressing granzyme A was 0.3% (Table 2). When the sample not expressing granzyme A was taken out, the median was still similar with 0.4% of cells expressing the immune protein granzyme A. In contrast, the median for granzyme B expression in all samples was 2.7% (Table 2) whereas when the samples not expressing granzyme B were taken out, the median increased to 3.01%. When looking at the different cell populations, a high presence of CD45 positive cells (51.5%) exists in cell population 1 (Table 2). Moreover this population included a large cell population expressing granzyme B (11.9%), granulysin (11.7%) and perforin (8.4%) positive cells (Table 3). Epithelial cell marker EPCAM was present in all three gated populations at a similar level (population 1: 18.2%, population 2: 20.2% and population 3: 19.9%, Table 2). All immune related proteins were more highly expressed in CD45 positive cells in comparison to EPCAM positive cells (Table 3), as shown for granzyme B (CD45: 5.2%, EPCAM: 0.5%) (Figure 5). Moreover, there seem to be a co-localization between granzyme B, granulysin and perforin with the highest percentage in population 1 (Table S5).

Table 2. Flow cytometric analysis of immune and epithelial cell proteins in HM cells (%) taken from healthy, mastitis and non-mammary post-surgery participants. Single marker expression.

	Healthy (n = 12)	Mastitis Sample (n = 1)		Non-Mammary Surgery Sample (n = 1)
	Median (Range)	Mastitis Breast	Non-Mastitic Adjacent Breast	
CD45⁺ (%)				
All single cells	7.8 (2.1–13.4)	12.2	8.4	26.7
Population 1	51.5 (1.5–66.7)	78.2	64.8	66.8
Population 2	11.8 (1.9–51.5)	69.6	73.5	71.8
Population 3	2.7 (1.2–8.7)	3.2	1.5	17.3
Granzyme A⁺ (%)				
All single cells	0.3 (0.0–10.6)		0.8	0
Population 1	1.9 (0.4–82.0)		7.1	4.3
Population 2	0.5 (0.0–19.2)		1.6	0
Population 3	0.9 (0.00–1.3)		0.4	0
Granzyme B⁺ (%)				
All single cells	2.7 (0.0–4.1)	0.4	1.2	2.6
Population 1	11.9 (0.3–39.6)	37.7	17.4	33.1
Population 2	0.8 (0.0–9.5)	1.1	1.7	7.8
Population 3	0.4 (0.0–4.3)	0.3	0.6	10.1
Granulysin⁺ (%)				
All single cells	1.6 (0.3–12.3)		1.6	2.2
Population 1	11.7 (1.2–18.8)		4.3	13
Population 2	2.0 (0.4–12.8)		4.5	12.4
Population 3	15.5 (0.6–30.3)		1.1	15.7
Perforin⁺ (%)				
All single cells	1.4 (0.5–2.5)	2.3	1.4	2.4
Population 1	8.4 (0.0–31.7)	37.4	8.6	27
Population 2	2.2 (0.5–13.9)	4.5	9.7	10.3
Population 3	1.3 (0.8–9.5)	0.3	0.6	1.1
EPCAM⁺ (%)				
All single cells	4.5 (3.8–12.8)	6.6	5.1	3.4
Population 1	18.2 (3.5–36.8)	18.2	11.4	13.4
Population 2	20.2 (5.8–26.0)	23.4	12.9	9.5
Population 3	19.9 (9.4–30.3)	19.3	16.5	7.1

3.2.2. Increased Number of Immune Cells and Higher Expression of Immune Proteins in Mastitic Milk Samples in Comparison to Healthy Milk Samples

HM cells taken from a single participant with mastitis from both the affected and tender adjacent breast were examined for protein expression of immune, antimicrobial and epithelial markers and compared to results from the healthy population (Tables 2 and 3, Figure 6). Cells taken from the mastitic breast were stained for the markers CD45, granzyme B, perforin and EPCAM due to the low cell number. CD45 positive cells were in a higher proportion in the mastitic sample (12.2% of the whole cell population, Table 2) compared to 8.4% and 7.8% in the adjacent breast and healthy population respectively (Table 2). Similarly, population 1 in healthy participant's milk showed the highest expression of immune components (Table 2). In this particular population (population 1), the mastitis sample contained a significantly higher number of CD45 positive cells (78.2%) and higher amount of granzyme B positive cells (37.7%) in comparison with the sample from the adjacent breast (64.8% $CD45^+$, 17.4% granzyme B^+) or healthy population (51.5% $CD45^+$, 11.9% granzyme B^+) (Table 2). It also appeared that the sample from the adjacent breast contained slightly higher amounts of CD45 positive cells as well as cells expressing the immune proteins granzyme A and B in comparison to the cohort of healthy population (n = 12) (Table 2). Colocalization of granzyme B and perforin in CD45 and EPCAM positive cells from population 1 is shown in Figure 6. In the mastitis sample, clear co-expression of granzyme B in CD45 cells (27.0%, Table 3) as well as perforin in CD45 cells (34.1%, Table 3) is evident. Interestingly, there was also expression of the immune proteins granzyme B (2.2%, Table 3) and perforin (2.1%, Table 3) in cells expressing the epithelial marker EPCAM.

Table 3. Flow cytometric analysis of immune and epithelial cell proteins in HM cells (%) taken from healthy, mastitis and non-mammary post-surgery participants. Double stainings between either CD45 or EPCAM positive cells and immune proteins.

	Healthy (n = 12)	**Mastitis Sample (n = 1)**		**Non-Mammary Surgery Sample (n = 1)**
	Median (Range)	**Mastitis Breast**	**Adjacent Breast**	
CD45–Granzyme A (%)				
All single cells	0.2 (0.0–14.9)		0.2	0.4
Population 1	1.0 (0.3–32.6)		10.9	5.4
Population 2	0.2 (0.0–50.0)		3.5	1.3
Population 3	0.2 (0.0–0.4)		0.2	0
CD45–Granzyme B (%)				
All single cells	0.7 (0.0–5.5)	0.5	0.4	4.4
Population 1	5.2 (0.0–26.8)	27	17.2	33.4
Population 2	0.3 (0.0–13.9)	0.3	4.2	20.3
Population 3	0.0 (0.0–0.3)	0	0.3	1.4
CD45–Granulysin (%)				
All single cells	0.7 (0.0–10.4)		0.3	4.1
Population 1	3.2 (0.8–21.1)		4.4	12.9
Population 2	3.6 (0.0–13.4)		5.8	34
Population 3	13.6 (0.2–27.1)		0.1	0.9
CD45–Perforin (%)				
All single cells	0.9 (0.6–8.3)	0.8	0.9	23.7
Population 1	11.0 (0.1–35.2)	34.1	8.2	27.7
Population 2	2.1 (0.1–26.8)	3.9	10.6	48.2
Population 3	0.7 (0.1–1.8)	0.7	0.1	4.8
EPCAM–Granzyme A (%)				
All single cells	0.0 (0.0–0.2)		0.1	0
Population 1	0.1 (0.0–35.2)		0.1	0.1
Population 2	0.4 (0.0–1.5)		0.6	0
Population 3	1.0 (0.2–1.8)		0.2	0
PCAM–Granzyme B (%)				
All single cells	0.2 (0.1–1.0)	1.3	0	1.5
Population 1	0.5 (0.3–3.5)	2.2	0.6	0.9
Population 2	1.4 (0.0–3.0)	0.3	0.5	6.1
Population 3	1.3 (0.2–2.3)	0	0.2	1.1
EPCAM–Granulysin (%)				
All single cells	0.2 (0.0–2.1)		0.1	2.4
Population 1	1.5 (0.2–3.1)		1.8	1
Population 2	0.6 (0.1–1.4)		1.4	7.9
Population 3	2.6 (0.2–5.0)		0.1	1.9
EPCAM–Perforin (%)				
All single cells	0.2 (0.0–5.5)	0.2	0.1	5.2
Population 1	3.3 (1.1–9.5)	2.1	0.5	2.2
Population 2	1.7 (0.3–8.4)	0.7	1.1	7.4
Population 3	0.4 (0.3–0.4)	0.3	0	1.8

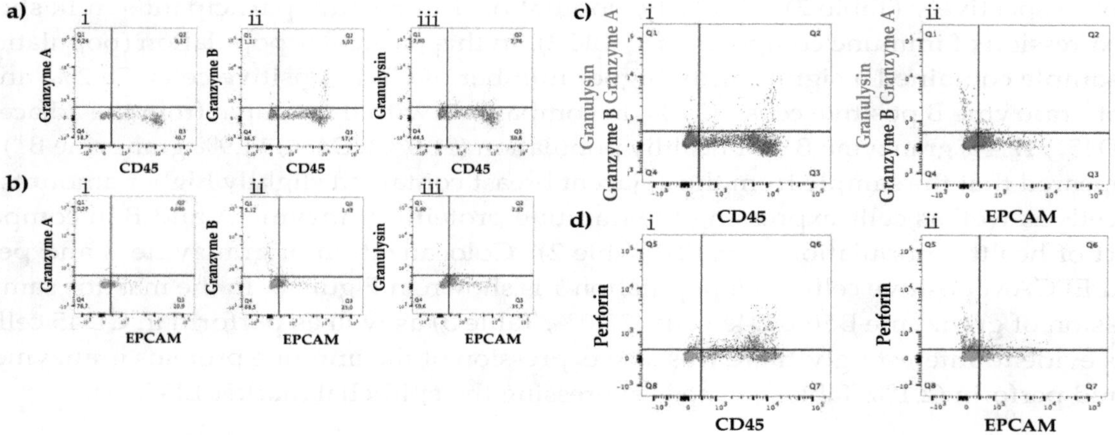

Figure 5. Co-expression of immune proteins granulysin, granzyme A, granzyme B and perforin with immune cell marker CD45 or epithelial marker EPCAM. Granzyme A, granzyme B and granulysin were all co-expressed with CD45 (0.3%, 5.0% and 2.8% respectively) positive cells (**a**(**i–iii**)), whereas little co-expression was found between the immune proteins and the epithelial cell marker EPCAM (0.1%, 1.4% and 2.8% respectively) (**b**(**i–iii**)). Superposition of the co-expression of granulysin, granzyme B and granzyme A in CD45$^+$ (**c**(**i**)) and EPCAM$^+$ (**c**(**ii**)). Perforin co-expression with CD45$^+$ (**d**(**i**)) cells at a level of 23.7% whereas only 5.2% with EPCAM$^+$ (**d**(**ii**)) cells.

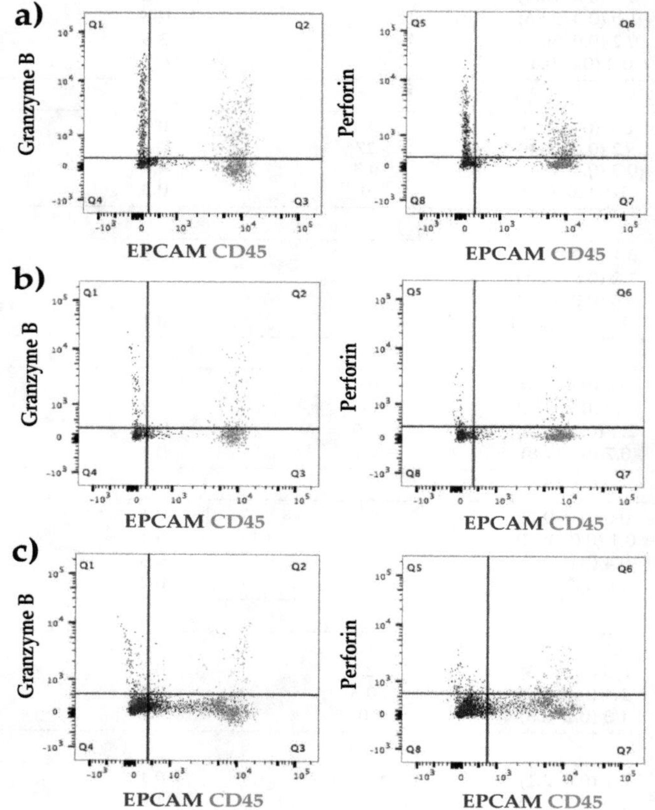

Figure 6. Flow cytometry analysis of human milk cells taken from a participant suffering from (**a**) mastitis with comparison sample of the (**b**) adjacent breast of the same participant and (**c**) compared to a healthy participant. Increased numbers of CD45 positive cells expressing of granzyme B and perforin, whereas no co-expression observed in EPCAM positive cells. Higher expression of immune proteins in CD45 cells was evident in the mastitis affected participant when compared to healthy participants.

3.2.3. Participant Recovering from Non-Mammary Surgery Shows Higher Expression of Immune Proteins Compared to Healthy Participants

HM cells (84 days post-partum) isolated from a participant recovering from a reparative surgery of the hand after a household accident, showed a higher expression of antimicrobial proteins (Figure 7) compared to the median expression of healthy HM cells (Table 2) indicative of heightened levels of activated or memory t-cells. Higher levels of granzyme B, granulysin and perforin were observed in HM cells from the participant that had undergone non-mammary surgery (Figure 7, Table 2). Curved gating was chosen for the double staining of CD45 and granzyme A, CD45 and granzyme B as well as CD45 and granulysin to better exclude the false positive measurements (Figure 7). CD45 positive cells expressed granzyme B (4.4%) as well as granulysin (4.1%) (Table 3). Similar to the mastitis sample, the presence of these immune proteins in EPCAM positive cells was minor. The same tendency is observed with perforin, where the protein was found in higher amounts in CD45 positive cells (23.7%) compared to EPCAM positive cells (5.2%) (Table 3).

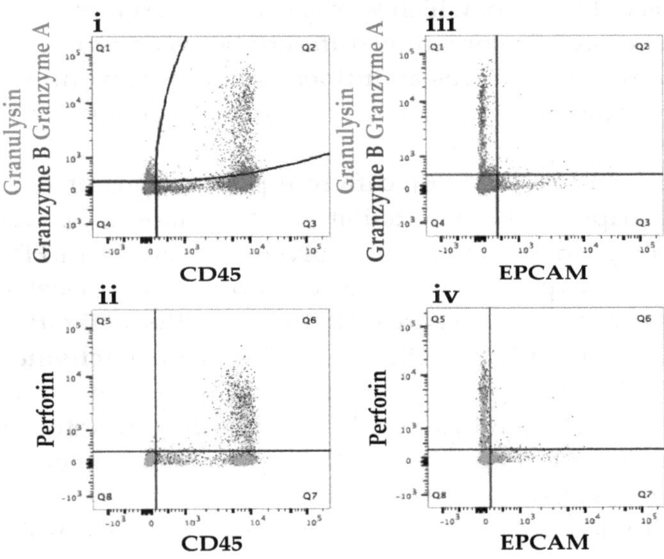

Figure 7. Expression of granzyme A, granyme B, granulysin and perforin in CD45 positive cells and EPCAM positive cells in population 1 in a participant recovering from a non-breast related surgery. Dot plots revealed increased number of CD45$^+$ cells (**i,ii**) expressing the immune proteins compared with EPCAM$^+$ cells (**iii,iv**). Expression of the immune proteins in the EPCAM positive cells was low and similar in both participant populations.

4. Discussion

Human milk is known to contain immune cells [7] and display antimicrobial properties [24], little is known about the purpose of the cells in the milk or the mechanisms involved in the antibacterial activity. To better understand the actions of immune cells in milk, this study examined the presence of the known antimicrobial proteins perforin, granzymes and granulysin in HM. This study confirms for the first time the expression of the genes GZMA, GZMB, GZMH, GZMM, GNLY and PRF1 in resting mammary tissue, prepartum secretion cells and human milk cells taken from a larger population of women at different stages of lactation. All HM cell samples within this study contained cells positive for the protein CD45 that co-stained with granulysin and perforin and in most cases for granzyme A and B. Whilst EPCAM positive cells were also identified in all samples, co-staining with the investigated immune proteins was minimal. Further investigation revealed that HM cells from participants with local or systemic inflammation had a higher protein expression of CD45 positive cells compared with healthy participants, which is consistent with data from previous studies [8]. The presence and variation of immunological factors in human milk cells in both healthy and participants with inflammation suggests a selected prevalence of activated immune T-cells in HM that also expresses the cytotoxic immune proteins, likely involved both in maternal mammary gland and overall infant protection.

Extending previous studies examining immune cells in human milk, antimicrobial proteins not previously identified in milk cells were found and varied depending on the stage of mammary gland maturation. Investigation of the immune cell related genes identified in mammary transcriptomic data revealed a similar expression pattern between milk leukocyte content and lactation stage with previous data, showing a decreased immune cell content over lactation period [3,7,8]. Pre-partum cells, resting mammary tissue extracts and milk cells at month 1 and 3 had the highest levels of perforin, granulysin and granzymes whilst lower levels were observed in milk samples of the later months. Despite this, gene expression analysis using qRT-PCR did not find a linear relationship between immune gene expression and lactation stage over the first four months except for GZMB where a significant decrease over lactation stage was found. This may reflect the elevated levels of immune cells naturally present in milk from the first 4 months of lactation, which was specifically examined in the qRT-PCR experiments or may suggest that immune protein content is different between women despite infant age in early lactation. It was found that participant was an influencing factor on antimicrobial protein expression but further investigation should consider a larger cohort of women with samples examined at the same lactation stage.

According to previous studies [3,25,26], different populations of T lymphocytes are present in the milk compared to the peripheral blood circulation. Associations between the expression of PRF1 and the genes encoding for granzymes and granulysin (Figure 3) in HM cells supports previous findings identifying increased expression of effector and memory T-cells in HM in comparison to peripheral blood [25,27], as these proteins are only present after activation of the lymphocytes [28]. Further investigations should include specific antibodies against activated T lymphocytes markers such as CD45RO+ or HLA-DR [29]. A linear association analysis of the immune related gene products showed a positive correlation between PRF1 and the genes encoding for granzymes and granulysin. This observation could mean that the expression of these proteins might be linked, possibly by the same expression control mechanisms. Co-expression of perforin with granulysin and granzymes in CD45 positive HM cells found with flow cytometry also confirms this theory as the efficiency of the proteins is higher when all three proteins are working together [11,12]. Surprisingly, some co-expression was found between EPCAM and the immune proteins (Figure 6) which may indicate low level expression of immune proteins in epithelial cells, epithelial cell uptake of exocytosed cytotoxic granules from activated leukocytes [28,30] or low levels of cell aggregates in the FACS data. Future studies should further investigate the presence of immunological proteins in epithelial cells or whether granules containing immune proteins are released into the milk in cases of infection. Results from this study suggest that leukocytes in the milk are increased not only in the case of mammary inflammation but also in the case of systemic inflammation.

Investigated immune components (cells and immune proteins) were not only more prevalent in HM taken from the breast affected by mastitis but also in the adjacent breast. Interestingly immune components were also elevated in a participant who had undergone non-mammary surgery, compared to HM cells from healthy participants. Mastitis, being an infection of the breast tissue [8], creates a local inflammation and a systemic response leading to an increase of circulating immune cells in the blood [31]. Consequently, a higher quantity of lymphocytes infiltrating mammary tissue likely being the cause of heightened immune cells in the milk during mastitis [8]. As shown by flow cytometry, there were a heightened number of CD45 positive HM cells with co-expression of granzymes, granulysin and perforin from a participant with mastitis (Figure 6). As mastitis is usually a bacterial infection, the increased presence of immune cells and increased expression of antimicrobial proteins having an antibacterial effect was an expected outcome. In addition, elevated levels of CD45 cells with co-expression of the investigated immune proteins was also found in the milk obtained from the non-mastitic adjacent breast, although they were at much lower levels (Figure 6). The presence of immune related proteins in healthy participants, may suggest that they might not only play a role in the fight against an infection, but also in the prevention of one. This indicates that immune cells may not only have a role in the development of the immune system of the infant [32], but also in the protection of the lactating breast [3]. Follow-up studies should consider including complimentary blood samples alongside with milk to have an appropriate comparison point between milk and blood leukocytes.

5. Conclusions

This study showed for the first time the expression of the antimicrobial proteins perforin, granulysin and different granzymes at the protein and mRNA level in HM cells, RMT and PS cells. Furthermore, it provided confirmation that HM from healthy women is enriched in cells that carry hallmarks of activated or memory T-cells, which are elevated in case of maternal infection. Presence of these cells may indicate a purpose in the protection of the vulnerable infant or as a mechanism to defend the maternal breast against infection however further investigations should done to clarify this.

Supplementary Materials:
Figure S1: Gating around single cells using forward scatter area (FSC-A) and forward scatter height (FSC-H). Three populations were then gated using only single cells. Figure S2: Relative quantitation (RQ) of the expression of the epithelial marker EPCAM, the immune cell marker PTPRC and the genes coding for granzyme A (GZMA), granzyme B (GZMB), granzyme H (GZMH), granzyme M (GZMM), granulysin (GNLY) and perforin (PRF1) distributed according to the time period post-partum. Table S1: Taqman probes from Life Technologies. Table S2: Antibodies used for FACS analysis. Table S3: Expression of selected genes in human milk cells (HMC) measured via RT-PCR, normalised to either lymphokine activated killer cells (LAK) or resting tissue (RT). Table S4: Univariate linear mixed modelling of days post-partum and antimicrobial protein genes, with participant as an influencing factor on gene expression. Table S5: Flow cytometric analysis of immune and epithelial cell proteins in HM cells (%) taken from healthy, mastitis and non-related surgical patient participants.

Author Contributions: Conceptualization, G.K.K., A.-J.T., D.T.G. and L.F.; Data curation, A.-J.T.; Formal analysis, G.K.K.; Funding acquisition, D.T.G. and L.F.; Investigation, G.K.K., A.-J.T. and L.F.; Methodology, G.K.K. and A.-J.T.; Project administration, A.-J.T., D.T.G. and L.F.; Resources, D.T.G. and L.F.; Supervision, A.-J.T., D.T.G. and L.F.; Visualization, G.K.K.; Writing–original draft, G.K.K. and A.-J.T.; Writing–review & editing, G.K. K., A.-J.T., D.T.G. and L.F.

Acknowledgments: Many thanks to the Australian Breastfeeding Association for their support and to all participating mothers of the study. The Centre for Microscopy, Characterisation & Analysis (UWA) provided access to facilities and technical assistance. Many thanks to Solange Kharoubi-Hess, Alethea Rea and Michelle Trevenen for their technical and statistical support.

References

1. Hale, T.W.; Hartmann, P.E. *Textbook of Human Lactation*, 1st ed.; Hale Publishing L.P.: Amarillo, TX, USA, 2007; p. 662.
2. Hanson, L.; Silfverdal, S.A.; Stromback, L.; Erling, V.; Zaman, S.; Olcen, P.; Telemo, E. The immunological role of breast feeding. *Pediatr. Allergy Immunol.* **2001**, *12* (Suppl. S14), 15–19. [CrossRef]
3. Hassiotou, F.; Geddes, D.T. Immune cell-mediated protection of the mammary gland and the infant during breastfeeding. *Adv. Nutr.* **2015**, *6*, 267–275. [CrossRef] [PubMed]
4. Liepke, C.; Zucht, H.D.; Forssmann, W.G.; Standker, L. Purification of novel peptide antibiotics from human milk. *J. Chromatogr. B Biomed. Sci. Appl.* **2001**, *752*, 369–377. [CrossRef]
5. Zhang, F.; Cui, X.; Fu, Y.; Zhang, J.; Zhou, Y.; Sun, Y.; Wang, X.; Li, Y.; Liu, Q.; Chen, T. Antimicrobial activity and mechanism of the human milk-sourced peptide casein201. *Biochem. Biophys. Res. Commun.* **2017**, *485*, 698–704. [CrossRef] [PubMed]

6. Hanson, L.A.; Korotkova, M.; Lundin, S.; Haversen, L.; Silfverdal, S.A.; Mattsby-Baltzer, I.; Strandvik, B.; Telemo, E. The transfer of immunity from mother to child. *Ann. N. Y. Acad. Sci.* **2003**, *987*, 199–206. [CrossRef] [PubMed]
7. Hassiotou, F.; Geddes, D.T.; Hartmann, P.E. Cells in human milk: State of the science. *J. Hum. Lact.* **2013**, *29*, 171–182. [CrossRef] [PubMed]
8. Hassiotou, F.; Hepworth, A.R.; Metzger, P.; Tat Lai, C.; Trengove, N.; Hartmann, P.E.; Filgueira, L. Maternal and infant infections stimulate a rapid leukocyte response in breastmilk. *Clin. Transl. Immunol.* **2013**, 2. [CrossRef] [PubMed]
9. Xu, Q.; Abdubek, P.; Astakhova, T.; Axelrod, H.L.; Bakolitsa, C.; Cai, X.; Carlton, D.; Chen, C.; Chiu, H.J.; Clayton, T.; et al. Structure of a membrane-attack complex/perforin (macpf) family protein from the human gut symbiont bacteroides thetaiotaomicron. *Acta Crystallogr. Sect. F Struct. Biol. Cryst. Commun.* **2010**, *66*, 1297–1305. [CrossRef] [PubMed]
10. Nobre, T.M.; Martynowycz, M.W.; Andreev, K.; Kuzmenko, I.; Nikaido, H.; Gidalevitz, D. Modification of salmonella lipopolysaccharides prevents the outer membrane penetration of novobiocin. *Biophys. J.* **2015**, *109*, 2537–2545. [CrossRef] [PubMed]
11. Walch, M.; Dotiwala, F.; Mulik, S.; Thiery, J.; Kirchhausen, T.; Clayberger, C.; Krensky, A.M.; Martinvalet, D.; Lieberman, J. Cytotoxic cells kill intracellular bacteria through granulysin-mediated delivery of granzymes. *Cell* **2014**, *157*, 1309–1323. [CrossRef] [PubMed]
12. Dotiwala, F.; Mulik, S.; Polidoro, R.B.; Ansara, J.A.; Burleigh, B.A.; Walch, M.; Gazzinelli, R.T.; Lieberman, J. Killer lymphocytes use granulysin, perforin and granzymes to kill intracellular parasites. *Nat. Med.* **2016**, *22*, 210–216. [CrossRef] [PubMed]
13. Lieberman, J. Granzyme a activates another way to die. *Immunol. Rev.* **2010**, *235*, 93–104. [CrossRef] [PubMed]
14. Stenger, S.; Hanson, D.A.; Teitelbaum, R.; Dewan, P.; Niazi, K.R.; Froelich, C.J.; Ganz, T.; Thoma-Uszynski, S.; Melian, A.; Bogdan, C.; et al. An antimicrobial activity of cytolytic t cells mediated by granulysin. *Science* **1998**, *282*, 121–125. [CrossRef] [PubMed]
15. Bryan, D.L.; Hart, P.H.; Forsyth, K.D.; Gibson, R.A. Immunomodulatory constituents of human milk change in response to infant bronchiolitis. *Pediatr. Allergy Immunol.* **2007**, *18*, 495–502. [CrossRef] [PubMed]
16. Twigger, A.J.; Kakulas, F. RNA-Sequencing of Milk Cells Extracted from Pre-Partum Secretions and Longitudinally from Mature Human Milk accros the First Year of Lactation. NCBI: Gene Expression Omnibus, 2016. Available online: https://www.ncbi.nlm.nih.gov/geo/ (accessed on 25 August 2016).
17. Twigger, A.J.; Hepworth, A.R.; Lai, C.T.; Chetwynd, E.; Stuebe, A.M.; Blancafort, P.; Hartmann, P.E.; Geddes, D.T.; Kakulas, F. Gene expression in breastmilk cells is associated with maternal and infant characteristics. *Sci. Rep.* **2015**, *5*. [CrossRef] [PubMed]
18. Hassiotou, F.; Beltran, A.; Chetwynd, E.; Stuebe, A.M.; Twigger, A.J.; Metzger, P.; Trengove, N.; Lai, C.T.; Filgueira, L.; Blancafort, P.; et al. Breastmilk is a novel source of stem cells with multilineage differentiation potential. *Stem Cells* **2012**, *30*, 2164–2174. [CrossRef] [PubMed]
19. Mortazavi, A.; Williams, B.A.; McCue, K.; Schaeffer, L.; Wold, B. Mapping and quantifying mammalian transcriptomes by rna-seq. *Nat. Methods* **2008**, *5*, 621–628. [CrossRef] [PubMed]
20. Wickham, H. *Ggplot2: Elegant Graphics for Data Analysis*; Springer: New York, NY, USA, 2009.
21. Sarkar, D. *Lattice: Multivariate Data Visualization with R*; Springer: New York, NY, USA, 2008.
22. Pinheiro, J.; Bates, D.; DebRoy, S.; Sarkar, D.; Team, R.C. Nlme: Linear and Nonlinear Mixed Effects Models. R Package Version 3.1-131 2017. Available online: https://mran.microsoft.com/snapshot/2017-02-20/web/packages/nlme/index.html (accessed on 20 February 2017).
23. Lê, S.; Josse, J.; Husson, F. Factominer: An r package for multivariate analysis. *J. Stat. Softw.* **2008**, *25*, 1–18. [CrossRef]
24. Chirico, G.; Marzollo, R.; Cortinovis, S.; Fonte, C.; Gasparoni, A. Antiinfective properties of human milk. *J. Nutr.* **2008**, *138*, 1801s–1806s. [CrossRef] [PubMed]
25. Sabbaj, S.; Ghosh, M.K.; Edwards, B.H.; Leeth, R.; Decker, W.D.; Goepfert, P.A.; Aldrovandi, G.M. Breast milk-derived antigen-specific cd8+ t cells: An extralymphoid effector memory cell population in humans. *J. Immunol.* **2005**, *174*, 2951–2956. [CrossRef] [PubMed]
26. Wirt, D.P.; Adkins, L.T.; Palkowetz, K.H.; Schmalstieg, F.C.; Goldman, A.S. Activated and memory t lymphocytes in human milk. *Cytometry* **1992**, *13*, 282–290. [CrossRef] [PubMed]

27. Peroni, D.G.; Chirumbolo, S.; Veneri, D.; Piacentini, G.L.; Tenero, L.; Vella, A.; Ortolani, R.; Raffaelli, R.; Boner, A.L. Colostrum-derived b and t cells as an extra-lymphoid compartment of effector cell populations in humans. *J. Matern. Fetal Neonatal Med.* **2013**, *26*, 137–142. [CrossRef] [PubMed]
28. Cullen, S.P.; Martin, S.J. Mechanisms of granule-dependent killing. *Cell Death Differ.* **2007**, *15*, 251–262. [CrossRef] [PubMed]
29. Costello, P.; Bresnihan, B.; O'Farrelly, C.; FitzGerald, O. Predominance of cd8+ t lymphocytes in psoriatic arthritis. *J. Rheumatol.* **1999**, *26*, 1117–1124. [PubMed]
30. Veugelers, K.; Motyka, B.; Goping, I.S.; Shostak, I.; Sawchuk, T.; Bleackley, R.C. Granule-mediated killing by granzyme b and perforin requires a mannose 6-phosphate receptor and is augmented by cell surface heparan sulfate. *Mol. Biol. Cell* **2006**, *17*, 623–633. [CrossRef] [PubMed]
31. Coutinho, A.E.; Chapman, K.E. The anti-inflammatory and immunosuppressive effects of glucocorticoids, recent developments and mechanistic insights. *Mol. Cell. Endocrinol.* **2011**, *335*, 2–13. [CrossRef] [PubMed]
32. Field, C.J. The immunological components of human milk and their effect on immune development in infants. *J. Nutr.* **2005**, *135*, 1–4. [CrossRef] [PubMed]

11

Breastfeeding Difficulties and Risk for Early Breastfeeding Cessation

Maria Lorella Gianni [1,2,*], Maria Enrica Bettinelli [2], Priscilla Manfra [1], Gabriele Sorrentino [1], Elena Bezze [1], Laura Plevani [1], Giacomo Cavallaro [1], Genny Raffaeli [1], Beatrice Letizia Crippa [1,2], Lorenzo Colombo [1], Daniela Morniroli [1,2], Nadia Liotto [1,2], Paola Roggero [1,2], Eduardo Villamor [3], Paola Marchisio [4,5] and Fabio Mosca [1,2]

1 Fondazione IRCCS Ca' Granda Ospedale Maggiore Policlinico, NICU, via Commenda 12, 20122 Milan, Italy; priscilla.manfra@gmail.com (P.M.); gabriele.sorrentino@mangiagalli.it (G.S.); elena.bezze@policlinico.mi.it (E.B.); laura.plevani@mangiagalli.it (L.P.); giacomo.cavallaro@mangiagalli.it (G.C.); genny.raffaeli@gmail.com (G.R.); beatriceletizia.crippa@gmail.com (B.L.C.); lorenzo.colombo@policlinico.mi.it (L.C.); daniela.morniroli@gmail.com (D.M.); nadia.liotto@mangiagalli.it (N.L.); paola.roggero@unimi.it (P.R.); fabio.mosca@mangiagalli.it (F.M.)

2 Department of Clinical Sciences and Community Health, University of Milan, Via San Barnaba 8, 20122 Milan, Italy; maria.bettinelli@unimi.it

3 Department of Pediatrics, Maastricht University Medical Center (MUMC+), School for Oncology and Developmental Biology (GROW), 6202 AZ Maastricht, The Netherlands; e.villamor@mumc.nl

4 Fondazione IRCCS Ca' Granda Ospedale Maggiore Policlinico, 20122 Milan, Italy; paola.marchisio@unimi.it

5 Department of Pathophysiology and Transplantation, University of Milan, 20122 Milan, Italy

* Correspondence: maria.gianni@unimi.it

Abstract: Although breast milk is the normative feeding for infants, breastfeeding rates are lower than recommended. We investigated breastfeeding difficulties experienced by mothers in the first months after delivery and their association with early breastfeeding discontinuation. We conducted a prospective observational study. Mothers breastfeeding singleton healthy term newborns at hospital discharge were enrolled and, at three months post-delivery, were administered a questionnaire on their breastfeeding experience. Association among neonatal/maternal characteristics, breastfeeding difficulties and support after hospital discharge, and type of feeding at three months was assessed using multivariate binary logistic regression analysis. We enrolled 792 mothers, 552 completed the study. Around 70.3% of mothers experienced breastfeeding difficulties, reporting cracked nipples, perception of insufficient amount of milk, pain, and fatigue. Difficulties occurred mostly within the first month. Half of mothers with breastfeeding issues felt well-supported by health professionals. Maternal perception of not having a sufficient amount of milk, infant's failure to thrive, mastitis, and the return to work were associated with a higher risk of non-exclusive breastfeeding at three months whereas vaginal delivery and breastfeeding support after hospital discharge were associated with a decreased risk. These results underline the importance of continued, tailored professional breastfeeding support.

Keywords: breastfeeding difficulties; early breastfeeding cessation; term infants; breastfeeding support

---

1. Introduction

Breastfeeding is associated with improvement of infants' survival and significant health benefits both for infants and mothers in a dose-response manner [1–3]. Consequently, promotion and support of breastfeeding initiation, duration, and exclusivity is a public health issue. However, the worldwide rates of breastfeeding are lower than international recommendations, especially in high-income countries [4]. Therefore, there is a need for increasing the health care professionals' awareness of the intrinsic factors associated with early breastfeeding cessation and for gaining further insight into the related modifiable risk factors [5]. Several determinants of breastfeeding have been described within a complex framework, including structural settings and individual factors that are involved at multiple levels [6]. Among the individual factors, the experience of breastfeeding difficulties greatly contributes to early breastfeeding cessation and causes mothers to be less likely to breastfeed a future child [7]. However, "breastfeeding difficulties" includes a wide range of different biological, psychological, and social factors [8]. Unpacking this issue to gain further insight into the modifiable barriers mothers experience during breastfeeding may help health professionals in overcoming them and in refining community support [5].

The aim of the present study was to investigate the breastfeeding difficulties experienced by mothers of healthy, singleton term-born infants in the first months after delivery and their association with early breastfeeding discontinuation.

2. Materials and Methods

We conducted a prospective, observational study in the nursery of Fondazione IRCCS Ca' Granda Ospedale Maggiore Policlinico in Milan, Lombardy, Italy. The hospital is a Level III center for neonatal care that covers around 6000 deliveries per year, admitting pregnant women prevalently resident in Lombardy but also those resident in other Italian regions.

All subjects gave their informed consent for inclusion before they participated in the study. The study was conducted in accordance with the Declaration of Helsinki, and the protocol was approved by the Ethics Committee of Milano (Comitato Etico Milano Area 2, n. 0120, atti n. 1580/2018).

Mothers with a low risk for early breastfeeding cessation, that is having delivered singleton, healthy, term (gestational age ≥37 weeks) newborns with the birthweight ≥10th percentile for gestational age, according to the Bertino's neonatal growth chart [9], and breastfeeding were enrolled at hospital discharge, which occurred within the completion of the first 72 h after delivery. Exclusion criteria included exclusive formula feeding, multiple pregnancy, non-Italian speaking mothers due to fact that the language barrier could have interfered with the accuracy of the answers, and mothers whose newborns were admitted to Neonatal Intensive Care Unit and/or were affected by any condition that could interfere with breastfeeding, such as congenital diseases, chromosomal abnormalities, lung disease, brain disease, metabolic disease, cardiac disease, or gastrointestinal diseases. Breastfeeding was promoted and supported in all mother-infant pairs throughout the hospital stay, following the Ten Steps to Successful Breastfeeding [10]. Socio-demographic maternal variables (age, marital status, education, mode of delivery, parity), basic infants' characteristics (gestational age, birth weight, length, head circumference, Apgar score), and the infants' mode of feeding at hospital discharge were collected. At discharge, mothers were instructed to record in a diary their infant's mode of feeding at seven days, one month, and three months after delivery. The mode of feeding was categorized according to the World Health Organization definition [11] as exclusive breastfeeding (infants are fed only breast milk and no other food or drink; not even water; oral rehydration solutions, drops and syrups such as vitamins, minerals and medicines are permitted); predominant breastfeeding (breast milk is the infant's predominant source of nourishment but liquids such as water and water-based drinks are permitted); complementary feeding (infants are mainly breastfed but also consume formula milk and other liquid or non-dairy foods); and exclusive formula feeding.

At three months post-delivery, mothers were contacted by phone in order to collect the recorded infant feeding data, and were reminded to access and complete the online questionnaire investigating their breastfeeding experience following hospital discharge within the subsequent 48 h. Specifically, mothers were asked whether they had encountered any difficulty with regard to breastfeeding. If the mothers answered yes, they had to report which difficulties they had encountered during their breastfeeding experience, when the encountered difficulties had arisen (discharge–1st month after delivery, 1st month–2nd month after delivery, 2nd month–3rd month after delivery) and how they had been solved. Mothers were also required to rate the breastfeeding support they had received by health care professionals after hospital discharge (excellent, very good, satisfactory, poor, very poor, or unacceptable).

Statistical Analysis

Data are presented as mean (SD) or number of observations (%). For analysis, maternal age was divided into two categories based on the median value; maternal educational age was categorized as ≤13 years or >13 years, while breastfeeding support after discharge was considered positive if mothers rated it either as excellent, very good, or satisfactory and negative if the mothers rated it either as poor, very poor or unacceptable. Mode of feeding was categorized as exclusive breastfeeding vs. non-exclusive breastfeeding. The latter category included complementary feeding and exclusive formula feeding. Association between socio-demographic characteristics, the mode of delivery, parity, the occurrence of breastfeeding difficulties at any time point of the study, having been supported after hospital discharge and the mode of infant's feeding at three months (reference group: non-exclusive breastfeeding) were first assessed using univariate binary logistic regression analysis. A multivariate binary logistic regression analysis was then conducted in order to identify which breastfeeding difficulties arisen through the study period were independently associated with the type of feeding at three months. When adjusting the model, we included the items that showed a significant association with type of feeding at univariate analysis. Statistical significance was set at the $\alpha = 0.05$ level. The statistical analyses were performed using SPSS (version 12, SPSS, Inc., Chicago, IL, USA).

3. Results

Of the 1843 mothers who delivered during the study period, 868 were eligible for the study. A total of 76 mothers refused to participate and 792 mother-infant pairs were enrolled. Among these, 552 (70%) completed the study and the online questionnaire whereas the remaining 240 mothers did not complete either the study or the online questionnaire since it was not possible to reach them by telephone after hospital discharge.

Basic characteristics of mother-infant pairs which completed the study are summarized in Table 1. Mother-infant pairs that have not completed the study did not significantly differ from the ones completing the study.

Table 1. Basic characteristics of the mother-infant pairs that completed ($n = 552$) and that not completed (240) the study.

Mothers that Completed the Study ($n = 552$)		Mothers Who did not Complete the Study ($n = 240$)
Maternal age, years (mean ± SD)	35.5 ± 4.6	34.9 ± 4.6
Marital status, n (%)		
Married or cohabitant	540 (98)	237 (99)
Single or divorced	12 (2)	3 (1)
Maternal education level, n (%)		
≤13 years	150 (27)	75 (31)
>13 years	402 (73)	165 (69)
Vaginal delivery, n (%)	369 (66.8)	157 (65.4)
Primiparous, n (%)	290 (52.5)	138 (57.5)

Table 1. *Cont.*

Mothers that Completed the Study (n = 552)		Mothers Who did not Complete the Study (n = 240)
Infants Born to Mothers that had Completed the Study (n = 552)		**Infants Born to Mothers Who did not Complete the Study (n = 240)**
Gestational age, weeks (mean ± SD)	39.2 ± 1.0	39.3 ± 0.9
Birth weight, g (mean ± SD)	3368 ± 350	3390 ± 332
Length, cm (mean ± SD)	50.1 ± 1.6	50.3 ± 1.5
Head circumference, cm (mean ± SD)	34.5 ± 1.4	34.3 ± 1.3

The mode of feeding at each time point of the study is reported in Table 2. At enrollment, 95% of the mothers practiced exclusive breastfeeding, whereas 5% of the mothers practiced complementary feeding. At one and three months, exclusive breastfeeding rates declined to 73% and 68%, respectively, whereas complementary feeding rates were 20% and 15%, respectively. Percentage of infants receiving exclusive formula feeding was 7% at one month, increasing up to 17% at three months.

Table 2. Mode of feeding at each time point of the study.

	Enrollment	Seven Days	One Month	Three Months
Exclusive breastfeeding	524 (95%)	447 (81%)	402 (73%)	375 (68%)
Predominant breastfeeding	0%	5 (1%)	5 (1%)	5 (1%)
Complementary feeding	28 (5%)	99 (18%)	105 (19%)	77 (14%)
Exclusive formula feeding	0%	0%	39 (7%)	94 (17%)

A total of 388 (70.3%) mothers experienced difficulties during breastfeeding. The difficulties most frequently reported by the mothers were cracked nipples, the perception of insufficient amount of milk, pain, and fatigue (Table 3).

Table 3. Breastfeeding difficulties arisen at any time point of the study according to mothers' experience.

Breastfeeding Difficulties	*N* (%)
Cracked nipples	159 (41.0)
Perception of an insufficient amount of milk	139 (35.8)
Pain not associated with cracked nipples	121 (31.2)
Fatigue	117 (30.2)
Breast engorgement	102 (26.3)
Infant's failure to thrive	79 (20.4)
Incorrect latching	74 (19.1)
Perception of own's milk limited nutritional value	68 (17.5)
Mastitis	27 (7.0)
Return to work	17 (4.4)
Prescription drugs	8 (2.1)

Most of the mothers (63%) reported the occurrence of difficulties within the first month after delivery whereas, in the second and third month after delivery, difficulties were experienced only by 9% and 10% of the enrolled mothers, respectively. A total of 189 (48.7%) mothers among those that have encountered difficulties in breastfeeding reported they were successfully supported by health professionals, whereas 78 (20.1%) mothers solved the difficulties by themselves and 45 (11.6%) mothers with the support of friends or relatives. Difficulties were not solved in 19.6% of cases; however, 7% of these latter mothers kept on breastfeeding.

After hospital discharge, the breastfeeding support received by health professionals was rated as either excellent, very good, or satisfactory in most cases (86.1%) whereas only in the 13.9% of cases the breastfeeding support was reported as either poor, very poor, or unacceptable. The mothers who rated the breastfeeding support after hospital discharge as negative were at higher risk of non-exclusive breastfeeding at three months than the mothers that rated the support after hospital discharge as positive (OR = 1.367, 95%CI 1.09–1.70, $p = 0.005$).

Univariate analysis showed that the absence of breastfeeding difficulties and having been supported in case of difficulties were significantly associated with a lower risk of non-exclusive breastfeeding at three months (OR = 0.051; 95% CI 0.022; 0.117, $p < 0.0001$; OR = 0.39; 95% CI 0.202–0.756, $p = 0.005$, respectively). When taking into account the type of breastfeeding difficulties, the perception of not having enough milk, pain perception, infant's failure to thrive, the perception of milk's limited nutritional value, the occurrence of mastitis, and the return to work were associated with a higher risk of non-exclusive breastfeeding at three months (Table 4). Primiparity and an incorrect latching tended to be associated with a higher risk of non-exclusive breastfeeding at three months whereas vaginal delivery resulted in being associated with a lower risk (Table 4). No significant association was found between maternal education level and age, breast engorgement, cracked nipples, fatigue, prescription drugs, and the infant's mode of feeding (Table 4).

Table 4. Association among maternal age and education, the mode of delivery, parity, and types of breastfeeding difficulties and the mode of infant's feeding at three months (univariate binary logistic regression analysis).

Reference Group: Non-Exclusive Breastfeeding			
	OR	**95%; CI**	***p***
Maternal age (≤35 vs. >35 years)	1.02	0.711; 1.465	0.913
Maternal education (≤13 vs. >13 years)	0.67	0.237; 1.93	0.465
Mode of delivery (spontaneous vs. caesarean delivery)	0.60	0.415; 0.881	0.009
Parity (primiparous vs. multiparous)	1.42	0.988; 2.051	0.058
Cracked nipples (yes vs. no)	1.38	0.933; 2.042	0.107
Perception of not having enough milk (yes vs. no)	9.23	5.961; 14.301	<0.0001
Pain not associated with cracked nipples (yes vs. no)	1.62	1.066; 2.487	0.024
Fatigue (yes vs. no)	1.22	0.790; 1.903	0.363
Breast engorgement (yes vs. no)	0.87	0.545; 1,412	0.590
Infant's failure to thrive (yes vs. no)	5.136	3.094; 8.525	<0.0001
Incorrect latching (yes vs. no)	1.58	0.949; 2.635	0.078
Perception of milk's limited nutritional value (yes vs. no)	3.44	2.015; 5.898	<0.0001
Mastitis (yes vs. no)	2.49	1.144; 5.420	0.022
Return to work (yes vs. no)	7.65	2.457; 23.830	<0.0001
Prescription drugs (yes vs. no)	2.29	0.266; 19.761	0.452

Multivariate binary logistic regression showed that the maternal perception of not having a sufficient amount of milk, infant's failure to thrive, mastitis, and the return to work were associated with a higher risk of non-exclusive breastfeeding at three months whereas vaginal delivery and breastfeeding support after hospital discharge were associated with a decreased risk (Table 5).

Table 5. Association among the mode of delivery, having been supported after discharge, the types of breastfeeding difficulties and the mode of infant's feeding at three months (multivariate binary logistic regression analysis).

	Reference Group: Non-Exclusive Breastfeeding			
	B	OR	95%; CI	*p*
Mode of delivery (spontaneous vs. caesarean delivery)	−0.57	0.56	0.329; 0.961	0.035
Having been supported after hospital discharge (yes vs. no)	−1.28	0.27	0.130; 0.594	0.001
Perception of not having enough milk (yes vs. no)	1.96	7.15	4.096; 12.499	<0.0001
Pain not associated with cracked nipples (yes vs. no)	0.25	1.29	0.737; 2.265	0.37
Infant's failure to thrive (yes vs. no)	1.00	2.73	1.441; 5.180	0.002
Perception of milk's limited nutritional value (yes vs. no)	0.59	1.81	0.912; 3.607	0.089
Mastitis (yes vs. no)	1.07	2.92	1.166; 7.314	0.022
Return to work (yes vs. no)	1.63	5.136	1.046; 25.204	0.044

4. Discussion

Increasing awareness of the modifiable barriers experienced by mothers during breastfeeding may help health professionals in the detection of mothers at risk for early cessation of breastfeeding and the implementation of targeted breastfeeding support [12,13].

Our findings contribute to the understanding of the specific breastfeeding difficulties experienced by mothers with a low risk for early breastfeeding cessation, which appear to be related to several major areas, including lactational, nutritional, psychosocial, lifestyle, and medical factors, towards which breastfeeding promotion and support at the community level should be directed. Indeed, although in our study, the mother–infant dyads were enrolled in only one hospital, the present results reflect the primary care provided by the national "family pediatrics" network at the community level since, according to the Italian Public Health Care System, all patients aged 0–16 years must have an identified primary care provider among those available in the different regional health districts [14].

The perception of not having enough milk, the infant's failure to thrive, and mastitis are well-known factors acting negatively on breastfeeding [15–19], according to our results. Moreover, in this study, the return to work was associated with early exclusive breastfeeding failure. As previously described, balancing work and exclusive breastfeeding is challenging and requires a strong support in the short and long term [20,21]. In this scenario, employers could play a critical role in providing encouragement for working mothers to continue breastfeeding after returning to work and workplaces should establish dedicated breastfeeding rooms [22–26].

The perception of milk's limited nutritional value and pain during lactation was associated with a higher risk of exclusive breastfeeding discontinuation only in univariate analysis. It can be speculated that these factors might be closely related to the perception of reduced milk supply and often mentioned together. Incorrect latching showed a tendency even though it did not reach statistical significance, possibly reflecting the provision of adequate education and support both during the hospital stay and after hospital discharge with regard to the improvement of mothers' breastfeeding technique.

The findings of the present study are consistent with previous studies in the literature. Poor breastfeeding technique has been reported among the individual factors associated with unsuccessful breastfeeding [6,15,24,27], indicating that adequate breastfeeding support, including evaluation of latching, position, and feeding at the breast, could prevent nipple cracks and thus mastitis. Accordingly, the impact on breastfeeding cessation of acute pain, fever, and other typical mastitis symptoms presented by 8–10% of breastfeeding mothers has been broadly described in literature [28–30]. Mosca et al. [31] found that lactational and nutritional factors were the most cited by mothers as determinants for breastfeeding discontinuation, particularly during the first three months after delivery. Remarkably, the authors reported that the evaluation by a health care professional was rated as important only in 29% to 51% of cases whereas the maternal perception of inadequate milk or insufficient milk supply was cited as important by 40% up to 99% of mothers through the six months' study duration.

The present findings highlight the importance of educating mothers on the criteria that have to be taken into account when considering the adequateness of breast milk supply. Moreover, in this study, our results confirm the association between infant's failure to thrive and discontinuation of exclusive breastfeeding at three months. Accordingly, it has also been described how infant's failure to thrive, objectively evaluated by a healthcare professional, was one of the reasons of exclusive breastfeeding discontinuation, reported throughout the first 6 months of lactation [31]. Interestingly, a study by Flaherman et al. [32] has reported how early and limited administration of small quantities of formula milk during hospital stay could improve breastfeeding rates at three months. The authors speculated that limiting infants' weight loss during the first days of life may reduce maternal milk supply concern, which has been associated with breastfeeding discontinuation. It is then crucial to enhance maternal confidence in her own abilities, enabling mothers to get further insight into the lactation process and the peculiar characteristics of infant growth that often take place in spurts [16]. Within this context, it has to be underlined that a previous negative breastfeeding experience and difficulty negatively affect the likelihood of subsequent breastfeeding success, leading to a potential fear of breastfeeding secondary to prior breastfeeding trauma [7].

In agreement with previous data [15,27,31], in the present study, mothers reported psychosocial factors, in terms of pain and fatigue as breastfeeding difficulties in a relatively high number of cases. The occurrence of physical difficulty during breastfeeding has been associated with a greater risk for developing depressive symptoms in the postnatal period. Hence, it is crucial to provide mothers with early adequate breastfeeding support, including emotional [8].

Accordingly, antenatal and postnatal support including mothers' counseling and education positively affects breastfeeding success [6,12]. Consistently, in the present study, the availability of adequate support at the community level was associated with exclusive breastfeeding at three months post-delivery. Moreover, our results confirm that the mode of delivery modulates breastfeeding success [33], although it must be considered that caesarean section does not seem to negatively impact breastfeeding outcomes at six months, once adequate breastfeeding support is provided [34].

On the contrary, no mention about lifestyle factors, previously reported by other authors, regarding body image, such as wish to lose weight or dislike of breast appearance and breastfeeding convenience [8,15], have been reported, suggesting a positive breastfeeding attitude within the enrolled mothers.

Remarkably, most of the reported breastfeeding difficulties occurred within the first month after delivery, highlighting the importance of offering continuity of care after hospital discharge as underlined in the third guiding principle of the Ten Steps to Successful Breastfeeding [10]. Moreover, the largest decrease in exclusive breastfeeding in the present study was registered between enrollment and seven days after birth.

Literature shows how global breastfeeding rates are far below the international targets, particularly for high-income countries [4], although Italy has one of the highest rates of early initiation of breastfeeding. Moreover, according to the Italian National Statistics Institute [35], in Italy, 48.7% of infants are being exclusively breastfed in the first month, with a drop to 43.9% within the first three months. A survey conducted in 2012 in Lombardy [36] reported a progressive reduction of exclusive breastfeeding rates from 67.3% at hospital discharge to 47.3% and 27% within 120 and 180 days, respectively. Our rates are higher and reflect a particular local context of a high-income country where the breastfeeding benefits are well known and mothers are also supported at the community level. It must be acknowledged that this study focused on mothers with a low risk for breastfeeding cessation and did not include non-Italian speaking mothers due to the potential language barrier that could have interfered with the accuracy of the results, even though they could actually represent a subgroup particularly in need of breastfeeding support structures.

The strength of the present study is that it enrolled a relatively large sample of breastfeeding mother-infant pairs even though the duration of follow up was relatively limited and the dropout rate was 30%, thus partially limiting the generalizability of the present findings. However, it has to be taken into account that, with regard to cohort studies, although the maximum follow-up rate possible should be achieved, dropout rates ranging from 20% up to 50% have been suggested as acceptable [37].

5. Conclusions

Our findings provide further insight into breastfeeding difficulties experienced by mothers through the first three months after delivery in a high-income country with a positive breastfeeding culture and attitude. We underline the importance of providing continued tailored professional support in the community in the attempt to overcome maternal breastfeeding difficulties after discharge from the hospital.

Author Contributions: Conceptualization, M.L.G., M.E.B., G.C., P.R., E.V., P.M. and F.M.; methodology, M.L.G., G.C., P.R., E.V., F.M.; validation, M.L.G., M.E.B., E.B., L.P., P.R. and F.M.; formal analysis, B.L.C. and N.L.; investigation, P.M., G.S., G.R., B.L.C., D.M. and N.L.; supervision, M.L.G., E.B., L.P., G.C., P.R., E.V., P.M., F.M.; resources, M.L.G., G.S., and D.M.; data curation, P.M., G.S., G.R., B.L.C., D.M., N.L.; visualization, E.B., L.P.; writing—original draft preparation, M.L.G. and M.E.B.; writing—review and editing, G.C., G.R., L.C., E.V., P.M., F.M.

Acknowledgments: We thank the mothers for participating in the study.

Abbreviations

SD	Standard Deviation,
OR	Odd Ratio,
CI	Confidence Interval

References

1. Shamir, R. The Benefits of Breast Feeding. *Nestle Nutr. Inst. Workshop Ser.* **2016**, *86*, 67–76. [CrossRef] [PubMed]
2. Mosca, F.; Giannì, M.L. Human milk: Composition and health benefits. *Pediatr. Med. Chir.* **2017**, *39*, 155. [CrossRef] [PubMed]
3. Brown, A. Breastfeeding as a public health responsibility: A review of the evidence. *J. Hum. Nutr. Diet.* **2017**, *30*, 759–770. [CrossRef] [PubMed]
4. Victora, C.G.; Bahl, R.; Barros, A.J.; França, G.V.; Horton, S.; Krasevec, J.; Murch, S.; Sankar, M.J.; Walker, N.; Rollins, N.C.; et al. Breastfeeding in the 21st century: Epidemiology, mechanisms, and lifelong effect. *Lancet* **2016**, *387*, 475–490. [CrossRef]
5. Sayres, S.; Visentin, L. Breastfeeding: Uncovering barriers and offering solutions. *Curr. Opin. Pediatr.* **2018**, *30*, 591–596. [CrossRef]
6. Rollins, N.C.; Bhandari, N.; Hajeebhoy, N.; Horton, S.; Lutter, C.K.; Martines, J.C.; Piwoz, E.G.; Richter, L.M.; Victoria, C.G. The Lancet Breastfeeding Series Group. Why invest, and what it will take to improve breastfeeding practices? *Lancet* **2016**, *387*, 491–504. [CrossRef]
7. Palmér, L. Previous breastfeeding difficulties: An existential breastfeeding trauma with two intertwined pathways for future breastfeeding-fear and longing. *Int. J. Qual. Stud. Health Well Being* **2019**, *14*, 1588034. [CrossRef]
8. Brown, A.; Rance, J.; Bennett, P.J. Understanding the relationship between breastfeeding and postnatal depression: The role of pain and physical difficulties. *J. Adv. Nurs.* **2016**, *72*, 273–282. [CrossRef]

9. Bertino, E.; Di Nicola, P.; Varalda, A.; Occhi, L.; Giuliani, F.; Coscia, A. Neonatal growth charts. *J. Matern. Neonatal Med.* **2012**, *25*, 67–69. [CrossRef]
10. Ten Steps to Successful Breastfeeding. Available online: https://www.who.int/nutrition/bfhi/ten-steps/en/ (accessed on 2 April 2019).
11. The World Health Organization's Infant Feeding Recommendation. Available online: https://www.who.int/nutrition/en/ (accessed on 2 April 2019).
12. McFadden, A.; Gavine, A.; Renfrew, M.J.; Wade, A.; Buchanan, P.; Taylor, J.L.; MacGillivray, S.; Veitch, E.; Rennie, A.M.; Crowther, S.A.; et al. Support for healthy breastfeeding mothers with healthy term babies. *Cochrane Database Syst. Rev.* **2017**, *2*, CD001141. [CrossRef]
13. Heidari, Z.; Kohan, S.; Keshvari, M. Empowerment in breastfeeding as viewed by women: A qualitative study. *J. Educ. Health Promot.* **2017**, *6*, 33. [CrossRef]
14. Corsello, G.; Ferrara, P.; Chiamenti, G.; Nigri, L.; Campanozzi, A.; Pettoello-Mantovani, M. The Child Health Care System in Italy. *J. Pediatr.* **2016**, *177S*, S116–S126. [CrossRef]
15. Odom, E.C.; Li, R.; Scanlon, K.S.; Perrine, C.G.; Grummer-Strawn, L. Reasons for earlier than desired cessation of breastfeeding. *Pediatrics* **2013**, *131*, e726–e732. [CrossRef] [PubMed]
16. Li, R.; Fein, S.B.; Chen, J.; Grummer-Strawn, L.M. Why Mothers Stop Breastfeeding: Mothers' Self-reported Reasons for Stopping During the First Year. *Pediatrics* **2008**, *122*, S69–S76. [CrossRef] [PubMed]
17. Brown, C.R.L.; Dodds, L.; Legge, A.; Bryanton, J.; Semenic, S. Factors influencing the reasons why mothers stop breastfeeding. *Can. J. Public Health* **2014**, *105*, e179–e185. [CrossRef] [PubMed]
18. Kirkland, V.L.; Fein, S.B. Characterizing reasons for breastfeeding cessation throughout the first year postpartum using the construct of thriving. *J. Hum. Lact.* **2003**, *19*, 278–285. [CrossRef] [PubMed]
19. Ahluwalia, I.B.; Morrow, B.; Hsia, J. Why do women stop breastfeeding? Findings from the pregnancy risk assessment and monitoring system. *Pediatrics* **2005**, *116*, 1408–1412. [CrossRef] [PubMed]
20. Thomas-Jackson, S.C.; Bentley, G.E.; Keyton, K.; Reifman, A.; Boylan, M.; Hart, S.L. In-hospital breastfeeding and intention to return to work influence mothers' breastfeeding intentions. *J. Hum. Lact.* **2016**, *32*, NP76–NP83. [CrossRef]
21. Pounds, L.; Fisher, C.M.; Barnes-Josiah, D.; Coleman, J.D.; Lefebvre, R.C. The role of early maternal support in balancing full-time work and infant exclusive breastfeeding: A qualitative study. *Breastfeed. Med.* **2017**, *12*, 33–38. [CrossRef]
22. Tsai, S.Y. Employee perception of breastfeeding-friendly support and benefits of breastfeeding as a predictor of intention to use breast-pumping breaks after returning to work among employed mothers. *Breastfeed. Med.* **2014**, *9*, 16–23. [CrossRef] [PubMed]
23. Bettinelli, M.E. Breastfeeding policies and breastfeeding support programs in the mother's workplace. *J. Matern. Fetal Neonatal Med.* **2012**, *25*, 81–82. [CrossRef] [PubMed]
24. Maharlouei, N.; Pourhaghighi, A.; Raeisi Shahraki, H.; Zohoori, D.; Lankarani, K.B. Factors affecting exclusive breastfeeding, using adaptive LASSO regression. *Int. J. Community Based Nurs. Midwifery* **2018**, *6*, 260–271.
25. Mirkovic, K.R.; Perrine, C.G.; Scanlon, K.S.; Grummer-Strawn, L.M. Maternity leave duration and full-time/part-time work status are associated with US mothers' ability to meet breastfeeding intentions. *J. Hum. Lact.* **2014**, *30*, 416–419. [CrossRef]
26. Dinour, L.M.; Szaro, L.M. Employer-based programs to support breastfeeding among working mothers: A Systematic review. *Breastfeed. Med.* **2017**, *12*, 131–141. [CrossRef] [PubMed]
27. Colombo, L.; Crippa, B.; Consonni, D.; Bettinelli, M.; Agosti, V.; Mangino, G.; Plevani, L.; Bezze, E.N.; Mauri, P.A.; Zanotta, L.; et al. Breastfeeding determinants in healthy term newborns. *Nutrients* **2018**, *10*, 48. [CrossRef]
28. Khanal, V.; Scott, J.A.; Lee, A.H.; Binns, C.W. Incidence of mastitis in the neonatal period in a traditional breastfeeding society: Results of a cohort study. *Breastfeed. Med.* **2015**, *10*, 481–487. [CrossRef] [PubMed]
29. Spencer, J.P. Management of mastitis in breastfeeding women. *Am. Fam. Physician* **2008**, *78*, 727–731. [PubMed]
30. Schwartz, K.; D'Arcy, H.J.; Gillespie, B.; Bobo, J.; Longeway, M.; Foxman, B. Factors associated with weaning in the first 3 months postpartum. *J. Fam. Pract.* **2002**, *51*, 439–444.
31. Mosca, F.; Roggero, P.; Garbarino, F.; Morniroli, D.; Bracco, B.; Morlacchi, L.; Consonni, D.; Marlladi, D.; Gianni, M.L. Determinants of breastfeeding discontinuation in an Italian cohort of mother-infant dyads in the first six months of life: A randomized controlled trial. *Ital. J. Pediatr.* **2018**, *44*, 134. [CrossRef]

32. Flaherman, V.J.; Aby, J.; Burgos, A.E.; Lee, K.A.; Cabana, M.D.; Newman, T.B. Effect of early limited formula on duration and exclusivity of breastfeeding in at-risk infants: An RCT. *Pediatrics* **2013**, *131*, 1059–1065. [CrossRef]
33. Cato, K.; Sylvén, S.M.; Lindbäck, J.; Skalkidou, A.; Rubertsson, C. Risk factors for exclusive breastfeeding lasting less than two months-identifying women in need of targeted breastfeeding support. *PLoS ONE* **2017**, *12*, e0179402. [CrossRef] [PubMed]
34. Prior, E.; Santhakumaran, S.; Gale, C.; Philipps, L.H.; Modi, N.; Hyde, M.J. Breastfeeding after cesarean delivery: A systematic review and meta-analysis of world literature. *Am. J. Clin. Nutr.* **2012**, *95*, 1113–1135. [CrossRef] [PubMed]
35. Istituto Nazionale di Statistica. Available online: https://www.istat.it/it/archivio/141431 (accessed on 29 July 2019).
36. Regione Lombardia Sanità. Available online: http://www.epicentro.iss.it/argomenti/allattamento/pdf/Report%20allattamento%20RL%202012.pdf (accessed on 29 July 2019).
37. Fewtrell, M.S.; Kennedy, K.; Singhal, A.; Martin, R.M.; Ness, A.; Hadders-Algra, M.; Koletzko, B.; Lucas, A. How much loss to follow-up is acceptable in long-term randomised trials and prospective studies? *Arch. Dis. Child.* **2008**, *93*, 458–461. [CrossRef] [PubMed]

12

Endocannabinoid Metabolome Characterization of Transitional and Mature Human Milk

Adriana V. Gaitán [1,*], JodiAnne T. Wood [2], Fan Zhang [1], Alexandros Makriyannis [2] and Carol J. Lammi-Keefe [1,3]

1 Louisiana State University and Louisiana State University Agricultural Center, Baton Rouge, LA 70803, USA; fzhan14@lsu.edu (F.Z.); clammi-keefe@agcenter.lsu.edu (C.J.L.-K.)
2 Center for Drug Discovery, Northeastern University, Boston, MA 02115, USA; j.wood@northeastern.edu (J.T.W.), a.makriyannis@northeastern.edu (A.M.)
3 Pennington Biomedical Research Center, Baton Rouge, LA 70803, USA
* Correspondence: gaitan.adri@gmail.com

Abstract: Recognized as the gold standard, human milk (HM) is an extremely complex yet fascinating biofluid tailored to meet an infant's nutritional requirements throughout development. Endocannabinoids and endocannabinoid-like compounds (endocannabinoid metabolome, ECM) are endogenous lipid mediators derived from long-chain polyunsaturated fatty acids that have been identified in HM. Previous research has shown that arachidonoylglycerol might play a role in establishing the infant's suckling response during lactation by activating the type 1 cannabinoid receptor in the infant's brain. The mechanisms of action and the role of the ECM in HM are not fully understood. Transitional and mature milk samples were collected from lactating women (n = 24) for ECM characterization, quantification, and to evaluate differences among the two stages. HM samples were analyzed by liquid chromatography-mass spectrometry. Identified members of the ECM were: arachidonoylethanolamine, palmitoylethanolamine, oleoylethanolamine, docosahexaenoylethanolamine, eicoapentaenoylethanolamine, eicosenoylethanolamine, arachidonoylglycerol, palmitoyglycerol, oleoylglycerol, docosahexaenoylglycerol, eicosapentaenoylglycerol, eiconenooylglycerol, arachidonic acid, docosahexaenoic acid, and eicosapentaenoic acid. Only docosahexaenoylglycerol was different across transitional and mature milk ($p \leq 0.05$). Data from this cohort suggest that bioactive constituents in HM may also play a role in infant health and development. Future studies can be developed based on this study's data to help elucidate specific roles for each ECM member in addition to understanding how the ECM modulates infant health.

Keywords: fatty acids; long-chain polyunsaturated fatty acids; endocannabinoids; infant health; breast milk

---

1. Introduction

According to the Center for Disease Control and Prevention (2018) [1], 83.2% of infants in the United States are breastfed, with almost 60% breastfeeding at six months, almost 36% breastfeeding at 12 months, and only 24.9% meeting the global recommendation to breastfeed exclusively for six months [2,3]. The recommendation for exclusive breastfeeding during the first months following delivery is based in part on the knowledge that breast milk provides the infant with nutrients that meet his requirements during development. These beneficial nutrients include the long-chain polyunsaturated fatty acids (LCPUFAs), docosahexaenoic acid (DHA, 22:6n3), and arachidonic acid (ARA, 20:4n6), that play a role in cognitive and retinal development and growth of the infant [4]. These nutrients are transferred to the infant across the placenta during pregnancy and through breast milk after birth.

It has been shown that LCPUFAs are precursors to endocannabinoids (EC) which are endogenous lipid mediators that bind to the same receptors as *Cannabis sativa* (marijuana) [5]. Endocannabinoids have been shown to play a role in appetite and food intake [6] by activating cannabinoid receptor 1 (CB1) which is present in the central nervous system [7]. Cannabinoid receptor 1 is activated by two different EC, arachidonoylethanolamide (anandamide, AEA) and arachidonoyl glycerol (AG), both derived from *n*-6 ARA. In particular, for infant feeding behavior, AG has been demonstrated to play a role in establishing the suckling response of the neonate when nursing [8]. Evidence in mouse pups suggest that CB1 activation by AG is needed to establish the suckling response by activating the oral-motor musculature behavior needed for milk suckling [8–10]. Establishment of this role for AG was demonstrated after administration of a CB1 antagonist (SR141716A) to mouse pups which resulted in growth inhibition and even death by day eight after birth [8].

Recent work has indicated that EC and EC-like compounds (collectively referred to as the endocannabinoid metabolome, ECM) are present in human milk [11–13]. Endocannabinoid-like compounds, referred to as entourage metabolites [14], may support the activity and physiologic responses of the EC system by interacting with AEA and AG, their enzymes, or their receptors. These entourage metabolites exert cannabimimetic effects (similar pharmacological effects to those of cannabis) [15]. The ECM encompasses 15 metabolites identified to date: (i) ethanolamide derivatives: AEA, palmitoyl ethanolamide (PEA), oleoyl ethanolamide (OEA), docosahexaenoyl ethanolamide (DHEA), eicosapentaenoyl ethanolamide (EPEA), and eicosenoyl ethanolamide (EEA); (ii) glycerol derivatives: AG, palmitoyl glycerol (PG), oleoyl glycerol (OG), docosahexaenoyl glycerol (DHG), eicosapenaenoyl glycerol (EPG), eicosenoyl glycerol (EG); and (iii) precursor LCPUFAs: ARA, DHA, and eicosapentaenoic acid (EPA, 20:5*n*3). There is limited information regarding the ECM of human milk and its role in infant development. Thus, in the present study, we characterized and quantified the ECM in human milk in transitional and mature milk and evaluated if the concentrations of these metabolites changed over time.

2. Materials and Methods

2.1. Study Design

This research project was an exploratory-longitudinal study to evaluate if there was a difference in the ECM of transitional milk (two weeks postpartum) and the ECM of mature milk (four weeks postpartum).

2.2. Subject Recruitment

Pregnant women from the greater Baton Rouge, Louisiana area who were planning to breastfeed for a minimum of four weeks were invited to participate in this study. Recruitment was based on intent to breastfeed. Subjects were invited to participate before delivery through private physicians' offices and hospital prenatal clinics or by posting flyers describing the study around the community. Women who demonstrated interest in participation in the study were contacted to explain the study and for pre-screening based on the inclusion criteria: maternal age of 18–40 years at the time of delivery, full term delivery ($\geq$37 gestational weeks), singleton birth, plan to breastfeed for at least 4 weeks, willing to provide a breast milk sample (complete breast emptying from one breast) during the morning (6–10 am), have not been breastfeeding or pregnant in the previous year. Before delivery, women were contacted again to schedule the consent process (thorough explanation of the study and for signature of the consent form). The exclusion criteria were discussed at the time of consent: any tobacco use during lactation, alcohol consumption (>1 drink per week), presumed or confirmed congenital birth defects.

Materials provided to the subjects for the study included two breast milk storage bags, instruction on how to collect the breast milk sample, and a schedule card for visits. These were provided the same day that the consent was obtained. The Louisiana State University Agricultural Center Institutional Review Board approved the study.

2.3. Sample Collection

Participants provided written consent and filled out a health history questionnaire that included questions about previous and current pregnancies, pregravid body mass index (BMI), and prior lactation experience. Details regarding infant birth weight and length were completed following the infant's birth. In addition, participants provided information about education and socioeconomic status. This information was confirmed by their health care providers.

Breast milk samples were collected at two and four weeks postpartum at the participants' homes. Participants were asked to provide a breast milk expression from a single breast (emptying a full mammary gland by collecting all the milk from that breast) [16] by using an electric breast pump. In preparation for milk collection, participants fasted for at least two hours and collections were made between 6 am and 10 am. The sample was stored under refrigeration at the participant's house (for a maximum of 24 h) in the breast milk storage bag provided by the researcher. Samples were transported on ice to the laboratory where the milk was warmed in a 37 °C water bath, manually gently swirled to mix, and ~15 mL aliquots were made in small glass vials with Teflon-lined caps and stored at −80 °C until analyses. Information including the breast pump brand used, exclusive breastfeeding, and use of formula for supplementation were also recorded. Samples were shipped overnight on dry ice to the Center for Drug Discovery, Northeastern University, Boston, MA, USA and kept at −80 °C until analysis.

2.4. Sample Analysis

The breast milk samples were analyzed by liquid chromatography-mass spectrometry (LC-MS) with a state-of-the-art methodology established at the Center for Drug Discovery at Northeastern University, Boston, MA, USA. Milk samples were thawed in a 37 °C water bath and vortexed at medium speed for 10 s at room temperature. Protein precipitation was carried out with chilled acetonitrile and PBS (pH 7.4) and the addition of an internal standard mixture containing the same 15 metabolites identified followed by centrifugation (14,000× g, 5 min, 4 °C). The resulting supernatant was diluted with four volumes of 5% phosphoric acid followed by solid phase extraction using OASIS HLB reverse-phase chromatography cartridges (Waters Corp., Mildford, MA, USA) which were previously rinsed with methanol and water prior to loading the diluted samples. Loaded cartridges were washed with 40% aqueous methanol prior to eluting the absorbed lipids with acetonitrile. The acetonitrile fraction was evaporated to dryness under nitrogen, reconstituted in ethanol, vortexed and sonicated, and centrifuged prior to LC-MS analysis. The autosampler was kept at 4 °C to prevent analyte degradation. A TSQ Quantum Ultra triple quadrupole mass spectrometer (Thermo Electron, San Jose, CA, USA) with an Agilent 1100 liquid chromatograph (Agilent Technologies, Wilmington, DE, USA) at the front end was used for identification and quantification. Separation of analytes was carried out using an Agilent 2.1 × 50 mm, 5 µm Zorbax SB-CN column [17,18] with gradient elution using 10 mM ammonium acetate (pH 7.3) and methanol (flow rate, 0.5 mL/min). Elution of fatty acids was achieved while the mass spectrometer was in negative ionization mode, followed by a change in the mass spectrometer to positive ionization mode for elution of ethanolamine and glycerol esters. Eluted peaks were ionized via atmospheric pressure chemical ionization in multiple reaction monitoring mode as previously described [18]. Deuterated internal standards were used to derive a standard curve for each analyte and concentrations (ng/mL) of breast milk were calculated. Each sample was analyzed in triplicate and concentrations were averaged.

2.5. Statistical Analyses

Statistical analyses were performed using SAS by SAS Institute, Inc., version 9.4 (Cary, NC, USA). The level of significance was set at $\leq$0.05. Descriptive statistics (mean, standard deviation, and range) were used for numeric variables. Repeated measures analysis of variance using proc mixed was used to assed the effect of time across the two different time points on the concentrations of members of the ECM.

3. Results

One hundred thirty-one potential participants were invited to participate in the study from which 31 consented to participate. Seven women dropped out during the study; thus, data from 24 participants was included in the study. Table 1 provides the participants' characteristics. Lactating women in the study were between 18 years old and 39 years old.

Table 2 shows the constituents of the ECM at two weeks (transitional milk) and four weeks (mature milk) postpartum. Standard curves for each metabolite were linear and had regression values $\geq$0.99, except for PG which was 0.98. Extraction efficiencies were greater than 80%, except for OG which was greater than 78%. The main metabolite present in the fatty acids group was ARA accounting for more than 60% of that fraction. In the ethanolamide group, OEA accounted for more than 50% of that portion, and PG in the glycerol group accounted for more than 90%. Eicosenoyl ethanolamide and EPG were present in the lowest concentrations in the ethanolamide and glycerol groups, respectively.

Table 1. Maternal-Infant Characteristics (n = 24).

Characteristic	Mean ± SD or % (Frequency)	
Maternal Characteristics		
Age (year)	30.5 ± 5.0	
Pre-pregnancy BMI (kg/m^2)	28.0 ± 5.8	
Race		
White	71 (17)	
Black	17 (4)	
Hispanic	8 (2)	
Asian	4 (1)	
Gestational age at delivery (weeks)	39.2 ± 1.3	
Previous breastfeeding experience		
No	71 (17)	
Education		
Some high school	4 (1)	
High school	4 (1)	
Some college	21 (5)	
4-year post-high school	25 (6)	
Post-graduate	46 (11)	
Marital Status		
Married	79 (19)	
WIC participation		
No	88 (21)	
Infant characteristics		
Sex		
Girls	33 (8)	
Mode of delivery		
Vaginal	75 (18)	
Birth weight (lbs)	7.4 ± 0.8	
Feeding type	2 weeks	4 weeks
Exclusively breastfed	83 (20)	67 (16)

BMI, body mass index; WIC, Woman, Infant, and Children Special Supplemental Nutrition Program.

Twenty-one percent of the samples for EPEA and 27% of the samples for EEA were below the standard curve and 21% of the samples for PG were above although values were close to the curve for the latter. Therefore, those results should be interpreted with caution. Only DHEA demonstrated a time effect ($p \leq 0.05$) across the two different time points postpartum (transitional (two weeks) versus mature (four weeks) milk) with higher concentrations in transitional milk. Overall, breast milk glycerol group concentrations were higher than those of the ethanolamides.

Table 2. Endocannabinoid Metabolome of Human Milk.

Metabolite	Transitional Milk [1]	Mature Milk [1]	*p* Value [2]
Fatty Acids			
ARA	2818.96 ± 580.77	7030.33 ± 3638.67	0.2451
DHA	2031.17 ± 486.39	2384.71 ± 1140.13	0.7569
EPA	381.49 ± 131.91	1362.93 ± 933.24	0.2979
Ethanolamides			
AEA	0.15 ± 0.05	0.08 ± 0.01	0.1772
PEA	0.90 ± 0.10	0.74 ± 0.08	0.1095
OEA	1.48 ± 0.24	1.12 ± 0.10	0.0841
DHEA	0.11 ± 0.01	0.07 ± 0.01	**0.0022**
EPEA [3]	0.07 ± 0.03	0.11 ± 0.04	0.5184
EEA [3]	0.03 ± 0.01	0.03 ± 0.00	0.2382
Glycerol esters			
AG	166.85 ± 36.30	312.11 ± 119.97	0.2550
PG [4]	37,477.67 ± 7296.61	110,091.70 ± 54,443.90	0.1905
OG	4059.33 ± 716.85	7719.96 ± 2269.68	0.1225
DHG	673.50 ± 198.01	866.30 ± 383.60	0.6352
EPG	24.70 ± 7.70	61.99 ± 28.85	0.2161
EG	242.48 ± 66.75	899.37 ± 509.86	0.2078

All data are presented in ng/mL and are mean ± SE. Significant difference marked in bold. [1] Two and four weeks postpartum. [2] *p* value represents the effect of time across the two time points. [3] Some values were below the standard curve. [4] Some values were above the standard curve. ARA, arachidonic acid; DHA, docosahexaenoic acid; EPA, eicosapentaenoic acid; AEA, Anandamide; PEA, palmitoyl ethanolamide; OEA, oleoyl ethanolamide; DHEA, docosahexaenoyl ethanolamide; EPEA, eicosapentaenoyl ethanolamide; EEA, eicosenoyl ethanolamide; AG, arachidonoyl glycerol; PG, palmitoyl glycerol; OG, oleoyl glycerol; DHG, docosahexaenoyl glycerol; EPG, eicosapenaenoyl glycerol; EG, eicosenoyl glycerol.

Combining the two time points together to evaluate relationships, it was observed that there were significant correlations between the precursor LCPUFA and its derived EC. Results are showed in Table 3.

Table 3. Correlations between the Parent Fatty Acid and its Derived Metabolites.

Fatty Acid	Metabolite	Pearson Correlation Coefficient [1]
ARA	AG	0.88
DHA	DHEA	0.69
DHA	DHG	0.95
EPA	EPEA	0.80
EPA	EPG	0.91

[1] $p \leq 0.01$. ARA, arachidonic acid; DHA, docosahexaenoic acid; EPA, eicosapentaenoic acid; AG, arachidonoyl glycerol; DHEA, docosahexaenoyl ethanolamide; DHG, docosahexaenoyl glycerol; EPEA, eicosapentaenoyl ethanolamide; EPG, eicosapenaenoyl glycerol.

4. Discussion

Our study has characterized the ECM in transitional and mature human milk to explore differences in the ECM concentrations at these two stages of breast milk production. The mechanisms of action and the roles of the ECM in both breast milk and for infant development are not fully described/understood. Understanding the bioactive components (i.e., ECM) in breast milk contributes to the body of research that supports the importance of breast milk for infant nourishment and development.

In this exploratory study, we have characterized the ECM of transitional and mature milk. Our results showed that only DHEA, a derivative of DHA conjugated with ethanolamine, was different across the two different time points ($p \leq 0.05$) with higher concentrations in transitional milk. Research evaluating the role of the endocannabinoid system (ECS) in infant feeding behavior has been focused on the activation of CB1 when binding to AG, which in turn activates the oral-motor musculature needed for milk suckling [8]. However, DHEA has also been shown to be an agonist to CB1 [19]. Although the role of DHEA in food intake has not been studied, it may be hypothesized that by binding to the same receptor as AG, DHEA exerts some of the same activities. In addition, as DHA plays a key role in infant cognitive development [20,21] and is a precursor to DHEA, it is plausible that DHEA also supports brain development. Moreover, the development of the hippocampus, a brain area related to learning and memory, has been shown to be supported by DHEA [22].

Scarce data are available for a comparison with our current results. However, the earliest study by Fride et al. (2001) [8] that established a role for the ECS in mouse pup suckling and growth, also analyzed milk from various sources including human milk. Even though the study by Fride et al. (2001) did not specify the number of milk samples analyzed, our results follow the same pattern in demonstrating that PG is present in human milk in higher concentrations than AG. Furthermore, a study by Di Marzo et al. (1998) [23] reported 330 ng/mL of AG in mature human milk, a concentration very similar to our result of 312.11 ng/mL, and indicated that AG is found in human milk in higher concentrations than AEA which is also demonstrated in our present results. Similarly, a study by Schuel et al. (2002) [24] in which ethanolamides were analyzed in human fluids, including mature milk, demonstrated that OEA was present in higher concentrations than PEA, and PEA in higher concentrations than AEA, as also shown in our results. In addition, our results are in line with preliminary data from our laboratory [11,12] that included the same members of the ECM that were investigated in the current study. Our results follow the same pattern in terms of the proportion of each member within each group: fatty acids, ethanolamides, and glycerols. In summary, there are only a few studies available for a comparison to the findings of our current study that support the presence of EC and EC-like metabolites in human milk.

Correlations between the precursor LCPUFAs and their ethanolamide- and glycerol-derivatives showed a more robust correlation for the precursor LCPUFA and its derived glycerol metabolites. This strong correlation between the precursor LCPUFA with its glycerol- but not its ethanolamide-derivatives, may support a more important role for the glycerols (AG, PG, OG, DHG, EPG, and EG) in establishing the suckling response of the newborn by modulating motor development and behavior. In addition, the presence of entourage metabolites (PEA, OEA, DHEA, EPEA, EEA, PG, OG, DHG, EPG, and EG), which exhibit cannabimimetic responses [14], may enhance the activity of the two most thoroughly studied EC, AG, and AEA. For example, PG has been shown to increase AG affinity to CB2 by acting as a lipid signaling mediator [18]; and PEA and OEA reduce enzymatic breakdown, cellular uptake, and degradation of AEA. These entourage metabolites may interfere with enzymatic activity as they can also act as substrates for catabolic and anabolic enzymes. In addition, the presence of these lipid mediators may prevent EC activation or deactivation. All of these interactions may also explain our finding that n-3 LCPUFA derivatives, both ethanolamides and glycerols, correlated with each other (DHEA-DHG ($r = 0.61$, $p \leq 0.01$) and EPEA-EPG ($r = 0.84$, $p \leq 0.01$)). The associations among the n-3 LCPUFA derivatives, but not for the n-6 derivatives (AEA and AG), leads to the speculation that they support the role of DHA in infant cognitive development, although their roles have not yet been fully elucidated.

To date, the mechanisms of action regarding how the ECM as a whole interacts with the ECS and its role in infant feeding behavior, and therefore infant development and growth, are still poorly understood. Our results provide evidence that there are metabolites similar to the previously described EC [5], i.e., AEA and AG, present in human milk. With an understanding of the role of the ECM and its interactions with the ECS in human milk and the infant's brain, potential interventions could be developed for infants with difficulties latching on and for preterm infants who could be aided by the countless benefits of breast milk to ensure continued development outside the womb. While this is out of the scope of this study, it merits further exploration.

This study was limited by its small sample size ($n = 24$). Having a relatively small group of participants did not allow for further explorations between the concentrations for some of the ECM members and demographic data such as BMI and race, for example. However, this study provides an opportunity to develop hypotheses for future studies to evaluate how the ECM of breast milk may be modulated on the basis of maternal and/or infant factors.

5. Conclusions

Our study provides evidence that EC and EC-like metabolites are present in human milk. The findings in this study not only support the role of AG in establishing the suckling response of the newborn by activating oral-motor musculature needed for milk suckling, but also suggest that other bioactive constituents in breast milk may also play a role in infant health and development. In addition, knowing that EC-like metabolites are present in breast milk, future studies can be developed to elucidate specific roles for each member of the ECM.

Author Contributions: Study conceptualization and design, A.G. and C.J.L.-K.; Participant recruitment and sample collections, A.G.; Sample methodology of analysis, J.T.W. and A.M.; Statistical analyses, F.Z. and A.G.; Writing-Original Draft Preparation, A.G.; Writing-Review & Editing, C.J.L.-K.; Supervision, C.J.L.-K.; Project Administration, A.G.; Funding Acquisition, C.J.L.-K. All authors read and approved the final manuscript.

Acknowledgments: We would like to thank the participants in this study and physicians' offices in the community, especially at Woman's Hospital of Baton Rouge. Thank you to Georgianna Tuuri of Louisiana State University who edited an initial version of this manuscript.

References

1. Centers for Disease Control and Prevention. Breastfeeding Report Card. Available online: https://www.cdc.gov/breastfeeding/pdf/2018breastfeedingreportcard.pdf (accessed on 26 August 2018).
2. World Health Organization. Infant and Young Child Feeding. Available online: http://www.who.int/mediacentre/factsheets/fs342/en/ (accessed on 13 February 2018).
3. American Academy of Pediatrics. Breastfeeding and the Use of Human Milk. *Pediatrics* **2012**, *129*, e827–e841. [CrossRef] [PubMed]
4. Koletzko, B. Human Milk Lipids. *Ann. Nutr. Metab.* **2016**, *69* (Suppl. S2), 27–40. [CrossRef] [PubMed]
5. Di Marzo, V. Endocannabinoids: Synthesis and degradation. *Rev. Physiol. Biochem. Pharmacol.* **2008**, *160*, 1–24. [CrossRef] [PubMed]
6. Cascio, M.G. PUFA-derived endocannabinoids: An overview. *Proc. Nutr. Soc.* **2013**, *72*, 451–459. [CrossRef] [PubMed]
7. Grant, I.; Cahn, B.R. Cannabis and endocannabinoid modulators: Therapeutic promises and challenges. *Clin. Neurosci. Res.* **2005**, *5*, 185–199. [CrossRef] [PubMed]
8. Fride, E.; Ginzburg, Y.; Breuer, A.; Bisogno, T.; Di Marzo, V.; Mechoulam, R. Critical role of the endogenous cannabinoid system in mouse pup suckling and growth. *Eur. J. Pharmacol.* **2001**, *419*, 207–214. [CrossRef]
9. Fride, E. The endocannabinoid-CB1 receptor system in pre- and postnatal life. *Eur. J. Pharmacol.* **2004**, *500*, 289–297. [CrossRef] [PubMed]
10. Fride, E.; Foox, A.; Rosenberg, E.; Faigenboim, M.; Cohen, V.; Barda, L.; Blau, H.; Mechoulam, R. Milk intake and survival in newborn cannabinoid CB1 receptor knockout mice: Evidence for a "CB3" receptor. *Eur. J. Pharmacol.* **2003**, *461*, 27–34. [CrossRef]
11. Durham, H.A.; Wood, J.T.; Vadivel, S.K.; Makriyannis, A.; Lammi-Keefe, C.J. Detection of the endocannabinoid metabolome in human plasma and breast milk. *FASEB J.* **2013**, *27* (Suppl. S1), 45.8.
12. Wood, J.T.; Durham, H.A.; Vadivel, S.K.; Makriyannis, A.; Lammi-Keefe, C.J. Postpartum changes in the endocannabinoid metabolome of human breast milk. *FASEB J.* **2013**, *27* (Suppl. S1), 629.15.

13. Wu, J.; Gouveia-Figueira, S.; Domellöf, M.; Zivkovic, A.M.; Nording, M.L. Oxylipins, endocannabinoids, and related compounds in human milk: Levels and effects of storage conditions. *Prostaglandins Other Lipid Mediat.* **2016**, *122*, 28–36. [CrossRef] [PubMed]
14. Ben-Shabat, S.; Fride, E.; Sheskin, T.; Tamiri, T.; Rhee, M.-H.; Vogel, Z.; Bisogno, T.; De Petrocellis, L.; Di Marzo, V.; Mechoulam, R. An entourage effect: Inactive endogenous fatty acid glycerol esters enhance 2-arachidonoyl-glycerol cannabinoid activity. *Eur. J. Pharmacol.* **1998**, *353*, 23–31. [CrossRef]
15. Mechoulam, R.; Fride, E.; Di Marzo, V. Endocannabinoids. *Eur. J. Pharmacol.* **1998**, *359*, 1–18. [CrossRef]
16. Miller, E.M.; Aiello, M.O.; Fujita, M.; Hinde, K.; Milligan, L.; Quinn, E.A. Field and laboratory methods in human milk research. *Am. J. Hum. Biol.* **2013**, *25*, 1–11. [CrossRef] [PubMed]
17. Williams, J.; Pandarinathan, L.; Wood, J.; Vouros, P.; Makriyannis, A. Endocannabinoid metabolomics: A novel liquid chromatography-mass spectrometry reagent for fatty acid analysis. *AAPS J.* **2006**, *8*, E655–E660. [CrossRef] [PubMed]
18. Williams, J.; Wood, J.; Pandarinathan, L.; Karanian, D.A.; Bahr, B.A.; Vouros, P.; Makriyannis, A. Quantitative Method for the Profiling of the Endocannabinoid Metabolome by LC-Atmospheric Pressure Chemical Ionization-MS. *Anal. Chem.* **2007**, *79*, 5582–5593. [CrossRef] [PubMed]
19. Brown, I.; Cascio, M.G.; Wahle, K.W.J.; Smoum, R.; Mechoulam, R.; Ross, R.A.; Pertwee, R.G.; Heys, S.D. Cannabinoid receptor-dependent and -independent anti-proliferative effects of omega-3 ethanolamides in androgen receptor-positive and -negative prostate cancer cell lines. *Carcinogenesis* **2010**, *31*, 1584–1591. [CrossRef] [PubMed]
20. Carlson, S.E.; Colombo, J. Docosahexaenoic Acid and Arachidonic Acid Nutrition in Early Development. *Adv. Pediatr.* **2016**, *63*, 453–471. [CrossRef] [PubMed]
21. Jensen, C.L.; Voigt, R.G.; Llorente, A.M.; Peters, S.U.; Prager, T.C.; Zou, Y.L.; Rozelle, J.C.; Turcich, M.R.; Fraley, J.K.; Anderson, R.E.; et al. Effects of Early Maternal Docosahexaenoic Acid Intake on Neuropsychological Status and Visual Acuity at Five Years of Age of Breast-Fed Term Infants. *J. Pediatr.* **2010**, *157*, 900–905. [CrossRef] [PubMed]
22. Kim, H.-Y.; Moon, H.-S.; Cao, D.; Lee, J.; Kevala, K.; Jun, S.B.; Lovinger, D.M.; Akbar, M.; Huang, B.X. *N*-Docosahexaenoylethanolamide promotes development of hippocampal neurons. *Biochem. J.* **2011**, *435*, 327–336. [CrossRef] [PubMed]
23. Di Marzo, V.; Sepe, N.; De Petrocellis, L.; Berger, A.; Crozier, G.; Fride, E.; Mechoulam, R. Trick or treat from food endocannabinoids? *Nature* **1998**, *396*, 636. [CrossRef] [PubMed]
24. Schuel, H.; Burkman, L.J.; Lippes, J.; Crickard, K.; Forester, E.; Piomelli, D.; Giuffrida, A. *N*-Acylethanolamines in human reproductive fluids. *Chem. Phys. Lipids* **2002**, *121*, 211–227. [CrossRef]

13

Lactoferrin: A Critical Player in Neonatal Host Defense

Sucheta Telang [1,2,*]

1 Division of Neonatology, Department of Pediatrics, University of Louisville, Louisville, KY 40202, USA
2 Division of Hematology/Oncology, Department of Medicine, James Graham Brown Cancer Center, University of Louisville, Louisville, KY 40202, USA

Abstract: Newborn infants are at a high risk for infection due to an under-developed immune system, and human milk has been shown to exhibit substantial anti-infective properties that serve to bolster neonatal defenses against multiple infections. Lactoferrin is the dominant whey protein in human milk and has been demonstrated to perform a wide array of antimicrobial and immunomodulatory functions and play a critical role in protecting the newborn infant from infection. This review summarizes data describing the structure and important functions performed by lactoferrin in protecting the neonate from infection and contributing to the maturation of the newborn innate and adaptive immune systems. We also briefly discuss clinical trials examining the utility of lactoferrin supplementation in the prevention of sepsis and necrotizing enterocolitis in newborn infants. The data reviewed provide rationale for the continuation of studies to examine the effects of lactoferrin administration on the prevention of sepsis in the neonate.

Keywords: lactoferrin; human milk; infection; immunity

---

1. Introduction

The neonatal period is an exceptionally vulnerable period of life, during which term and preterm infants are at high risk for morbidity and mortality. According to recent data from the World Health Organization, 2.6 million neonates died globally in 2016 alone—accounting for 46% of the deaths under the age of five years [1]. Infections are responsible for approximately 36% of the deaths that occur in the newborn period [1], and there thus exists an urgent need for better strategies and approaches to improve neonatal outcomes worldwide.

The increased susceptibility of the newborn infant to infection is largely due to the immaturity of the neonatal immune system. Limited antigenic exposure in the predominantly sterile in utero environment is a dominant factor contributing to the underdevelopment of the adaptive immune response. Additional contributory factors are deficiencies in the cells responsible for adaptive immunity themselves—they are present in smaller numbers and show great variability in their adaptive responses [2]. As a result, to combat early infectious threats, newborn rely on their innate immune response, which is also not yet fully developed [3,4].

Neonatal deficiencies in immunity and host defense are compensated by several mechanisms. An early mechanism is the acquisition of antibodies passively transferred through the placenta from the mother [5]. Since this transfer occurs largely in the third trimester, the term infant is able to benefit from these antibodies but the preterm infant is unfortunately deprived of their protection.

A critical component of the armamentarium of the term and preterm neonate against infection is contributed by human milk. Human milk contains a wide array of bioactive proteins, growth factors, cells, and other constituents that modulate the development of a competent immune system to defend the term and preterm newborn against infections [6]. Of the bioactive factors present in human milk, lactoferrin has emerged as a key player that performs wide-ranging functions to directly and indirectly protect the neonate against infection.

2. Lactoferrin Distribution and Properties

Lactoferrin (or lactotransferrin, Lf) is a glycoprotein from the transferrin family of proteins. Lf was first identified in bovine milk by Sørensen and Sørensen in 1939 [7], then isolated from human and bovine milk by several investigators in 1960 [8–10]. Human Lf is a ~78 kDa glycoprotein which contains 691 amino acids and is expressed and secreted by epithelial cells in many exocrine secretions, including saliva, tears, and milk [11,12].

In human milk, Lf is the most abundant protein in the whey fraction, with a concentration varying from 1 gm/L to 7 gm/L (in colostrum) [12]. Multiple studies have evaluated Lf concentrations in colostrum and mature milk and in term and preterm milk. An early study that compared Lf levels between colostrum and mature milk in 30–32 week and >39 week neonates found trends towards higher initial Lf levels in the term infant group and higher sustained Lf levels in the preterm mature milk, but the differences did not reach significance [13]. A recent and comprehensive study has examined maternal milk samples from 24 week to term infants, and from birth to >10 days after birth, and found that Lf levels were highest in milk samples from mothers with infants <1400 g and that the levels varied significantly over time and with gestation [14]. Interestingly, the variation between samples within groups appeared fairly uniform, indicating that Lf concentrations in maternal milk at similar gestations may be relatively similar [14].

Lf levels are also sensitive to low and high temperatures. Studies (from our group) found that refrigeration of human milk samples (at 4 °C) for up to 5 days did not significantly lower Lf levels, but freezing (to −18 to −20 °C) decreased Lf dramatically to ~35% of the levels in fresh milk by 6 months, with a similarly significant decrease in its activity (by ~43%, measured by nitric oxide production) [15,16]. Heating also appears to decrease Lf levels, indicated by data showing that pasteurization (62.5 °C for 30 min, Holder method) significantly decreased the total protein (and thus presumably Lf) in human milk samples [17,18]. Further studies, in donor milk samples, showed an even more dramatic decrease (up to 88%) in Lf levels due to pasteurization [19]. This, when coupled with the freezing that these samples are exposed to, may indicate why donor milk has not shown the advantages of fresh maternal milk in terms of reduction in sepsis and necrotizing enterocolitis [18–20]. The detrimental effects of Holder pasteurization on immunological proteins in human milk have led to the active exploration of alternative methods to process donor human milk. Of these methods, exposure to 72 °C for 15 s (high temperature/short time or HTST pasteurization) has been demonstrated to preserve the integrity of Lf to a greater extent than the Holder method, although a significant decline in Lf relative to untreated milk is still noted [21–24]. Interestingly, studies have found that human Lf exposure to HTST conditions had only mild effects on its anti-bacterial activity [25], which may indicate that isolated and recombinant Lf may be less susceptible to temperature variations. Non-thermal alternatives to process donor milk are also under evaluation, such as high pressure processing, which has been shown to efficiently destroy microorganisms and allow greater retention of the immune components of human milk, including Lf [21,24]. A highly promising method that is currently under study is ultraviolet-C (UV-C) radiation. Recent data have indicated that UV-C radiation causes significant retention of Lf relative to Holder pasteurization and additionally induces greater resistance to bacterial infections in vivo [26–28]. In addition, these studies have described a technique to deliver UV-C radiation that has successfully overcome the limitations imposed by the high absorption coefficient of human milk [27]. These alternative processing methods will require extensive further investigation before reaching clinical application but certainly carry great promise.

The crystal structure of human Lf (hLf) was first solved in 1987 [29] and the protein has since been well described [30]. HLf contains two homologous lobes, each of which binds one ferric iron (Fe^{3+}) with high affinity, making hLf a strong scavenger of iron. Lf is also able to retain bound iron down to a pH of ~3.5 [31] due to interactions between the 2 lobes, allowing it to be an effective anti-oxidant and bacteriostatic agent. Depending on its metal ion status, Lf can adopt either an iron-bound closed (holo-Lf) or a metal-free open conformation (apo-Lf)—both states have been demonstrated to perform functions in host defense. Lf additionally carries a high positive charge, with an isoelectric point of 9–10 that provides a high propensity for binding to negatively charged molecules on cell surfaces or in solution. Of particular importance are the basic residues at the N-terminus of Lf, at which proteolytic cleavage releases a potent antimicrobial peptide termed lactoferricin (Lfc) [32] that is highly exposed in both apo- and holo-Lf and may enable binding to bacterial cell membranes. A second peptide sequence, lactoferrampin, also has been identified as a major binding site with potential antibacterial properties. Additional data indicate that the glycan chains of Lf may mediate certain anti-bacterial and anti-viral activities as well [30].

Human Lf shares ~70% sequence homology with bovine Lf (bLf) [33], which has a molecular weight of ~76 kDa [34] and consists of 689 amino acids, and is both folded into N and C lobes and has antigenic determinants highly similar to its human counterpart [35]. Bovine Lf has a lower iron affinity than hLf, potentially due to altered interdomain interactions in its structure driven by the orientation and domains of its lobes and by its oligosaccharide units (particularly a glycan chain at Asn 545) [35,36]. Despite this difference, near-identical functions of human and bovine Lf [11] against multiple pathogenic organisms have been well documented [11]. Similar to human Lf, bovine Lf generates Lfc by cleavage at the cationic N-terminal region, which has been shown to cause a rapid loss of colony-forming capability [37]. Interestingly, the bovine Lf-generated Lfc was observed to have greater efficacy than human Lf against Gram-negative and Gram-positive bacteria [37]. Since bovine Lf is generally recognized as safe by the United States Food and Drug Administration (GRAS), it is easily available commercially and has therefore been widely used in vitro and in vivo for the examination of the various functions of this protein. In a recent study, commercial bLf added to infant formula was compared with hLf in an intestinal enterocyte model [38]. Commercial bLf was found to bind to the cells, be taken up by the human lactoferrin receptor, internalize, and promote proliferation and differentiation, indicating that it will likely exert bioactivities similar to hLf if supplemented in infant formula [38]. Several clinical trials examining the effects of bLf on infection have been conducted in preterm and term neonates, where bLf has been tolerated well (see Section 7). Bovine Lf-containing formula is also currently under active study in a clinical trial (NCT#02103205) evaluating the effects of the addition of bLf on the immune system, the microbiota composition, metabolomics, growth, body composition, and cognitive development.

The variable Lf levels in maternal milk likely indicate the evolving requirement for this protein with gestational and post-natal age, and these data form an important basis for the development of optimal strategies for infants who require supplementation. Although the susceptibility of Lf in milk to heat and cold may hamper the use of stored human milk for such strategies, the stability of isolated hLf and the similarities between hLf and bLf structure and function indicate the potential utility of these proteins in formula supplementation.

3. Direct Anti-Microbial Effects

The anti-microbial effects attributed to Lf (Figure 1) were initially believed to be entirely due to the ability of unsaturated Lf to avidly bind iron and thereby cause bacteriostatic effects in iron-requiring pathogens. Early studies indicated that human milk and Lf purified from human milk had bacteriostatic effects on the growth of *E. coli* that were lost on saturation with iron [39]. These investigators went on to examine the effects of Lf against *E. coli* in vivo by gavage-feeding guinea pig pups with *E. coli*, and then either allowing the pups to suckle or feeding them with a milk substitute diet. They found that the suckled pups had substantially lower intestinal *E. coli* counts, interestingly with a corresponding increase in *Lactobacillus* numbers, and that the decrease in counts was reversed by feeding the pups hematin [39]. Iron-dependent anti-microbial effects of human and bovine Lf have been observed against a number of pathogens, including *S. mutans*, *V. cholerae*, and also *P. aeruginosa*, where iron chelation by Lf was found to stimulate a form of cell motility that inhibited biofilm formation by these bacteria [40–44].

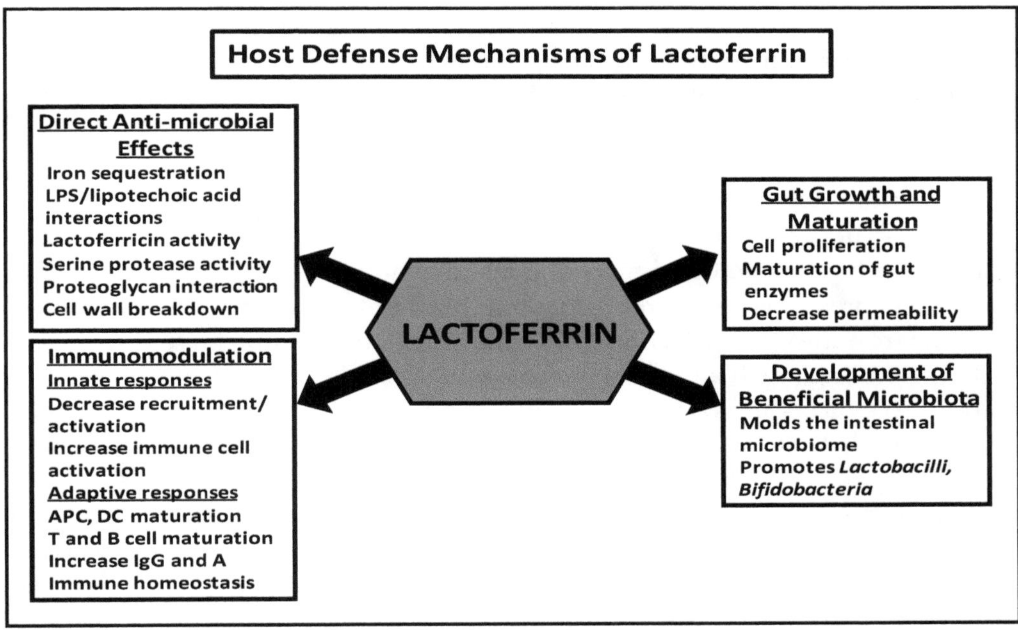

Figure 1. Functions of Lactoferrin in Neonatal Host Defense.

Several studies demonstrate that, independent of its iron-binding capabilities, Lf is bactericidal to several pathogens [45,46] through interactions with the lipopolysaccharide (LPS) of Gram negative and the lipotechoic acid of Gram-positive bacteria [11]. In *E. coli*, Lf inhibits adherence and biofilm formation potentially by binding to lipid portions of the LPS layer, with a resultant increase in membrane permeability and disruption of virulence proteins anchored to the outer membrane [47]. These activities may be due to the action of Lfc—the peptide formed by the cleavage of Lf [32]. Further studies have determined another distinct anti-microbial function of the N-lobe of Lf due to the formation of a catalytic dyad by Ser259 and Lys73 that has a serine protease activity shown to successfully cleave and remove adherence elements of *H. influenzae*, thus attenuating its pathogenic potential [48,49]. An additional potential anti-bacterial mechanism has been proposed for Lf wherein it may enhance anoikis of infected enterocytes [50], but this activity requires significant further investigation. Taken together, these data indicate that the ability of Lf to affect bacterial attachment and invasion proteins may play a role in protecting suckling animals from infection by preventing the attachment and colonization of bacteria in the intestinal epithelium. In support of this hypothesis, studies have demonstrated that neonatal rodents pretreated with Lf had less bacteremia and less severe disease due to intestinal *E. coli* infection [51]. In addition, Lf has shown potent synergistic activity in killing Gram-negative bacteria in vitro with lysozyme—a second important component of the human milk whey fraction that is able to degrade bacterial membrane peptidoglycans. By binding LPS and removing it from the outer cell membrane, Lf allows lysozyme to access and degrade the inner membrane proteoglycans and kill the bacteria [52]. The bactericidal activity against Gram-positive bacteria appears to be caused by the same residues as with Gram-negative bacteria [53]. Of interest, a recent study examined the effects of *S. aureus* bacteremia in piglets pre-treated with dietary bovine Lf [54] and found that bLf pretreatment effectively reduced *S. aureus* systemic infection. BLf additionally decreased IL-10 and increased interferon-γ mRNA in these animals, indicating a type 1 T helper (Th1) immune response and, thus, effects on the innate and adaptive immunity of these animals. These results may explain some of the beneficial effects of bLf observed in preterm infants.

Lf also has direct inhibitory effects on viruses and other microbes. Against viruses, these effects may involve the attachment of Lf to surface proteoglycans, such as heparan sulfate, to which Lf has a high affinity through its N-terminus glycosaminoglycan-binding domains [55], thus blocking the entry of certain viruses, e.g., HSV. Other mechanisms may involve direct interactions of Lf with viral envelope proteins [56]. In fungi such as *Candida*, Lf has been shown to have effects as well, and was observed to cause cell wall perturbations, with the formation of surface blebs, swelling, and the collapse of the cell [57].

Variable responses to Lf-driven inhibition have been observed in different micro-organisms that are likely driven by differences in their iron requirement and their strategies to increase iron uptake and, additionally, by structural variations that may serve to limit direct access by Lf. As examples, several bacterial species have developed mechanisms to evade the iron-limiting effects of Lf. *Neisseria* and *Moraxella* species express specific Lf receptors that bind Lf to induce a conformational change in its structure and release iron into the bacteria [58]. Other micro-organisms have developed strategies to resist direct Lf-driven killing, such as *S. pneumoniae*, which binds Lf by pneumococcal surface protein A (PspA) and thereby evades the bactericidal effects of Lf [59], and *V. vulnificus*, which expresses a metalloprotease (Vvpe) that destroys Lf and facilitates the ability of the bacteria to invade the mucosa [60].

The studies indicate that further investigation into the anti-microbial functions of Lf is required. The examples described above notwithstanding, the available scientific evidence demonstrates the widespread inhibitory effects of Lf on the proliferation and survival of pathogenic micro-organisms—either by the sequestration of iron or direct activity on virulence factors—and strongly supports a protective role for Lf against infection in the newborn.

4. Immunomodulatory Functions of Lactoferrin

Lf plays a key role in neonatal host defense by modulating the innate and adaptive immune response of the neonate to infections (Figure 1). In addition, a growing body of evidence suggests that Lf facilitates mechanisms whereby adaptive immune changes may influence the innate immune system.

4.1. Mechanisms of Interaction of Lactoferrin with Immune Cells

The effects of Lf on immune cells are modulated by binding to a variety of targets. Among the most abundant are the glycosaminoglycans on membrane peptidoglycans [61], which are critical for the binding of many cytokines and factors, and it has been postulated that Lf may alter immune cell function by displacing these factors [62]. Other receptors described include lectins (e.g., TLR-4) which recognize the glycan chains of Lf, receptors recognizing the Lfc or N1 domain, intelectin-1 (found on enterocytes and immune cells), and nucleolin which may serve the additional function of transporting Lf to the nucleus [61,63]. All these receptors may potentially internalize Lf with downstream activation of signaling pathways e.g., the phosphoinositide 3-kinase (PI3K)/Akt and the mitogen activated protein kinase (MAPK)/extracellular signal-regulated kinase (ERK) signaling pathways, whereby Lf has been shown to activate cell cycle progression, proliferation, and downstream cellular responses [64–66] or, following nuclear localization, the NFkB pathway [61,67]. In addition, Lf has been found to bind to a receptor on (transformed) hematopoietic cells and translocate to the nucleus, leading to transcriptional activation with downstream effects [68,69].

4.2. Innate Immune Effects of Lactoferrin

The effects of Lf on the innate immune response are related in part to its ability to bind to conserved structures, termed pathogen-associated molecular patterns (PAMPs), present on pathogens (e.g., LPS on Gram-negative bacteria and peptidoglycans on Gram-positive bacteria). PAMPs are recognized by pattern recognition receptors or PRRs such as Toll-like receptors (TLRs) [70], that are critical for the activation of innate immunity. TLR4 has been demonstrated to bind and transfer LPS, with the assistance of the transfer molecule LPS-binding protein (LBP), to CD14. CD14 is a glycosylphosphatidylinositol-anchored membrane protein present on myeloid cells which leads to their activation and the release of pro-inflammatory cytokines e.g., TNF-α, IL-6, and IL-1β [71,72]. Lf is demonstrated to bind to several PAMPs, including LPS, and thereby compete with LBP to inhibit the release of pro-inflammatory cytokines [62,73]. Lf may also modulate recruitment of immune cells by interfering with the expression of endothelial cell adhesion molecules required for the recruitment of these cells to sites of inflammation as shown by data indicating that the interference of Lf in the LPS-CD14 interaction may inhibit the expression of E-selectin, ICAM-1, and IL-8 by human umbilical vein endothelial cells (HUVECs) [62,74]. Lf may cause further suppressive effects on immune cells by binding to other molecular cell surface targets, as evident by its function in competing with the chemokine IL-8 for binding to endothelial cell proteoglycans to inhibit the activation and recruitment of leukocytes to sites of inflammation [74].

Lf is also capable of enhancing the activation of immune cells. Following bacterial invasion, LPS binds to TLR4 on sentinel cells to cause the release of potent cytokines including TNF-α, IL-1β, and IL-6 [62,75]. These molecules will activate and modify the permeability of endothelial cells to allow the passage of complement and antibodies and recruit neutrophils to the site of inflammation. Activated neutrophils will release Lf from their secondary granules to exert its direct microbicidal effects [62]. Lf may also enhance the cytotoxic functions of NK and lymphokine-activated killer cells, potentially through binding to RNA and DNA [76].

Promotion of lytic cell activity is a key role played by Lf. Lf receptors are found on macrophages [77] and Lf is shown to activate macrophages to release pro-inflammatory molecules e.g., TNF-α, IL-8, and nitric oxide [15,78] and to increase their phagocytic activity when infected [79]. Lf is also expressed on the membranes of resting PMNs and may enable interaction between Lf-bound microbes and PMNs [80]. Bovine Lf was noted to increase phagocytic killing of *S. aureus*—potentially by activation of the alternate complement pathway by its Lfc domain [81,82].

4.3. Effects on Adaptive Immune Responses

Lf plays an important immunomodulatory role in activation and antigen presentation by antigen-presenting cells (APCs) and in their functions in the adaptive immune response by affecting T cell development. Macrophages function as APCs to stimulate the development of antigen-specific CD4+ T cells, and Lf enhances their ability to function as APCs by stimulating the production of cytokines, such as IL-12, responsible for modulating development of Th1 cells [83,84].

Lf also assists in the maturation of dendritic cells (DCs)—by enhancing their release of IL-8 and CXCL10, decreasing antigen internalization, increasing their capacity to trigger proliferation and release IFN-γ in the presence of allogeneic human T cells, and to prime naïve T cells in response to several antigenic stimuli [85]. Recent studies indicate that Lf may function similarly to an alarmin to promote the activation of APCs and antigen-specific immune responses [86,87]. These studies demonstrate that, similar to the previous study, Lf is able to chemoattract and cause the maturation of monocyte-derived DCs, and also stimulate the production of pro-inflammatory cytokines. Lf additionally may prompt Th1 polarized antigen-specific immune responses in immunized mice and the recruitment of macrophages and neutrophils when injected into the mouse peritoneal cavity [86].

More recent data indicate a role for Lf in immune homeostasis as well. Studies indicate that DCs differentiated in the presence of Lf showed decreased responsiveness towards TLR ligands [88,89] and reduced cytokine production demonstrating a potential role for Lf in immune homeostasis. These results indicate a potent anti-inflammatory function for Lf by skewing monocyte differentiation into DCs with impaired capacity for activation and for promotion of Th1 responses and may represent a strategy to block excessive DC activation upon TLR-induced inflammation, adding further evidence for a critical role of Lf in directing host immune function.

Lf has been shown to modulate the production of pro-inflammatory cytokines, such as TNF-α, IL-1β, and IL-6, from leukocyte populations, which may be increased or decreased depending on the condition recognized by the immune system. In addition, Lf may increase the production of IL-12 by APCs when presented with pathogens. IL-12 enhances IFN-γ production and proliferation, augments cytotoxic activity of lymphocytes responsible for innate (NK cells) and adaptive (CD4+and CD8+ T-cells) immunity, and is a major driver of Th1 cell development [83,84].

Lf also influences T and B lymphocyte maturation. Lf is able to bind to surface receptors and be internalized by human Jurkat lymphoblastic T cells [90], where it accelerates T cell maturation by induction of CD4 via activation of the MAPK pathway [91]. Human milk-derived Lf is observed to cause maturation of $CD4^-CD8^-$ murine T-cells, with a preference towards expression of CD4 [92]. When administered orally, Lf has the ability to restore the host T cell compartment, evident by an increase in splenic cellularity and enrichment of CD3+ CD4+ T cells, and suggesting a possible role for Lf in the reconstitution of the cellular immune response [93]. As noted with other cell types, Lf also appears to exert anti-inflammatory effects. The addition of Lf to mitogen-activated T-cells decreases overall cytokine production demonstrated by the decreased production of IFN-γ and IL-2 by ConA-stimulated murine splenocytes cultured with Lf [94]. Similarly, Lf is able to promote the maturation of immature B lymphocytes, shown by an increase in surface Ig D and complement receptor expression. In addition, Lf was shown to enable B cells from normal newborn and adult immunodeficient mice to present antigen to an antigen-specific T-helper type 2 (Th2) cell line [95]. Orally administered Lf has been demonstrated to increase the pool of CD4+ T cells, immunoglobulin levels (G and A), as well as proliferation in the Peyer's patches of the intestine, suggesting that Lf may act as an immunostimulatory factor on the mucosal immune system [96–98]. In addition, in a chemotherapy-induced immune suppression murine model, Lf administered intraperitoneally was able to decrease the suppression of antibody forming cells and facilitate the restoration of the immune response [99].

Taken together, these studies illustrate the multiple activities performed by Lf to modulate the nascent neonatal immune system and highlight the importance of this protein in the development of a mature immune response. The growing body of scientific evidence suggests that the effects of Lf vary depending on the threat faced by the immune system and thereby emphasizes the importance of this glycoprotein in the protection of the newborn from infection.

5. Effects of Lactoferrin on the Development of Beneficial Microbiota

The bacterial flora colonizing human milk fed infants have been demonstrated to be different from those of formula-fed infants. Higher concentrations of *Lactobacillus* and *Bifidobacteria* species are observed with comparatively fewer bacteria with high pathogenic potential e.g., *E. coli*, *Campylobacter*, and *Bacteroides* [100]. In vitro studies have demonstrated that Lf from human and bovine milk promotes the growth of intestinal bifidobacteria without the requirement for binding of the Lf molecule to the bacterial cell surface or a dependence on the acquisition and utilization of iron [101]. Bifidogenic peptides have been isolated from human milk (derived from hLf) that demonstrate strong bifidogenic effects on several bifidobacterial species (*B. bifidum*, *B. breve*, and *B. longum)* and are resistant to digestive enzymes [102,103]. The importance of Lf in the development of beneficial bacteria is underscored by data from breastfed term and preterm infants, showing high fecal Lf levels and a significant association of bifidobacteria and lactobacilli with fecal Lf levels on day three of life, suggesting that Lf may be a key factor in the initiation, development, and composition of the neonatal gut microbiota [104]. These data indicate that Lf is a tremendously important influence on the development of the intestinal microbiome (Figure 1). The importance of this function of Lf is magnified in critically ill and hospitalized term and preterm infants who are at risk for colonization and infection with highly pathogenic bacteria [105], and where Lf administration may be able to play a critical role in decreasing invasive infection and necrotizing enterocolitis. Interestingly, recent studies have examined the effect of Lf on probiotic bacterial growth in vitro and found that both hLf and bLf may retard the growth of certain bifidobacteria [106,107]. In view of the importance of the development of beneficial gut bacteria and ongoing clinical examination of Lf supplementation with probiotics, the further delineation of the precise effects of Lf in probacterial growth is a critical avenue of investigation.

6. Effects on Gut Growth and Maturation

Lf has been found to directly stimulate intestinal growth and proliferation [108,109] (Figure 1). Studies conducted on Caco-2 (transformed) enterocytes in vitro have found that exposure to high Lf concentrations led to a dose-dependent increase in cell proliferation, while low Lf levels stimulated intestinal cell differentiation [108]. These data suggest that Lf may actively modulate enterocyte growth and development in vivo due to variations in its concentration from colostrum to mature milk, in addition to its stimulatory effects on intestinal enzyme maturation [108]. Of interest, these studies found that bLf was a more potent effector of growth than hLf, which provides rationale for its supplementation in infant formula [108]. Beneficial effects of bLf administration were also noted in vivo. Neonatal piglets fed formula that contained physiological levels of bLf relative to controls fed low bLf showed an increase in intestinal cellular proliferation and, additionally, increased β-catenin levels, indicating a potential role for Wnt signaling in gut proliferation [110]. Other studies have observed that Lf is taken up by enterocytes via the Lf receptor and stimulates enterocyte proliferation through the Ras-MAPK pathway [68], the strong mitogenic effect of which also may drive the rapid development of the intestinal mucosa in newborns fed maternal milk. An additional possible function for Lf in intestinal maturation is in regulation of gut permeability. In its support, studies have shown that preterm infants fed maternal milk had decreased gastrointestinal permeability relative to formula-fed controls, which indicates a potential role for components of human milk in intestinal maturation [111]. This mechanism of action will require further examination in the newborn population.

The functions performed by Lf in the growth and maturation of the gut are critical for the development and maintenance of the intestinal barrier to infection. The breakdown of this barrier may expose the newborn to potentially highly pathogenic bacteria. These findings therefore support the importance of early and continued exposure of the newborn gut to Lf in human milk or as a supplement in formula.

7. Examination for Clinical Efficacy of Lf in Neonates

An overwhelming body of experimental evidence supports the beneficial anti-infective properties of Lf, providing strong rationale for its use against infection in newborn infants.

Based on the significant anti-microbial and immunomodulatory effects caused by Lf, this protein may be particularly useful in host defense in critically ill and very low birth weight (VLBW) neonates. VLBW infants carry an enhanced risk for bacterial sepsis and potentially devastating sequelae [112] and are frequently unable to tolerate feeds, thus depriving them of the protective benefits of maternal milk. Based on this rationale, several studies have examined the efficacy of Lf supplementation against sepsis [113] in the neonatal period. An early study where healthy, formula-fed infants ($\geq$34 weeks gestation and $\leq$4 weeks old) were fed formula supplemented with bovine Lf vs. cow milk-based formula and followed for 12 months found significantly fewer lower respiratory tract illnesses in the Lf-fed group [114] (Table 1). In 2009, Manzoni's group performed a multicenter, double-blinded, placebo-controlled, randomized trial in VLBW infants (<1500 g) comparing administration of bLf alone or in combination with *Lactobacillus rhamnosus* GG (LGG) to placebo [115]. They found significantly lower invasive infections in the treatment groups, with an effect on infection-related mortality (0% for bLf and 0.7% for bLf plus LGG, vs. 4.8% for placebo). A follow-up study from the same group in 2014 found that bLf supplementation alone or in combination with LGG significantly reduced the incidence of $\geq$stage 2 necrotizing enterocolitis (NEC), and of death-and/or $\geq$stage 2 NEC in VLBW neonates [116]. Apart from these, several other studies (Table 1) have also examined bovine Lf and found that treatment with bLf led to a reduction in infection in both VLBW and 500–2500 g neonates [117,118]. Importantly, none of these investigations noted any adverse effects or intolerance with bovine Lf. BLf has also been evaluated in a recent study that confirmed that it was well tolerated [119]. Several other studies examining the efficacy of bovine Lf are currently underway [113]. Of note, a multicenter trial of enteral bovine Lf in 2200 <32 week infants (the ELFIN trial UK) that has recently completed recruitment, will primarily evaluate effects on late onset invasive infection but also mortality, NEC, and several later sequelae [120]. The results of this large trial may serve to further validate the utility of bovine Lf supplementation in this vulnerable population.

Table 1. Clinical Studies of Lactoferrin in Neonates. The *n* values denote the number of patients in the treatment groups. Significant study outcomes are in bold type. LOS, Late-onset sepsis.

Year	Study Population	Study Design	Lf Type	Outcomes	Investigator, Site
2007	Neonates ≥34 weeks, ≤4 weeks of life (*n* = 26)	Formula + Lf (850 mg/L) vs. cow—milk formula + Lf (102 mg/L) (≤4 weeks–12 months)	Bovine	**Lower incidence of lower respiratory tract infections**	King, USA
2009, 2012	VLBW Neonates <1500 g (Lf, *n* = 153, Lf +LGG, *n* = 151)	Lf (100 mg/day) ± LGG vs. placebo, 0–30 days (0–45 days for <1000g at birth)	Bovine	**Lower incidence of first LOS episode (in Lf ± LGG) Lower incidence of *Candida* LOS**	Manzoni, Italy
2014	VLBW neonates <1500 g (Lf, *n* = 247, Lf + LGG, *n* = 238)	Lf (100 mg/day) ± LGG vs. placebo, 0–30 days (0–45 days for <1000 g at birth)	Bovine	**Reduced incidence of ≥stage 2 NEC and of death and/or ≥stage 2 NEC**	Manzoni, Italy and New Zealand
2014	VLBW neonates, <1500 g or <32 weeks (*n* = 25)	Lf (200 mg/day) vs. placebo, through hospitalization period	Bovine	Decreased nosocomial sepsis episodes	Akin, Turkey
2015	Neonates, 500–2500 g (*n* = 95)	200 mg/kg/day vs. placebo from 2–28 days	Bovine	Sepsis less frequent in Lf group (Primary outcome: incidence of LOS, no statistical significance but CI suggestive of effect)	Ochoa, Peru
2015	Neonates <2000 g (*n* = 65)	Lf (80–140 mg/kg/day) vs. placebo from 1–28 days	Bovine	**Lower incidence of first LOS episode, reduction in sepsis-attributable mortality**	Kaur, India
2016	Neonates 750–1500 g (*n* = 60)	Lf (150 mg/kg q12h) vs. placebo from 1–28 days	Human	Trend towards decreased infectious morbidities (primary outcomes: bacteremia, NEC pneumonia, UTI, meningitis)	Sherman, USA
2016	Neonates <32 weeks (*n* = 40)	Lf (100 mg/day) vs. placebo, until 36 weeks PMA or discharge	Bovine	No difference in feeding tolerance	Barrington, Canada

Multiple in vitro and animal studies have demonstrated potent anti-microbial and immunomodulatory effects with Lf isolated from human milk. A recombinant human lactoferrin, generated in *Aspergillus oryzae*, was demonstrated to have an amino acid structure and functions highly similar to the human milk molecule [121]. Based on this expression system, commercial amounts of this protein were generated, leading to the development of a clinical candidate (talactoferrin) that differs from the native human protein in its glycosylation due to the fungal expression system but is otherwise unchanged [122,123]. Studies have demonstrated that talactoferrin is well tolerated in adult patients [124]. A single multicenter trial was conducted using talactoferrin in 750–1500 g neonates, which examined 120 infants and showed a trend towards decreased infectious morbidity but did not achieve statistical significance [125] (Table 1). Further trials with this protein, however, currently appear to be on hold following recent data showing no benefit in a trial in adult ICU patients [126].

Based on the pre-clinical data, the potential benefits of Lf supplementation are clear—with strong evidence supporting its direct anti-microbial and immune-boosting properties and effects on gut proliferation, maturation, and the development of beneficial bacteria. The clinical studies done thus far have shown uniformly positive results that have reached statistical significance in certain studies (Table 1). Based on the clinical data, early commencement of Lf may be associated with greater clinical benefits, demonstrated by examining study results from Ochoa et al. (Lf started with enteral feeds at 4 ± 1.4 days [118]), Akin et al. (with feeds at 20 mL/kg/day [117]), and Manzoni et al. (at <72 h [115]). Early supplementation may mimic the higher Lf in human colostrum and, as shown in vitro, may allow for early gut proliferation. The addition of a probiotic [115,116] appeared to substantially improve outcomes and should be further explored. However, as indicated by recent in vitro data described above [106,107], the administration of Lf in conjunction with a probiotic requires further careful study. Additionally, the use of a standard dose of Lf for all patients may not be optimal for delivering adequate concentrations of Lf to each patient and weight-based dosing regimens should be evaluated for clinical efficacy. Last, although the results with recombinant human Lf were not significant, the use of a human Lf might be revisited in the future.

8. Conclusions

Taken together, the experimental and pre-clinical studies examining the functions of Lf present overwhelming evidence, supporting a pivotal role for this multifaceted glycoprotein in preventing infection, in immunomodulation, and bolstering host defense. Many questions remain to be answered regarding the function of this glycoprotein at the molecular level and the extent of direct and immune modulatory effects caused by supplementation of Lf in the diet. Several of these questions are best addressed by in vivo studies in patients. These are challenging studies, particularly as they are targeted towards the critical VLBW infant. However, the clinical data obtained thus far have been promising and certainly support the utility of continuation of studies to examine the effects of Lf supplementation on modulating the immune response and decreasing life-threatening infections in the highly vulnerable neonatal population. Several studies are currently underway, and their results will serve to clarify the benefits of Lf supplementation in the diet of the term and preterm infant, and potentially pave the way to using Lf in the clinical setting.

Author Contributions: S.T. researched and wrote the manuscript.

Acknowledgments: We thank John Eaton and Paula Radmacher for helpful discussions.

References

1. UNIGME. *Inter-Agency Group for Child Mortality Estimation: Levels and Trends in Child Mortality, Report 2017*; UNICEF: New York, NY, USA, 2017.
2. Adkins, B.; Leclerc, C.; Marshall-Clarke, S. Neonatal adaptive immunity comes of age. *Nat. Rev. Immunol.* **2004**, *4*, 553–564. [CrossRef] [PubMed]
3. Strunk, T.; Currie, A.; Richmond, P.; Simmer, K.; Burgner, D. Innate immunity in human newborn infants: Prematurity means more than immaturity. *J. Matern. Fetal. Neonatal Med.* **2011**, *24*, 25–31. [CrossRef] [PubMed]
4. De Jong, E.; Strunk, T.; Burgner, D.; Lavoie, P.M.; Currie, A. The phenotype and function of preterm infant monocytes: Implications for susceptibility to infection. *J. Leukocyte Biol.* **2017**, *102*, 645–656. [CrossRef] [PubMed]
5. Fouda, G.G.; Martinez, D.R.; Swamy, G.K.; Permar, S.R. The Impact of IgG Transplacental Transfer on Early Life Immunity. *ImmunoHorizons* **2018**, *2*, 14–25. [CrossRef] [PubMed]
6. Ballard, O.; Morrow, A.L. Human milk composition: Nutrients and bioactive factors. *Pediatr. Clin. N. Am.* **2013**, *60*, 49–74. [CrossRef] [PubMed]
7. Sorensen, M.; Sorensen, S.P.L. The proteins in whey. *C. R. Trav. Lab. Carlsberg* **1939**, *23*, 55–99.
8. Groves, M.L. The isolation of a red protein from milk. *J. Am. Chem. Soc.* **1960**, *83*, 3345–3350. [CrossRef]
9. Johansson, B. Isolation of an iron-containing red protein from human milk. *Acta Chem. Scand.* **1960**, *14*, 510–512. [CrossRef]
10. Montreuil, J.; Tonnelat, J.; Mullet, S. Preparation and properties of lactosiderophilin (lactotransferrin) of human milk. *Biochim. Biophys. Acta* **1960**, *45*, 413–421. [CrossRef]

11. Rosa, L.; Cutone, A.; Lepanto, M.S.; Paesano, R.; Valenti, P. Lactoferrin: A Natural Glycoprotein Involved in Iron and Inflammatory Homeostasis. *Int. J. Mol. Sci.* **2017**, *18*, 1985. [CrossRef] [PubMed]
12. Liao, Y.; Alvarado, R.; Phinney, B.; Lonnerdal, B. Proteomic characterization of human milk whey proteins during a twelve-month lactation period. *J. Proteome Res.* **2011**, *10*, 1746–1754. [CrossRef] [PubMed]
13. Ronayne de Ferrer, P.A.; Baroni, A.; Sambucetti, M.E.; Lopez, N.E.; Ceriani Cernadas, J.M. Lactoferrin levels in term and preterm milk. *J. Am. Coll. Nutr.* **2000**, *19*, 370–373. [CrossRef] [PubMed]
14. Albenzio, M.; Santillo, A.; Stolfi, I.; Manzoni, P.; Iliceto, A.; Rinaldi, M.; Magaldi, R. Lactoferrin Levels in Human Milk after Preterm and Term Delivery. *Am. J. Perinatol.* **2016**, *33*, 1085–1089. [PubMed]
15. Raoof, N.A.; Adamkin, D.H.; Radmacher, P.G.; Telang, S. Comparison of lactoferrin activity in fresh and stored human milk. *J. Perinatol. Off. J. Calif. Perinat. Assoc.* **2016**, *36*, 207–209. [CrossRef] [PubMed]
16. Rollo, D.E.; Radmacher, P.G.; Turcu, R.M.; Myers, S.R.; Adamkin, D.H. Stability of lactoferrin in stored human milk. *J. Perinatol. Off. J. Calif. Perinat. Assoc.* **2014**, *34*, 284–286. [CrossRef] [PubMed]
17. Koenig, Á.; Diniz, E.M.D.A.; Barbosa, S.F.C.; Vaz, F.A.C. Immunologic Factors in Human Milk: The Effects of Gestational Age and Pasteurization. *J. Hum. Lact.* **2005**, *21*, 439–443. [CrossRef] [PubMed]
18. Manzoni, P. Clinical Benefits of Lactoferrin for Infants and Children. *J. Pediatr.* **2016**, *173*. [CrossRef] [PubMed]
19. Meier, P.P.; Patel, A.L.; Esquerra-Zwiers, A. Donor Human Milk Update: Evidence, Mechanisms and Priorities for Research and Practice. *J. Pediatr.* **2017**, *180*, 15–21. [CrossRef] [PubMed]
20. Underwood, M.A.; Scoble, J.A. *Human Milk and the Premature Infant: Focus on Use of Pasteurized Donor Human Milk in the NICU*; Springer: New York, NY, USA, 2015; pp. 795–806.
21. Picaud, J.C.; Buffin, R. Human Milk-Treatment and Quality of Banked Human Milk. *Clin. Perinatol.* **2017**, *44*, 95–119. [CrossRef] [PubMed]
22. Mayayo, C.; Montserrat, M.; Ramos, S.J.; Martínez-Lorenzo, M.J.; Calvo, M.; Sánchez, L.; Pérez, M.D. Kinetic parameters for high-pressure-induced denaturation of lactoferrin in human milk. *Int. Dairy J.* **2014**, *39*, 246–252. [CrossRef]
23. Baro, C.; Giribaldi, M.; Arslanoglu, S.; Giuffrida, M.G.; Dellavalle, G.; Conti, A.; Tonetto, P.; Biasini, A.; Coscia, A.; Fabris, C.; et al. Effect of two pasteurization methods on the protein content of human milk. *Front. Biosci. (Elite Ed.)* **2011**, *3*, 818–829. [CrossRef] [PubMed]
24. Peila, C.; Emmerik, N.E.; Giribaldi, M.; Stahl, B.; Ruitenberg, J.E.; van Elburg, R.M.; Moro, G.E.; Bertino, E.; Coscia, A.; Cavallarin, L. Human Milk Processing: A Systematic Review of Innovative Techniques to Ensure the Safety and Quality of Donor Milk. *J. Pediatr. Gastroenterol. Nutr.* **2017**, *64*, 353–361. [CrossRef] [PubMed]
25. Conesa, C.; Rota, C.; Castillo, E.; PÉRez, M.-D.; Calvo, M.; SÁNchez, L. Antibacterial Activity of Recombinant Human Lactoferrin from Rice: Effect of Heat Treatment. *Biosci. Biotechnol. Biochem.* **2009**, *73*, 1301–1307. [CrossRef] [PubMed]
26. Li, Y.; Nguyen, D.N.; de Waard, M.; Christensen, L.; Zhou, P.; Jiang, P.; Sun, J.; Bojesen, A.M.; Lauridsen, C.; Lykkesfeldt, J.; et al. Pasteurization Procedures for Donor Human Milk Affect Body Growth, Intestinal Structure, and Resistance against Bacterial Infections in Preterm Pigs. *J. Nutr.* **2017**, *147*, 1121–1130. [CrossRef] [PubMed]
27. Christen, L.; Lai, C.T.; Hartmann, B.; Hartmann, P.E.; Geddes, D.T. Ultraviolet-C Irradiation: A Novel Pasteurization Method for Donor Human Milk. *PLoS ONE* **2013**, *8*, e68120. [CrossRef] [PubMed]
28. Christen, L.; Lai, C.T.; Hartmann, B.; Hartmann, P.E.; Geddes, D.T. The Effect of UV-C Pasteurization on Bacteriostatic Properties and Immunological Proteins of Donor Human Milk. *PLoS ONE* **2013**, *8*, e85867. [CrossRef] [PubMed]
29. Anderson, B.F.; Baker, H.M.; Dodson, E.J.; Norris, G.E.; Rumball, S.V.; Waters, J.M.; Baker, E.N. Structure of human lactoferrin at 3.2-A resolution. *Proc. Natl. Acad. Sci. USA* **1987**, *84*, 1769–1773. [CrossRef] [PubMed]
30. Baker, H.M.; Baker, E.N. A structural perspective on lactoferrin function. *Biochem. Cell Biol.* **2012**, *90*, 320–328. [CrossRef] [PubMed]
31. Mazurier, J.; Spik, G. Comparative study of the iron-binding properties of human transferrins. I. Complete and sequential iron saturation and desaturation of the lactotransferrin. *Biochim. Biophys. Acta* **1980**, *629*, 399–408. [CrossRef]
32. Tomita, M.; Bellamy, W.; Takase, M.; Yamauchi, K.; Wakabayashi, H.; Kawase, K. Potent antibacterial peptides generated by pepsin digestion of bovine lactoferrin. *J. Dairy Sci.* **1991**, *74*, 4137–4142. [CrossRef]

33. Pierce, A.; Colavizza, D.; Benaissa, M.; Maes, P.; Tartar, A.; Montreuil, J.; Spik, G. Molecular Cloning and Sequence Analysis of Bovine Lactoferrin. *Eur. J. Biochem.* **2005**, *196*, 177–184. [CrossRef]
34. Castellino, F.J.; Fish, W.W.; Mann, K.G. Structural Studies on Bovine Lactoferrin. *J. Biol. Chem.* **1970**, *245*, 4269–4275. [PubMed]
35. Moore, S.A.; Anderson, B.F.; Groom, C.R.; Haridas, M.; Baker, E.N. Three-dimensional structure of diferric bovine lactoferrin at 2.8 Å resolution11Edited by D. Rees. *J. Mol. Biol.* **1997**, *274*, 222–236. [CrossRef] [PubMed]
36. Magnuson, J.S.; Henry, J.F.; Yip, T.T.; Hutchens, T.W. Structural homology of human, bovine, and porcine milk lactoferrins: Evidence for shared antigenic determinants. *Pediatr. Res.* **1990**, *28*, 176–181. [CrossRef] [PubMed]
37. Bellamy, W.; Takase, M.; Yamauchi, K.; Wakabayashi, H.; Kawase, K.; Tomita, M. Identification of the bactericidal domain of lactoferrin. *Biochim. Biophys. Acta Protein Struct. Mol. Enzymol.* **1992**, *1121*, 130–136. [CrossRef]
38. Lonnerdal, B.; Jiang, R.; Du, X. Bovine lactoferrin can be taken up by the human intestinal lactoferrin receptor and exert bioactivities. *J. Pediatr. Gastroenterol. Nutr.* **2011**, *53*, 606–614. [CrossRef] [PubMed]
39. Bullen, J.J.; Rogers, H.J.; Leigh, L. Iron-binding proteins in milk and resistance to Escherichia coli infection in infants. *Br. Med. J.* **1972**, *1*, 69–75. [CrossRef] [PubMed]
40. Acosta-Smith, E.; Viveros-Jimenez, K.; Canizalez-Roman, A.; Reyes-Lopez, M.; Bolscher, J.G.M.; Nazmi, K.; Flores-Villasenor, H.; Alapizco-Castro, G.; de la Garza, M.; Martinez-Garcia, J.J.; et al. Bovine Lactoferrin and Lactoferrin-Derived Peptides Inhibit the Growth of Vibrio cholerae and Other Vibrio species. *Front. Microbiol.* **2017**, *8*, 2633. [CrossRef] [PubMed]
41. Allison, L.M.; Walker, L.A.; Sanders, B.J.; Yang, Z.; Eckert, G.; Gregory, R.L. Effect of Human Milk and its Components on Streptococcus Mutans Biofilm Formation. *J. Clin. Pediatr. Dent.* **2015**, *39*, 255–261. [CrossRef] [PubMed]
42. Berlutti, F.; Ajello, M.; Bosso, P.; Morea, C.; Petrucca, A.; Antonini, G.; Valenti, P. Both lactoferrin and iron influence aggregation and biofilm formation in Streptococcus mutans. *Biometals* **2004**, *17*, 271–278. [PubMed]
43. Singh, P.K.; Parsek, M.R.; Greenberg, E.P.; Welsh, M.J. A component of innate immunity prevents bacterial biofilm development. *Nature* **2002**, *417*, 552–555. [CrossRef] [PubMed]
44. Arnold, R.R.; Cole, M.F.; McGhee, J.R. A bactericidal effect for human lactoferrin. *Science* **1977**, *197*, 263–265. [CrossRef] [PubMed]
45. Arnold, R.R.; Russell, J.E.; Champion, W.J.; Brewer, M.; Gauthier, J.J. Bactericidal activity of human lactoferrin: Differentiation from the stasis of iron deprivation. *Infect. Immun.* **1982**, *35*, 792–799. [PubMed]
46. Arnold, R.R.; Russell, J.E.; Champion, W.J.; Gauthier, J.J. Bactericidal activity of human lactoferrin: Influence of physical conditions and metabolic state of the target microorganism. *Infect. Immun.* **1981**, *32*, 655–660. [PubMed]
47. Ochoa, T.J.; Brown, E.L.; Guion, C.E.; Chen, J.Z.; McMahon, R.J.; Cleary, T.G. Effect of lactoferrin on enteroaggregative *E. coli* (EAEC). *Biochem. Cell Biol.* **2006**, *84*, 369–376. [CrossRef] [PubMed]
48. Qiu, J.; Hendrixson, D.R.; Baker, E.N.; Murphy, T.F.; St Geme, J.W., 3rd; Plaut, A.G. Human milk lactoferrin inactivates two putative colonization factors expressed by Haemophilus influenzae. *Proc. Natl. Acad. Sci. USA* **1998**, *95*, 12641–12646. [CrossRef] [PubMed]
49. Hendrixson, D.R.; Qiu, J.; Shewry, S.C.; Fink, D.L.; Petty, S.; Baker, E.N.; Plaut, A.G.; St Geme, J.W., 3rd. Human milk lactoferrin is a serine protease that cleaves Haemophilus surface proteins at arginine-rich sites. *Mol. Microbiol.* **2003**, *47*, 607–617. [CrossRef] [PubMed]
50. Sherman, M.P.; Petrak, K. Lactoferrin-enhanced anoikis: A defense against neonatal necrotizing enterocolitis. *Med. Hypotheses* **2005**, *65*, 478–482. [CrossRef] [PubMed]
51. Edde, L.; Hipolito, R.B.; Hwang, F.F.; Headon, D.R.; Shalwitz, R.A.; Sherman, M.P. Lactoferrin protects neonatal rats from gut-related systemic infection. *Am. J. Physiol. Gastrointest. Liver Physiol.* **2001**, *281*, G1140–G1150. [CrossRef] [PubMed]
52. Ellison, R.T., 3rd; Giehl, T.J. Killing of gram-negative bacteria by lactoferrin and lysozyme. *J. Clin. Investig.* **1991**, *88*, 1080–1091. [CrossRef] [PubMed]
53. Valenti, P.; Antonini, G. Lactoferrin: An important host defence against microbial and viral attack. *Cell. Mol. life Sci.* **2005**, *62*, 2576–2587. [CrossRef] [PubMed]

54. Reznikov, E.A.; Comstock, S.S.; Hoeflinger, J.L.; Wang, M.; Miller, M.J.; Donovan, S.M. Dietary Bovine Lactoferrin Reduces Staphylococcus aureus in the Tissues and Modulates the Immune Response in Piglets Systemically Infected with *S. aureus*. *Curr. Dev. Nutr.* **2018**, *2*, nzy001. [CrossRef] [PubMed]
55. Wu, H.F.; Monroe, D.M.; Church, F.C. Characterization of the glycosaminoglycan-binding region of lactoferrin. *Arch. Biochem. Biophys.* **1995**, *317*, 85–92. [CrossRef] [PubMed]
56. Jenssen, H.; Hancock, R.E.W. Antimicrobial properties of lactoferrin. *Biochimie* **2009**, *91*, 19–29. [CrossRef] [PubMed]
57. Xu, Y.Y.; Samaranayake, Y.H.; Samaranayake, L.P.; Nikawa, H. In vitro susceptibility of Candida species to lactoferrin. *Med. Mycol.* **1999**, *37*, 35–41. [CrossRef] [PubMed]
58. Beddek, A.J.; Schryvers, A.B. The lactoferrin receptor complex in Gram negative bacteria. *Biometals* **2010**, *23*, 377–386. [CrossRef] [PubMed]
59. Shaper, M.; Hollingshead, S.K.; Benjamin, W.H., Jr.; Briles, D.E. PspA protects Streptococcus pneumoniae from killing by apolactoferrin, and antibody to PspA enhances killing of pneumococci by apolactoferrin [corrected]. *Infect. Immun.* **2004**, *72*, 5031–5040. [CrossRef] [PubMed]
60. Kim, C.M.; Park, R.Y.; Chun, H.J.; Kim, S.Y.; Rhee, J.H.; Shin, S.H. Vibrio vulnificus metalloprotease VvpE is essentially required for swarming. *FEMS Microbiol. Lett.* **2007**, *269*, 170–179. [CrossRef] [PubMed]
61. Legrand, D. Overview of Lactoferrin as a Natural Immune Modulator. *J. Pediatr.* **2016**, *173*, S10–S15. [CrossRef] [PubMed]
62. Legrand, D.; Mazurier, J. A critical review of the roles of host lactoferrin in immunity. *BioMetals* **2010**, *23*, 365–376. [CrossRef] [PubMed]
63. Losfeld, M.E.; Khoury, D.E.; Mariot, P.; Carpentier, M.; Krust, B.; Briand, J.P.; Mazurier, J.; Hovanessian, A.G.; Legrand, D. The cell surface expressed nucleolin is a glycoprotein that triggers calcium entry into mammalian cells. *Exp. Cell Res.* **2009**, *315*, 357–369. [CrossRef] [PubMed]
64. Lee, S.H.; Pyo, C.W.; Hahm, D.H.; Kim, J.; Choi, S.Y. Iron-saturated lactoferrin stimulates cell cycle progression through PI3K/Akt pathway. *Mol. Cells* **2009**, *28*, 37–42. [CrossRef] [PubMed]
65. Liu, M.; Fan, F.; Shi, P.; Tu, M.; Yu, C.; Yu, C.; Du, M. Lactoferrin promotes MC3T3-E1 osteoblast cells proliferation via MAPK signaling pathways. *Int. J. Biol. Macromol.* **2018**, *107*, 137–143. [CrossRef] [PubMed]
66. Oh, S.-M.; Hahm, D.H.; Kim, I.-H.; Choi, S.-Y. Human Neutrophil Lactoferrin trans-Activates the Matrix Metalloproteinase 1 Gene through Stress-activated MAPK Signaling Modules. *J. Biol. Chem.* **2001**, *276*, 42575–42579. [CrossRef] [PubMed]
67. Oh, S.M.; Pyo, C.W.; Kim, Y.; Choi, S.Y. Neutrophil lactoferrin upregulates the human p53 gene through induction of NF-kappaB activation cascade. *Oncogene* **2004**, *23*, 8282–8291. [CrossRef] [PubMed]
68. Jiang, R.; Lopez, V.; Kelleher, S.L.; Lonnerdal, B. Apo- and holo-lactoferrin are both internalized by lactoferrin receptor via clathrin-mediated endocytosis but differentially affect ERK-signaling and cell proliferation in Caco-2 cells. *J. Cell. Physiol.* **2011**, *226*, 3022–3031. [CrossRef] [PubMed]
69. He, J.; Furmanski, P. Sequence specificity and transcriptional activation in the binding of lactoferrin to DNA. *Nature* **1995**, *373*, 721–724. [CrossRef] [PubMed]
70. Akira, S.; Hemmi, H. Recognition of pathogen-associated molecular patterns by TLR family. *Immunol. Lett.* **2003**, *85*, 85–95. [CrossRef]
71. Elass-Rochard, E.; Legrand, D.; Salmon, V.; Roseanu, A.; Trif, M.; Tobias, P.S.; Mazurier, J.; Spik, G. Lactoferrin Inhibits the Endotoxin Interaction with CD14 by Competition with the Lipopolysaccharide-Binding Protein. *Infect. Immun.* **1998**, *66*, 486–491. [PubMed]
72. Lee, W.J.; Farmer, J.L.; Hilty, M.; Kim, Y.B. The Protective Effects of Lactoferrin Feeding against Endotoxin Lethal Shock in Germfree Piglets. *Infect. Immun.* **1998**, *66*, 1421–1426. [PubMed]
73. Appelmelk, B.J.; An, Y.Q.; Geerts, M.; Thijs, B.G.; de Boer, H.A.; MacLaren, D.M.; de Graaff, J.; Nuijens, J.H. Lactoferrin is a lipid A-binding protein. *Infect. Immun.* **1994**, *62*, 2628–2632. [PubMed]
74. Elass, E.; Masson, M.; Mazurier, J.; Legrand, D. Lactoferrin inhibits the lipopolysaccharide-induced expression and proteoglycan-binding ability of interleukin-8 in human endothelial cells. *Infect. Immun.* **2002**, *70*, 1860–1866. [CrossRef] [PubMed]
75. Andonegui, G.; Zhou, H.; Bullard, D.; Kelly, M.M.; Mullaly, S.C.; McDonald, B.; Long, E.M.; Robbins, S.M.; Kubes, P. Mice that exclusively express TLR4 on endothelial cells can efficiently clear a lethal systemic Gram-negative bacterial infection. *J. Clin. Investig.* **2009**, *119*, 1921–1930. [CrossRef] [PubMed]

76. Shau, H.; Kim, A.; Golub, S.H. Modulation of natural killer and lymphokine-activated killer cell cytotoxicity by lactoferrin. *J. Leukocyte Biol.* **1992**, *51*, 343–349. [CrossRef] [PubMed]
77. Roseanu, A.; Chelu, F.; Trif, M.; Motas, C.; Brock, J.H. Inhibition of binding of lactoferrin to the human promonocyte cell line THP-1 by heparin: The role of cell surface sulphated molecules. *Biochim. Biophys. Acta* **2000**, *1475*, 35–38. [CrossRef]
78. Sorimachi, K.; Akimoto, K.; Hattori, Y.; Ieiri, T.; Niwa, A. Activation of macrophages by lactoferrin: Secretion of TNF-alpha, IL-8 and NO. *Biochem. Mol. Biol. Int.* **1997**, *43*, 79–87. [CrossRef] [PubMed]
79. Tanida, T.; Rao, F.; Hamada, T.; Ueta, E.; Osaki, T. Lactoferrin peptide increases the survival of Candida albicans-inoculated mice by upregulating neutrophil and macrophage functions, especially in combination with amphotericin B and granulocyte-macrophage colony-stimulating factor. *Infect. Immun.* **2001**, *69*, 3883–3890. [CrossRef] [PubMed]
80. Deriy, L.V.; Chor, J.; Thomas, L.L. Surface Expression of Lactoferrin by Resting Neutrophils. *Biochem. Biophys. Res. Commun.* **2000**, *275*, 241–246. [CrossRef] [PubMed]
81. Miyauchi, H.; Hashimoto, S.; Nakajima, M.; Shinoda, I.; Fukuwatari, Y.; Hayasawa, H. Bovine lactoferrin stimulates the phagocytic activity of human neutrophils: Identification of its active domain. *Cell. Immunol.* **1998**, *187*, 34–37. [CrossRef] [PubMed]
82. Kai, K.; Komine, K.I.; Komine, Y.; Kuroishi, T.; Kozutsumi, T.; Kobayashi, J.; Ohta, M.; Kitamura, H.; Kumagai, K. Lactoferrin stimulates A Staphylococcus aureus killing activity of bovine phagocytes in the mammary gland. *Microbiol. Immunol.* **2002**, *46*, 187–194. [CrossRef] [PubMed]
83. Actor, J.K.; Hwang, S.A.; Kruzel, M.L. Lactoferrin as a natural immune modulator. *Curr. Pharm. Des.* **2009**, *15*, 1956–1973. [CrossRef] [PubMed]
84. Trinchieri, G. Interleukin-12 and the regulation of innate resistance and adaptive immunity. *Nat. Rev. Immunol.* **2003**, *3*, 133–146. [CrossRef] [PubMed]
85. Spadaro, M.; Caorsi, C.; Ceruti, P.; Varadhachary, A.; Forni, G.; Pericle, F.; Giovarelli, M. Lactoferrin, a major defense protein of innate immunity, is a novel maturation factor for human dendritic cells. *FASEB J.* **2008**, *22*, 2747–2757. [CrossRef] [PubMed]
86. De la Rosa, G.; De, Y.; Tewary, P.; Varadhachary, A.; Oppenheim, J.J. Lactoferrin acts as an alarmin to promote the recruitment and activation of antigen-presenting cells and antigen-specific immune responses. *J. Immunol.* **2008**, *180*, 6868–6876. [CrossRef] [PubMed]
87. Kruzel, M.L.; Zimecki, M.; Actor, J.K. Lactoferrin in a Context of Inflammation-Induced Pathology. *Front. Immunol.* **2017**, *8*, 1438. [CrossRef] [PubMed]
88. Perdijk, O.; van Neerven, R.J.J.; van den Brink, E.; Savelkoul, H.F.J.; Brugman, S. Bovine Lactoferrin Modulates Dendritic Cell Differentiation and Function. *Nutrients* **2018**, *10*, 848. [CrossRef] [PubMed]
89. Puddu, P.; Carollo, M.G.; Belardelli, F.; Valenti, P.; Gessani, S. Role of endogenous interferon and LPS in the immunomodulatory effects of bovine lactoferrin in murine peritoneal macrophages. *J. Leukocyte Biol.* **2007**, *82*, 347–353. [CrossRef] [PubMed]
90. Bi, B.Y.; Liu, J.L.; Legrand, D.; Roche, A.C.; Capron, M.; Spik, G.; Mazurier, J. Internalization of human lactoferrin by the Jurkat human lymphoblastic T-cell line. *Eur. J. Cell Biol.* **1996**, *69*, 288–296. [PubMed]
91. Dhennin-Duthille, I.; Masson, M.; Damiens, E.; Fillebeen, C.; Spik, G.; Mazurier, J. Lactoferrin upregulates the expression of CD4 antigen through the stimulation of the mitogen-activated protein kinase in the human lymphoblastic T Jurkat cell line. *J. Cell. Biochem.* **2000**, *79*, 583–593. [CrossRef]
92. Zimecki, M.; Mazurier, J.; Machnicki, M.; Wieczorek, Z.; Montreuil, J.; Spik, G. Immunostimulatory activity of lactotransferrin and maturation of CD4- CD8- murine thymocytes. *Immunol. Lett.* **1991**, *30*, 119–123. [CrossRef]
93. Artym, J.; Zimecki, M.; Kruzel, M.L. Reconstitution of the cellular immune response by lactoferrin in cyclophosphamide-treated mice is correlated with renewal of T cell compartment. *Immunobiology* **2003**, *207*, 197–205. [CrossRef] [PubMed]
94. Kobayashi, S.; Sato, R.; Inanami, O.; Yamamori, T.; Yamato, O.; Maede, Y.; Sato, J.; Kuwabara, M.; Naito, Y. Reduction of concanavalin A-induced expression of interferon-gamma by bovine lactoferrin in feline peripheral blood mononuclear cells. *Vet. Immunol. Immunopathol.* **2005**, *105*, 75–84. [CrossRef] [PubMed]
95. Zimecki, M.; Mazurier, J.; Spik, G.; Kapp, J.A. Human lactoferrin induces phenotypic and functional changes in murine splenic B cells. *Immunology* **1995**, *86*, 122–127. [PubMed]

96. Siqueiros-Cendón, T.; Arévalo-Gallegos, S.; Iglesias-Figueroa, B.F.; García-Montoya, I.A.; Salazar-Martínez, J.; Rascón-Cruz, Q. Immunomodulatory effects of lactoferrin. *Acta Pharmacol. Sin.* **2014**, *35*, 557–566. [CrossRef] [PubMed]
97. Debbabi, H.; Dubarry, M.; Rautureau, M.; Tome, D. Bovine lactoferrin induces both mucosal and systemic immune response in mice. *J. Dairy Res.* **1998**, *65*, 283–293. [CrossRef] [PubMed]
98. Sfeir, R.M.; Dubarry, M.; Boyaka, P.N.; Rautureau, M.; Tome, D. The mode of oral bovine lactoferrin administration influences mucosal and systemic immune responses in mice. *J. Nutr.* **2004**, *134*, 403–409. [CrossRef] [PubMed]
99. Artym, J.; Zimecki, M.; Kuryszko, J.; Kruzel, M.L. Lactoferrin accelerates reconstitution of the humoral and cellular immune response during chemotherapy-induced immunosuppression and bone marrow transplant in mice. *Stem Cells Dev.* **2005**, *14*, 548–555. [CrossRef] [PubMed]
100. Kleessen, B.; Bunke, H.; Tovar, K.; Noack, J.; Sawatzki, G. Influence of two infant formulas and human milk on the development of the faecal flora in newborn infants. *Acta Paediatr.* **1995**, *84*, 1347–1356. [CrossRef] [PubMed]
101. Petschow, B.W.; Talbott, R.D. Response of bifidobacterium species to growth promoters in human and cow milk. *Pediatr. Res.* **1991**, *29*, 208–213. [CrossRef] [PubMed]
102. Liepke, C.; Adermann, K.; Raida, M.; Magert, H.J.; Forssmann, W.G.; Zucht, H.D. Human milk provides peptides highly stimulating the growth of bifidobacteria. *Eur. J. Biochem.* **2002**, *269*, 712–718. [CrossRef] [PubMed]
103. Oda, H.; Wakabayashi, H.; Yamauchi, K.; Abe, F. Lactoferrin and bifidobacteria. *Biometals* **2014**, *27*, 915–922. [CrossRef] [PubMed]
104. Mastromarino, P.; Capobianco, D.; Campagna, G.; Laforgia, N.; Drimaco, P.; Dileone, A.; Baldassarre, M.E. Correlation between lactoferrin and beneficial microbiota in breast milk and infant's feces. *Biometals* **2014**, *27*, 1077–1086. [CrossRef] [PubMed]
105. Claud, E.C.; Walker, W.A. Hypothesis: Inappropriate colonization of the premature intestine can cause neonatal necrotizing enterocolitis. *FASEB J.* **2001**, *15*, 1398–1403. [CrossRef] [PubMed]
106. Woodman, T.; Strunk, T.; Patole, S.; Hartmann, B.; Simmer, K.; Currie, A. Effects of lactoferrin on neonatal pathogens and Bifidobacterium breve in human breast milk. *PLoS ONE* **2018**, *13*, e0201819. [CrossRef] [PubMed]
107. Chen, P.W.; Ku, Y.W.; Chu, F.Y. Influence of bovine lactoferrin on the growth of selected probiotic bacteria under aerobic conditions. *Biometals* **2014**, *27*, 905–914. [CrossRef] [PubMed]
108. Buccigrossi, V.; de Marco, G.; Bruzzese, E.; Ombrato, L.; Bracale, I.; Polito, G.; Guarino, A. Lactoferrin induces concentration-dependent functional modulation of intestinal proliferation and differentiation. *Pediatr. Res.* **2007**, *61*, 410–414. [CrossRef] [PubMed]
109. Nichols, B.L.; McKee, K.S.; Henry, J.F.; Putman, M. Human lactoferrin stimulates thymidine incorporation into DNA of rat crypt cells. *Pediatr. Res.* **1987**, *21*, 563–567. [CrossRef] [PubMed]
110. Reznikov, E.A.; Comstock, S.S.; Yi, C.; Contractor, N.; Donovan, S.M. Dietary bovine lactoferrin increases intestinal cell proliferation in neonatal piglets. *J. Nutr.* **2014**, *144*, 1401–1408. [CrossRef] [PubMed]
111. Shulman, R.J.; Schanler, R.J.; Lau, C.; Heitkemper, M.; Ou, C.-N.; Smith, E.O.B. Early Feeding, Antenatal Glucocorticoids, and Human Milk Decrease Intestinal Permeability in Preterm Infants. *Pediatr. Res.* **1998**, *44*, 519. [CrossRef] [PubMed]
112. Stoll, B.J.; Hansen, N.I.; Adams-Chapman, I.; Fanaroff, A.A.; Hintz, S.R.; Vohr, B.; Higgins, R.D. Neurodevelopmental and growth impairment among extremely low-birth-weight infants with neonatal infection. *JAMA* **2004**, *292*, 2357–2365. [CrossRef] [PubMed]
113. Pammi, M.; Suresh, G. Enteral Lactoferrin Supplementation for Prevention of Sepsis and Necrotizing Enterocolitis in Preterm Infants. *Cochrane Database Syst. Rev.* **2017**, *6*, CD007137.
114. King, J.C.J.; Cummings, G.E.; Guo, N.; Trivedi, L.; Readmond, B.X.; Keane, V.; Feigelman, S.; De Waard, R. A Double-Blind, Placebo-Controlled, Pilot Study of Bovine Lactoferrin Supplementation in Bottle-fed Infants. *J. Pediatr. Gastroenterol. Nutr.* **2007**, *44*, 245–251. [CrossRef] [PubMed]
115. Manzoni, P.; Rinaldi, M.; Cattani, S.; Pugni, L.; Romeo, M.G.; Messner, H.; Stolfi, I.; Decembrino, L.; Laforgia, N.; Vagnarelli, F.; et al. Bovine lactoferrin supplementation for prevention of late-onset sepsis in very low-birth-weight neonates: A randomized trial. *JAMA* **2009**, *302*, 1421–1428. [CrossRef] [PubMed]

116. Manzoni, P.; Meyer, M.; Stolfi, I.; Rinaldi, M.; Cattani, S.; Pugni, L.; Romeo, M.G.; Messner, H.; Decembrino, L.; Laforgia, N.; et al. Bovine lactoferrin supplementation for prevention of necrotizing enterocolitis in very-low-birth-weight neonates: A randomized clinical trial. *Early Hum. Dev.* **2014**, *90* (Suppl. 1), S60–S65. [CrossRef]
117. Akin, I.M.; Atasay, B.; Dogu, F.; Okulu, E.; Arsan, S.; Karatas, H.D.; Ikinciogullari, A.; Turmen, T. Oral lactoferrin to prevent nosocomial sepsis and necrotizing enterocolitis of premature neonates and effect on T-regulatory cells. *Am. J. Perinatol.* **2014**, *31*, 1111–1120. [PubMed]
118. Ochoa, T.J.; Zegarra, J.; Cam, L.; Llanos, R.; Pezo, A.; Cruz, K.; Zea-Vera, A.; Carcamo, C.; Campos, M.; Bellomo, S. Randomized controlled trial of lactoferrin for prevention of sepsis in peruvian neonates less than 2500 g. *Pediat. Infect. Dis. J.* **2015**, *34*, 571–576. [CrossRef] [PubMed]
119. Barrington, K.J.; Assaad, M.A.; Janvier, A. The Lacuna Trial: A double-blind randomized controlled pilot trial of lactoferrin supplementation in the very preterm infant. *J. Perinatol.* **2016**, *36*, 666–669. [CrossRef] [PubMed]
120. Summary Protocol for a Multi-Centre Randomised Controlled Trial of Enteral Lactoferrin Supplementation in Newborn Very Preterm Infants (ELFIN). *Neonatology* **2018**, *114*, 142–148. [CrossRef] [PubMed]
121. Ward, P.P.; Lo, J.Y.; Duke, M.; May, G.S.; Headon, D.R.; Conneely, O.M. Production of biologically active recombinant human lactoferrin in *Aspergillus oryzae*. *Biotechnology (N. Y.)* **1992**, *10*, 784–789. [CrossRef]
122. Ward, P.P.; Cunningham, G.A.; Conneely, O.M. Commercial production of lactoferrin, a multifunctional iron-binding glycoprotein. *Biotechnol. Genet. Eng. Rev.* **1997**, *14*, 303–319. [CrossRef] [PubMed]
123. Sun, X.L.; Baker, H.M.; Shewry, S.C.; Jameson, G.B.; Baker, E.N. Structure of recombinant human lactoferrin expressed in *Aspergillus awamori*. *Acta Crystallogr. Sect. D Biol. Crystallogr.* **1999**, *55*, 403–407. [CrossRef]
124. Lyons, T.E.; Miller, M.S.; Serena, T.; Sheehan, P.; Lavery, L.; Kirsner, R.S.; Armstrong, D.G.; Reese, A.; Yankee, E.W.; Veves, A. Talactoferrin alfa, a recombinant human lactoferrin promotes healing of diabetic neuropathic ulcers: A phase 1/2 clinical study. *Am. J. Surg.* **2007**, *193*, 49–54. [CrossRef] [PubMed]
125. Sherman, M.P.; Adamkin, D.H.; Niklas, V.; Radmacher, P.; Sherman, J.; Wertheimer, F.; Petrak, K. Randomized Controlled Trial of Talactoferrin Oral Solution in Preterm Infants. *J. Pediatr.* **2016**, *175*, 68–73.e63. [CrossRef] [PubMed]
126. Vincent, J.L.; Marshall, J.C.; Dellinger, R.P.; Simonson, S.G.; Guntupalli, K.; Levy, M.M.; Singer, M.; Malik, R. Talactoferrin in Severe Sepsis: Results From the Phase II/III Oral tAlactoferrin in Severe sepsIS Trial. *Crit. Care Med.* **2015**, *43*, 1832–1838. [CrossRef] [PubMed]

14

Supporting Mothers of Very Preterm Infants and Breast Milk Production: A Review of the Role of Galactogogues

Elizabeth V. Asztalos

Department of Newborn and Developmental Paediatrics, Sunnybrook Health Sciences Centre, University of Toronto, M4N 3M5 Toronto, ON, Canada; elizabeth.asztalos@sunnybrook.ca

Abstract: Human milk, either mother's own milk or donor human milk, is recommended as the primary source of nutrition for very preterm infants. Initiatives should be in place in neonatal units to provide support to the mother as she strives to initiate and maintain a supply of breast milk for her infant. The use of galactogogues are considered when these initiatives alone may not be successful in supporting mothers in this endeavor. Although there are non-pharmacologic compounds, this review will focus on the pharmacologic galactogogues currently available and the literature related to their use in mothers of very preterm infants.

Keywords: breast milk; galactogogues; mothers of preterm infants

1. Introduction

The very preterm infant (<30 weeks gestation) is faced with an array of serious morbidities, which can include sepsis (late-onset), necrotizing enterocolitis (NEC), retinopathy of prematurity, bronchopulmonary dysplasia (BPD), and intracranial white matter injury [1–6]. Human milk is the recommended nutritional support for the very preterm infant as it aids in reducing these morbidities and improves the neurodevelopmental outcomes for these infants [7–10]. The bioactive components found in breast milk are thought to promote gastrointestinal development, provide substrate for brain development and reduce the incidence of sepsis and necrotizing enterocolitis, both of which are linked in part to a negative impact on neurodevelopment [11–14]. Based on these clinical information, it is recommended that very preterm infants receive breast milk, preferably mother's own milk, as the primary source of nutrition rather than rely on preterm formula [15]. Consequently, mothers are encouraged to initiate hand expression and pumping within hours of giving birth to provide breast milk for their infants. With very preterm infants requiring hospitalization for anywhere from 10–16 weeks, continued and sustained breast milk volumes can prove to be a challenge to even the most dedicated of mothers. Many mothers of very preterm infants, for a variety of reasons such as illness, stress and other factors related to preterm birth, are unable to exclusively feed their children [16–21].

2. Breast Milk Production in Mothers of Preterm Infants

Lactogenesis (milk synthesis) is noted to start around mid-pregnancy and has been referred to as having 2 stages (lactogenesis I and II) which are under the influence of hormones, namely estrogen, insulin, cortisol, progesterone, prolactin, and human placental lactogen [22–25]. Lactogenesis I represents the secretory differentiation phase where the mammary epithelial cells differentiate into secretory mammary epithelial cells with the capacity to synthesize milk constituents such as lactose, total proteins and immunoglobulins. After parturition, the secretory phase of lactogenesis or lactogenesis II is triggered by the rapid decline of serum maternal progesterone that occurs with the expulsion of the placenta; in addition, this leads to a drop in estrogen levels while prolactin levels remain high along with insulin and cortisol [24,25]. Colostrum is produced during the first 4 days postpartum, followed by transitional milk secretion for the next 10 days followed by mature milk production [26]. Milk volume rapidly increases after the first 24 h postpartum and stabilizes after 1 month postpartum to an average volume of 750–800 mL/24 h for the term infant [27,28]. Milk production is increased by efficient and timely removal of milk, with adequate milk removal by day 3 postpartum being critical to the establishment of ongoing successful lactation [29]. Milk production is regulated by endocrine hormones (prolactin and oxytocin) as well as adequate and regular milk removal. Prolactin is required to maintain milk yield while oxytocin is released in response to suckling and induces the contraction of myoepithelial cells surrounding mammary alveoli triggering milk ejection, "milk let-down" [25]. Once milk secretion is established, hormone levels are maintained at low levels and ongoing production is regulated by consistent and regular milk removal (autocrine control); in the term infant, the volume of milk produced is determined by how the breast is emptied at feedings which, in turn, is determined by the infant's appetite [29–32].

Preterm birth may alter the normal sequence of lactogenesis. A delay in secretory activation can be associated with a negative impact on successful lactation [33,34]. Mothers of preterm infants can have problems at this stage as a result of their preterm delivery, antenatal corticosteroids, stress, maternal illness and operative delivery [19–21]. Mothers of very preterm infants must establish their milk supply through mechanical expression as the normal mechanism of infant suckling is limited in the very preterm infant [29,35].

Studies have emphasized the importance of establishing an adequate milk production in the early postpartum period for mothers of preterm infants. In a study involving 95 mothers from four tertiary care centers in the Midwest United States, the milk volume expressed on day 4 postpartum was found to be predictive of an inadequate milk supply at 6 weeks postpartum. Mothers producing less than 140 mL/day on day 4 were found to be 9.5 times more at risk of low or inadequate milk production by 6 weeks postpartum [36].

Maintaining a milk volume in amounts sufficient to meet the nutritional needs of their very preterm infants can be challenging for many mothers [17,18,37,38]. A volume of 500 mL/day or 3500 mL/week (equivalent to a mother pumping 80–100 mL/pumping, six times a day) has been identified as the minimum milk volume a mother of a preterm infant should pump in order to meet the needs of her infant at discharge [39]. If a mother is producing >3500 mL by week 2, it can be expected that she will produce this ongoing adequate amount in weeks 4 and 5. If a mother is producing ≥1700 mL/week but <3500 mL by week 2, she has approximately a 50% likelihood of reaching the minimum of 3500 mL/week by week 5 postpartum. For a mother who is producing <1700 mL/week (<40 mL/pumping), the outlook is grim with 100% not achieving the goal of 500 mL/day by weeks 4–5 postpartum.

The inadequate milk volume and declining production over the subsequent weeks pose challenges for the mother eager to provide milk for her infant Additional approaches may need to be explored for those mothers who show a decline in production and will likely stop expression of breast milk for their infant.

3. Use of Galactogogues for Breast Milk Production—A Review of the Literature

Many non-pharmacological measures have been found to contribute to variable levels of success in augmenting the breast milk production in mothers of preterm infants [38]. While these approaches may be helpful, it is critical to emphasize that the primary effective strategy for optimizing breast milk volume is frequent and effective breast emptying [29]. In the setting of reduced breast milk volume, galactogogues can be added to an increased pumping regime to augment breast milk volume.

Medications which have galactogogue capabilities generally augment lactation by exerting its effects through either oxytocin or prolactin [40,41]. Oxytocin nasal spray has been evaluated in

3 clinical trials, but negative clinical experience and low use led to the spray being discontinued in many countries thereby limiting its use on a widespread nature [41]. Sulpiride is a substituted benzamide antipsychotic medication. It is an antagonist of dopamine that increases serum prolactin levels similar to other galactogogues. It has poor bioavailability (35%) and has many of the same side effects and complications as other antipsychotics including sedation, extrapyramidal effects, tardive dyskinesia, and neuroleptic malignant syndrome making its use less appealing [41].

The primary medications used today for prolactin production are, like sulpiride, dopamine antagonists. They increase serum prolactin by counteracting the inhibitory influence of dopamine on prolactin secretion. The medications studied most widely for their galactogogue capabilities have been metoclopramide and domperidone. Both medications are used in an "off-label" capacity, i.e., they have not been authorized for use in lactation support. In addition, availability of these medications vary; domperidone, in particular, is available in most countries but not in the United States. A search in the common literature databases (Medline, CINAHL, EMBASE, OVID, Cochrane Library) was done to identify studies or trials evaluating these two pharmacologic galactogogues in mothers of preterm infants.

Metoclopromide augments lactation by antagonizing the release of dopamine in the central nervous system. Because the medication exerts its effects centrally, it can cause extrapyramidal side effects which may include tremor, bradykinesia and other dystonic reactions [40,41].

Seventeen studies were identified evaluating metoclopromide to improve breast milk production (Table 1).

Table 1. Studies evaluating metoclopromide and breast milk production.

Study	Year	N	Placebo	Randomization	Intervention	Findings
Guzmán [42]	1979	21	Y	Y	20 mg TID 4 weeks	↑ BM, PRL
Lewis [43]	1980	20	Y	Y	10 mg TID 4 days	↑ BM
Tolino [44]	1981	10	N	N	10 mg TID 7 days	↑ BM, PRL
Kauppila [45]	1981	37	Y	Y	5–15 mg TID 2 weeks	↑ BM, PRL
Kauppila [46]	1981	17	N	N	10 mg TID 5 weeks	↑ BM, PRL
Kauppila [47]	1983	5	N	N	10 mg TID 5 days	↑ plasma levels in infant
de Gezelle [48]	1983	13	Y	Y	10 mg TID 8 days	↑ BM
Kauppila [49]	1985	24	Y	Y	10 mg TID 3 weeks	↑ BM
Gupta [50]	1985	32	N	N	10 mg TID	↑ lactation
Ehrenkranz [51]	1986	23	N	N	10 mg TID 7 days	↑ BM, basal PRL
Ertl [52]	1991	22	N	N	10 mg TID 5 days	↑ BM
Nemba [53]	1994	37	N	N	10 mg QID 5–11 days	↑ lactation
Toppare [54]	1994	60	N	N	10 mg TID	↑ lactation
Seema [55]	1997	50	N	N	10 mg TID 10 days	↑ lactation
Hansen [56]	2005	57	Y	Y	10 mg TID 10 days	No difference
Sakha [57]	2008	20	Y	Y	10 mg TID 8 days	No difference
Fife [58]	2011	19	Y	Y	10 mg TID 8 days	No difference

BM = breast milk; PRL = prolactin; TID = three times daily; Y = yes; N = no.

Many studies were done well before 2000 and mostly in mothers with term infants. However, three were conducted with mothers of preterm infants, Ehrenkranz et al. [51], Hansen et al. [56], and Fife et al. [58]. Although not a randomized clinical trial (RCT), Ehrenkranz demonstrated an increase in daily breast milk production with metoclopramide from 93.3 ± 18.0 mL/day to 197.4 ± 32.3 mL/day between the first and seventh day of therapy [51]. The other two, Hansen et al. [56] and Fife [58], found no difference in breast milk volume. These two studies had methodological concerns in that all mothers were enrolled without any evaluation of their ability to produce milk. The inclusion of mothers who would not have had any difficulty in breast milk production may have minimized differences between the groups.

Domperidone is a potent dopamine D_2 receptor antagonist and was developed and marketed as a prokinetic and antiemetic agent. By blocking dopamine D_2 receptors in the anterior pituitary, domperidone stimulates the release of prolactin. Domperidone is less lipid soluble, has a higher molecular weight and has lower protein binding (>90%) than metoclopromide (40%). These characteristics appear to prevent domperidone from crossing the blood brain barrier and therefore less likely to cause the extra pyramidal effects often seen with metoclopromide [59,60]. This characteristic made domperidone more appealing in use compared to metoclopramide. In addition, early studies in the 1980's evaluating its efficacy in augmenting breast milk production [50,51] made this medication more enticing to consider, particularly in mothers of preterm infants.

Nine studies involving domperidone are outlined in Table 2. Seven of these studies were conducted in mothers of preterm infants. All of the studies were small in terms of number of mothers enrolled.

Table 2. Studies evaluating domperidone and breast milk production.

Study	Year	N	Placebo	Randomization	Intervention	Findings
De Leo [61]	1986	15	Y	N	10 mg TID 4 days	↑ lactation
Petraglia [62]	1985	17	Y	N	10 mg TID 10 days	↑ PRL, BM
da Silva [63]	2001	20	Y	Y	10 mg TID 7 days	↑ PRL, BM
Wan [64]	2008	6	N	Y	10 mg vs. 20 mg TID 1–2 weeks	↑ PRL, BM
Campbell-Yeo [65]	2010	46	Y	Y	10 mg TID 14 days	↑↑ PRL, BM
Ingram [66]	2012	80	N	Y	10 mg TID 10d or Metoclopramide 10 mg TID 10 days	↑ BM
Knoppert [67]	2013	15	N	Y	10 mg vs. 20 mg TID 4 weeks	↑ BM
Rai [68]	2016	32	Y	N	Unknown dose for 8 days	↑ BM
Asztalos [69]	2017	90	Y	Y	10 mg TID 14 days	↑ BM

BM = breast milk; PRL = prolactin; TID = three times daily; Y = yes; N = no.

da Silva et al. was the first RCT to evaluate the efficacy of domperidone in mothers of preterm infants [63]. In this study, there was a mean increase in breast milk yield from days 2 to 7 in the domperidone group (49.5 mL, standard deviation 29.4 mL) compared to the placebo group (8.0 mL, standard deviation 39.5 mL) ($p < 0.05$) as well as an increase in serum prolactin ($p = 0.008$). Wan et al. evaluated a dose-response relationship between 30 and 60 mg daily [64]. Serum prolactin increased for both doses but was not dose-dependent. In addition, only two-thirds of the mothers (4 out of 6) were identified as "responders" and showed a significant increase in milk production which was also dose-dependent. Campbell-Yeo et al. randomized 46 mothers to either domperidone 10 mg three times daily or placebo equivalent for 14 days [65]. Although the study's primary goal was to evaluate the effect of domperidone on the nutrient composition of preterm human milk compared to those mothers having received a placebo, there was a significant increase in serum prolactin ($p = 0.07$) and breast milk volumes ($p = 0.005$) in the domperidone group. The mean within-subject increase by day 14 was 267% in the domperidone group (184 to 380 mL) compared to 19% in placebo group (218 to 250 mL). This trial did suggest that a larger yield in breast milk production could be achieved with the additional week as compared to the earlier trial.

Ingram et al. compared the effects of domperidone and metoclopramide on breast milk output in mothers of preterm infants and found no significant differences between the two galactogogues [66]. Both groups showed an increase in breast milk volume. Mothers in the domperidone group achieved a mean of 96.3% in milk volume compared to 93.7% increase for metoclopramide.

Knoppert et al. enrolled 12 mothers between 14–21 days post-delivery to evaluate the effectiveness of two dosing strategies, 10 mg compared to 20 mg three times daily for 28 days, on milk production in mothers of preterm infants [67]. Both dosing strategies showed breast milk volumes increasing with a clinically higher amount in the higher dosing approach, but the actual volumes were not given.

More recently, the EMPOWER trial by Asztalos et al. enrolled 90 mothers, who gave birth to preterm infants <30 weeks gestation, to receive domperidone 30 mg daily compared to a placebo for 14 days followed by all mothers receiving domperidone 30 mg daily for another 14 days [69]. More mothers achieved a 50% increase in milk volume after 14 days in the treated group (77.8%) compared to placebo (57.8%) (odds ratios 2.56; 95% confidence interval 1.02, 6.25; $p = 0.04$) ; however, the gain in actual volume was modest and not significantly different.

Each of the described studies evaluating domperidone as a means to augment breast milk production were significantly different in design and did not allow a more direct comparison. The studies were different in dosing approaches, timing and duration of treatment and the use or non-use of a placebo as well as outcome measures. The response to the interventions in the individual studies were different. Most, but not all, provided 24-h volumes as a measure for determining a response to domperidone. Two studies did not give actual values [64,67].

4. Clinical Efficacy

Overall, study findings indicate that metoclopramide is less efficacious than domperidone in augmenting breast milk production in mothers of preterm infants. Domperidone studies showed a modest increase in breast milk production but the approaches in dosing, timing and duration of treatment varied considerably in each trial. The cumulative dose in the trial by da Silva varied greatly compared to the trial by Knoppert [63,67]. In addition, even within a trial, mothers varied with respect to the cumulative dose [69]. Because the objectives of the individual studies varied, how breast milk volume was measured varied as well: 24-h volumes vs. percentages vs. volume per pump session.

Despite the varied approaches in outcome measures, the studies all demonstrated an increase in breast milk volume. However, it is important to note that 24-h volumes on average still remained below the target of 500 mL/day [63,65,66,68,69]. Recently, Grzeskowiak et al. conducted a meta-analysis which pooled five trials [63,65,68–70] which showed that short-term use of domperidone resulted in a modest 86 mL/day increase in expressed breast milk [71]. For a mother of a preterm infant weighing 1000 g and receiving enteral feeds at 160 mL/kg/day, this represents an opportunity to meet half of her infant's feeds with her own breast milk, if not more, depending what her starting baseline volume had been. However, this modest volume increase may still fall short of the volume that an infant will need by term corrected age.

Whether there is a sustained effect on volume maintenance with galactogogues, and, in particular domperidone, is not clear. The EMPOWER study did follow the mothers to 6 weeks post term gestation. However, regardless of the assigned grouping, almost 60% of the study participants attempted to continue to provide breast milk and continued with some form of lactation inducing compounds at term gestation with the numbers dropping to just over 40% for the combined groups at 6 weeks post term gestation suggesting there was no sustained effect on breast milk production for the mothers in the trial [69]. At present, there are no studies that have looked at long-term use of domperidone beyond two or four weeks and whether it has an effect on sustained breast milk provision post initial hospital discharge.

5. Safety Issues

As noted earlier, metoclopromide exerts its effects centrally and can cause extrapyramidal side effects which may include tremor, bradykinesia and other dystonic reactions which are both dose and duration related [40,41]. These centrally-based side effects have prompted many clinicians to use domperidone rather than metoclopramide as their primary galactogogue. Domperidone's use has grown exponentially for supporting mothers in breast milk production [72,73]. However, over the past decade, concerns have risen regarding the increased risk of prolongation of the Q-Tc interval, the risk of cardiac arrhythmias, and sudden cardiac death in the general adult population [74–77]. The relevance of these findings to women who are receiving this medication for lactation support is not clear and has been questioned [75]. However, given the wide use of domperidone to augment breast milk volumes, these concerns have led regulatory agencies, in particular the European Medicines Agency and Health Canada, to recommend caution in the use of domperidone and have provided dosing recommendations [78,79]. The most recent study to demonstrate these concerns, Smolina et al. identified 45,518 women from a provincial database who were dispensed domperidone in the first 6 months of their postpartum period [80]. Of these women, there were 21 women hospitalized for ventricular arrhythmia. The authors concluded that that there was a possible association between exposure to domperidone and hospitalization for ventricular arrhythmia (adjusted HR = 2.25, 95% CI 0.84–6.01), but that further research was needed to confirm this association. More recent studies have attempted to demonstrate an element of reassurance. In the EMPOWER trial, all of the 90 women enrolled had an ECG at study entry and at the end of the 4-week study period. Although not powered to detect a significant increase in cardiac arrhythmias, no women demonstrated any evidence of a QTc prolongation [69]. In addition, a recent review assessing QTc prolongation concluded that domperidone was not associated with QTc prolongation in healthy female volunteers [81]. A second major concern for safety related to domperidone is that of sudden cardiac death. Domperidone has been shown to have a 2.8-fold increased risk for sudden cardiac death in the general population [82,83]. However, no data to date demonstrates the risk specific to postpartum women. At present, recommendations from regulatory agencies suggest that a very small risk of cardiac arrhythmias and sudden cardiac death is associated with domperidone and clinician. If clinicians do prescribe domperidone for a non-authorized use such as lactation support, they should only use the established dosing guidelines of 30 mg daily [78,79].

As with any medication, there is always concern of transfer into breast milk. Lewis et al. evaluated the extent to which metoclopramide passed into breast milk in 10 mothers with full term infants. Maternal blood and milk samples collected 2 h after a single oral dose of 10 mg had plasma concentration of 69 $\pm$ 30 ng/mL and milk concentration 126 $\pm$ 42 ng/mL. The authors calculated that the average intake of metoclopramide by an infant would be less than 0.045 mg/kg/day which is well below the therapeutic doses used in preterm and term newborn infants [43]. Similarly, when evaluating 30 and 60 mg total daily doses of domperidone, the amounts transferred to breast milk were extremely low with median infant dose via milk being 0.04 and 0.07 μg/kg/day, respectively; this is far below the dose of 100–300 μg 3–4 times-a-day infants receive for gastrointestinal stasis [64]. With oral bioavailability at 15%, it is unlikely that pharmacologically meaningful amounts of domperidone reach the infant through the breast milk. No measures of infant serum concentrations of domperidone have been reported.

6. Summary

Following preterm delivery of an infant that is unable to breastfeed, measures should be in place to facilitate breast milk expression within one to six hours of birth as well as maintaining milk production [84,85]. The use of a galactogogue can be considered if additional support in breast milk production is needed especially in the presence of optimized pumping strategies. Although the trials demonstrate a modest efficacy in augmenting breast milk production at any point during the first 5 weeks of the postpartum period, earlier initiation by the end of the first week postpartum can be considered in order to optimize support for the mother. Based on the current literature and recommendations, domperidone, where available, should be the galactogogue of choice, with the dose of 10 mg three time daily for 14 days. There is inadequate evidence to guide treatment beyond 14 days. Careful history-taking and assessment are required to ensure domperidone is not administered to mothers at risk of cardiac arrhythmia. Mothers need to maintain pumping to facilitate the autocrine regulatory mechanism. Mothers should be assessed after 48–72 h of initiating domperidone to determine a response as evidence by an increase in breast milk volume.

Author Contributions: The author was responsible for the conception and design of this review.

Acknowledgments: The author received funding from the Canadian Institutes of Health Research (CIHR) grant MOP#114980 for the conduct of the EMPOWER trial and costs to publish in open access.

References

1. Maffei, D.; Schanler, R.J. Human milk is the feeding strategy to prevent necrotizing enterocolitis! *Semin. Perinatol.* **2017**, *41*, 36–40. [CrossRef] [PubMed]

2. Abrams, S.A.; Schanler, R.J.; Lee, M.L.; Rechtman, D.J. Greater mortality and morbidity in extremely preterm infants fed a diet containing cow milk protein products. *Breastfeed. Med.* **2014**, *9*, 281–285. [CrossRef] [PubMed]
3. Schanler, R.J. Mother's own milk, donor human milk, and preterm formulas in the feeding of extremely premature infants. *J. Pediatr. Gastroenterol. Nutr.* **2007**, *45*, 175S–177S. [CrossRef] [PubMed]
4. Morales, Y.; Schanler, R.J. Human milk and clinical outcomes in VLBW infants: How compelling is the evidence of benefit? *Semin. Perinatol.* **2007**, *31*, 83–88. [CrossRef] [PubMed]
5. Porcelli, P.J.; Weaver, R.G., Jr. The influence of early postnatal nutrition on retinopathy of prematurity in extremely low birth weight infants. *Early Hum. Dev.* **2010**, *86*, 391–396. [CrossRef] [PubMed]
6. Furman, L.; Taylor, G.; Minich, N.; Hack, M. The effect of maternal milk on neonatal morbidity of very low-birth-weight infants. *Arch. Pediatr. Adolesc. Med.* **2003**, *157*, 66–71. [CrossRef] [PubMed]
7. Lucas, A.; Morley, R.; Cole, T.J. Randomised trial of early diet in preterm babies and later intelligence quotients. *BMJ* **1996**, *317*, 1481–1487. [CrossRef]
8. Horwood, L.J.; Darlow, B.A.; Mogridge, N. Breast milk feeding and cognitive ability at 7–8 years. *Arch. Dis. Child. Fetal Neonatal Ed.* **2001**, *84*, 23F–27F. [CrossRef]
9. Vohr, B.R.; Poindexter, B.B.; Dusick, A.M.; McKinley, L.T.; Wright, L.L.; Langer, J.C.; Poole, W.K. NICHD Neonatal Research Network. Beneficial effects of breast milk in the neonatal intensive care unit on the developmental outcome of extremely low birth weight infants at 18 months of age. *Pediatrics* **2006**, *118*, e115–e123. [CrossRef] [PubMed]
10. Vohr, B.R.; Poindexter, B.B.; Dusick, A.M.; McKinley, L.T.; Higgins, R.D.; Langer, J.C.; Poole, W.K. NICHD Neonatal Research Network. Persistent beneficial effects of breast milk ingested in the neonatal intensive care unit on outcomes of extremely low birth weight infants at 30 months of age. *Pediatrics* **2007**, *12*, e953–e959. [CrossRef] [PubMed]
11. O'Connor, D.L.; Jacobs, J.; Hall, R.; Adamkin, D.; Auestad, N.; Castillo, M.; Connor, W.E.; Connor, S.L.; Fitzgerald, K.; Groh-Wargo, S.; et al. Growth and development of premature infants fed predominantly human milk, predominantly premature infant formula, or a combination of human milk and premature formula. *J. Pediatr. Gastroenterol. Nutr.* **2003**, *37*, 437–446. [CrossRef] [PubMed]
12. Ehrenkranz, R.A.; Dusick, A.M.; Vohr, B.R.; Wright, L.L.; Wrage, L.A.; Poole, W.K. Growth in the neonatal intensive care unit influences neurodevelopmental and growth outcomes of extremely low birth weight infants. *Pediatrics* **2006**, *117*, 1253–1261. [CrossRef] [PubMed]
13. Chirico, G.; Marzollo, R.; Cortinovis, S.; Fonte, C.; Gasparoni, A. Antiinfective properties of human milk. *J. Nutr.* **2008**, *138*, 1801S–1806S. [CrossRef] [PubMed]
14. Victora, C.G.; Bahl, R.; Barros, A.J.; França, G.V.; Horton, S.; Krasevec, J.; Murch, S.; Sankar, M.J.; Walker, N.; Rollins, N.C. Lancet Breastfeeding Series Group. Breastfeeding in the 21st century: Epidemiology, mechanisms, and lifelong effect. *Lancet* **2016**, *387*, 475–490. [CrossRef]
15. Moro, G.E.; Arslanoglu, S.; Bertino, E.; Corvaglia, L.; Montirosso, R.; Picaud, J.C.; Polberger, S.; Schanler, R.J.; Steel, C.; van Goudoever, J.; et al. American Academy of Pediatrics; European Society for Pediatric Gastroenterology, Hepatology, and Nutrition. Human milk in feeding premature infants: Consensus statement. *J. Pediatr. Gastroenterol. Nutr.* **2015**, *61*, S16–S19. [CrossRef] [PubMed]
16. Callen, J.; Pinelli, J. A review of the literature examining the benefits and challenges, incidence and duration, and barriers to breastfeeding in preterm infants. *Adv. Neonatal Care* **2005**, *5*, 72–88. [CrossRef] [PubMed]
17. Hill, P.D.; Ledbetter, R.J.; Kavanaugh, K.L. Breastfeeding patterns of low-birth-weight infants after hospital discharge. *J. Obstet. Gynecol. Neonatal Nurs.* **1997**, *26*, 189–197. [CrossRef] [PubMed]
18. Hill, P.D.; Aldag, J.C.; Chatterton, R.T.; Zinaman, M.J. Comparison of milk production between mothers of preterm and term mothers: The first six weeks after birth. *J. Hum. Lact.* **2005**, *21*, 22–30. [CrossRef] [PubMed]
19. Sievers, E.; Haase, S.; Oldigs, H.D.; Schaub, J. The impact of peripartum factors on the onset and duration of lactation. *Biol. Neonatol.* **2003**, *83*, 246–252. [CrossRef] [PubMed]
20. Houston, M.J.; Howie, P.W.; McNeilly, A.S. Factors affecting the duration of breast feeding: 1. Measurement of breast milk intake in the first week of life. *Early Hum. Dev.* **1983**, *8*, 49–54. [CrossRef]
21. Henderson, J.J.; Hartmann, P.E.; Newnham, J.P.; Simmer, K. Effects of preterm birth and antenatal corticosteroid treatment on lactogenesis II in women. *Pediatrics* **2008**, *121*, e92–e100. [CrossRef] [PubMed]
22. Neville, M.C.; McFadden, T.B.; Forsyth, I. Hormonal regulation of mammary differentiation and milk secretion. *J. Mammary Gland Biol. Neoplasia* **2002**, *7*, 49–66. [CrossRef] [PubMed]

23. Neville, M.C.; Morton, J. Physiology and endocrine changes underlying human lactogenesis II. *J. Nutr.* **2001**, *131*, 3005S–3008S. [CrossRef] [PubMed]
24. Pang, W.W.; Hartman, P.E. Initiation of human lactation: Secretory differentiation and secretory activation. *J. Mammary Gland Biol. Neoplasia* **2007**, *12*, 211–231. [CrossRef] [PubMed]
25. Truchet, S.; Honvo-Houéto, E. Physiology of milk secretion. *Best Pract. Res. Clin. Endocrinol. Metab.* **2017**, *31*, 367–384. [CrossRef] [PubMed]
26. Kulski, J.K.; Hartmann, P.E. Changes in human milk composition during the initiation of lactation. *Aust. J. Exp. Biol. Med. Sci.* **1981**, *59*, 101–114. [CrossRef] [PubMed]
27. Neville, M.C.; Allen, J.C.; Archer, P.C.; Casey, C.E.; Seacat, J.; Keller, R.P.; Lutes, V.; Rasbach, J.; Neifert, M. Studies in human lactation: Milk volume and nutrient composition during weaning and lactogenesis. *Am. J. Clin. Nutr.* **1991**, *54*, 81–92. [CrossRef] [PubMed]
28. Kent, J.C. How breastfeeding works. *J. Midwifery Womens Health* **2007**, *52*, 564–570. [CrossRef] [PubMed]
29. Kent, J.C.; Prime, D.K.; Garbin, C.P. Principles for maintaining or increasing breast milk production. *J. Obstet. Gynecol. Neonatal Nurs.* **2012**, *41*, 114–121. [CrossRef] [PubMed]
30. Daly, S.E.; Owens, R.A.; Hartmann, P.E. The short-term synthesis and infant-regulated removal of milk in lactating women. *Exp. Physiol.* **1993**, *78*, 209–220. [CrossRef] [PubMed]
31. Peaker, M.; Wilde, C.J. Feedback control of milk secretion from milk. *J. Mammary Gland Biol Neoplasia* **1996**, *1*, 307–315. [CrossRef] [PubMed]
32. DeCoopman, J. Breastfeeding after pituitary resection: Support for a theory of autocrine control of milk supply? *J. Hum. Lact.* **1993**, *9*, 35–40. [CrossRef] [PubMed]
33. Whichelow, M.J. Factors associated with the duration of breast feeding in a privileged society. *Early Hum. Dev.* **1982**, *7*, 273–280. [CrossRef]
34. Chapman, D.J.; Pérez-Escamilla, R. Identification of risk factors for delayed onset of lactation. *J. Am. Diet. Assoc.* **1999**, *99*, 450–454. [CrossRef]
35. Case-Smith, J.; Cooper, P.; Scala, V. Feeding efficiency of premature neonates. *Am. J. Occup. Ther.* **1989**, *43*, 245–250. [CrossRef] [PubMed]
36. Hill, P.D.; Aldag, J.C. Milk volume on day 4 and income predictive of lactation adequacy at 6 weeks of mothers of non-nursing preterm infants. *J. Perinat. Neonatal Nurs.* **2005**, *19*, 273–282. [CrossRef] [PubMed]
37. Ehrenkranz, R.A.; Ackerman, B.A.; Mesger, J.; Bracken, M.B. Breast-feeding and premature infants: Incidence and success. *Pediatr. Res.* **1985**, *19*, 199A. [CrossRef]
38. Meier, P.P.; Johnson, T.J.; Patel, A.L.; Rossman, B. Evidence-Based Methods That Promote Human Milk Feeding of Preterm Infants: An Expert Review. *Clin. Perinatol.* **2017**, *44*, 1–22. [CrossRef] [PubMed]
39. Hill, P.D.; Aldag, J.C.; Chattertoon, R.T. Effects of pumping style on milk production in mothers of non-nursing preterm infants. *J. Hum. Lact.* **1993**, *15*, 209–216. [CrossRef] [PubMed]
40. Gabay, P.G. Galactogogues: Medications that induce lactation. *J. Hum. Lact.* **2002**, *18*, 274–279. [CrossRef] [PubMed]
41. Forinash, A.B.; Yancey, A.M.; Barnes, K.N.; Myles, T.D. The use of galactogogues in the breastfeeding mother. *Ann. Pharmacother.* **2012**, *46*, 1392–1404. [CrossRef] [PubMed]
42. Guzmán, V.; Toscano, G.; Canales, E.S.; Zárate, A. Improvement of defective lactation by using oral metoclopramide. *Acta Obstet. Gynecol. Scand.* **1979**, *58*, 53–55. [CrossRef] [PubMed]
43. Lewis, P.J.; Devenish, C.; Kahn, C. Controlled trial of metoclopromide in the initiation of breastfeeding. *Br. J. Clin. Pharmacol.* **1980**, *9*, 217–219. [CrossRef] [PubMed]
44. Tolino, A.; Tedeschi, A.; Farace, R.; Granata, P. The relationship between metoclopramide and milk secretion in puerperium. *Clin. Exp. Obstet. Gynecol.* **1981**, *8*, 93–95. [PubMed]
45. Kauppila, A.; Kivinen, S.; Ylikorkala, O. A dose response relation between improved lactation and metoclopromide. *Lancet* **1981**, *1*, 1175–1177. [CrossRef]
46. Kauppila, A.; Kivinen, S.; Ylikorkala, O. Metoclopromide increases prolactin release and ilk secretion in puerperium without stimulating the secretion of thyrotropin and thyroid hormones. *J. Clin. Endocrinol. Metab.* **1981**, *52*, 436–439. [CrossRef] [PubMed]
47. Kauppila, A.; Arvela, P.; Koivisto, M.; Kivinen, S.; Ylikorkala, O.; Pelkonen, O. Metoclopramide and breast feeding: Transfer into milk and the newborn. *Eur. J. Clin. Pharmacol.* **1983**, *25*, 819–823. [CrossRef] [PubMed]
48. de Gezelle, H.; Ooghe, W.; Thierry, M.; Dhont, M. Metoclopramide and breast milk. *Eur. J. Obstet. Gynecol. Reprod. Biol.* **1983**, *15*, 31–36. [CrossRef]

49. Kauppila, A.; Anunti, P.; Kivinen, S.; Koivisto, M.; Ruokonen, A. Metoclopramide and breast feeding: Efficacy and anterior pituitary responses of the mother and the child. *Eur. J. Obstet. Gynecol. Reprod. Biol.* **1985**, *19*, 19–22. [CrossRef]
50. Gupta, A.P.; Gupta, P.K. Metoclopromide as a galactogogue. *Clin. Pediatr.* **1985**, *24*, 269–272. [CrossRef] [PubMed]
51. Ehrenkranz, R.A.; Ackerman, B.A. Metoclopromide effect of faltering milk production by mothers of premature infants. *Pediatrics* **1986**, *78*, 614–620. [PubMed]
52. Ertl, T.; Sulyok, E.; Ezer, E.; Sárkány, I.; Thurzó, V.; Csaba, I.F. The influence of metoclopramide on the composition of human breast milk. *Acta Paediatr. Hung.* **1991**, *31*, 415–422. [PubMed]
53. Nemba, K. Induced lactation: A study of 37 non-puerperal mothers. *J. Trop. Pediatr.* **1994**, *40*, 240–242. [CrossRef] [PubMed]
54. Toppare, M.F.; Laleli, Y.; Senses, D.A.; Kitapci, F.; Kaya, I.S.; Dilmen, U. Metoclopromide for breast milk production. *Nutr. Res.* **1994**, *14*, 1019–1029. [CrossRef]
55. Seema; Patwari, A.K.; Satyanarayana, I. Relactation: An effective intervention to promote exclusive breastfeeding. *J. Trop. Pediatr.* **1997**, *43*, 213–216. [CrossRef] [PubMed]
56. Hansen, W.F.; McAndrew, S.; Harris, K.; Zimmerman, M.B. Metoclopromide effect on breastfeeding the preterm infants: A randomized trial. *Obstet. Gynecol.* **2005**, *105*, 383–389. [CrossRef] [PubMed]
57. Sakha, K.; Behbahan, A.G. Training for perfect breastfeeding or metoclopramide: Which one can promote lactation in nursing mothers? *Breastfeed. Med.* **2008**, *3*, 120–123. [CrossRef] [PubMed]
58. Fife, S.; Gill, P.; Hopkins, M.; Angello, C.; Boswell, S.; Nelson, K.M. Metoclopramide to augment lactation, does it work? A randomized trial. *J. Matern. Fetal Neonatal Med.* **2011**, *24*, 1317–1320. [CrossRef] [PubMed]
59. Brogden, R.N.; Carmine, A.A.; Heel, R.C.; Speight, T.M.; Avery, G.S. Domperidone: A review of it pharmacological activity, pharmacokinetics and therapeutic efficacy in the symptomatic treatment of chronic dyspepsia and as an antiemetic. *Drugs* **1982**, *24*, 360–400. [CrossRef] [PubMed]
60. Barone, J. Domperidone: A peripherally acting dopamine2-receptor antagonist. *Ann. Pharmacother.* **1999**, *33*, 429–440. [CrossRef] [PubMed]
61. De Leo, V.; Petraglia, F.; Sardelli, S.; Pieroni, M.L.; Bruno, G.; Gioffrè, W.R.; Genazzani, A.R.; D'Antona, N. Use of domperidone in the induction and maintenance of maternal breast feeding. *Minerva Ginecol.* **1986**, *38*, 311–315. [PubMed]
62. Petraglia, F.; De Leo, V.; Sardelli, S.; Pieroni, M.L.; D'Antona, N.; Genazzani, A.R. Domperidone in defective and insufficient lactation. *Eur. J. Obstet. Gynecol. Reprod. Biol.* **1985**, *19*, 281–287. [CrossRef]
63. da Silva, O.P.; Knoppert, D.C.; Angelini, M.M.; Forret, P.A. Effect of domperidone on milk production in mothers of premature newborn: A randomized, double-blind, placebo-controlled trial. *Can. Med. Assoc. J.* **2001**, *164*, 17–21.
64. Wan, E.W.; Davey, K.; Page-Sharp, M.; Hartmann, P.E.; Simmer, K.; Ilett, K.F. Dose-effect study of domperidone as a galactagogue in preterm mothers with insufficient milk supply, and its transfer into milk. *Br. J. Clin. Pharmacol.* **2008**, *66*, 283–289. [CrossRef] [PubMed]
65. Campbell-Yeo, M.; Allen, A.C.; Joseph, K.S.; Ledwidge, J.; Allen, V.; Dooley, K. Effect of Domperidone on the Composition of Preterm Human Breast Milk: Randomized, Double Blind, Placebo-Controlled Trial. *Pediatrics* **2010**, *125*, e107–e114. [CrossRef] [PubMed]
66. Ingram, J.; Taylor, H.; Churchill, C.; Pike, A.; Greenwood, R. Metoclopramide or domperidone for increasing maternal breast milk output: A randomized controlled trial. *Arch. Dis. Child. Fetal Neonatal Ed.* **2012**, *97*, F241–F245. [CrossRef] [PubMed]
67. Knoppert, D.C.; Page, A.; Warren, J.; Seabrook, J.A.; Carr, M.; Angelini, M.; Killick, D.; DaSilva, O.P. The effect of two different doses on maternal milk production. *J. Hum. Lact.* **2013**, *29*, 38–44. [CrossRef] [PubMed]
68. Rai, R.; Mishra, N.; Singh, D. Effect of domperidone in 2nd week postpartum on milk output in mothers of preterm infants. *Indian J. Pediatr.* **2016**, *83*, 894–895. [CrossRef] [PubMed]
69. Asztalos, E.V.; Campbell-Yeo, M.; da Silva, O.P.; Ito, S.; Kiss, A.; Knoppert, D. EMPOWER Study Collaborative Group. Enhancing Human Milk Production with Domperidone in Mothers of Preterm Infants. *J. Hum. Lact.* **2017**, *33*, 181–187. [CrossRef] [PubMed]
70. Blank, C.; Eaton, V.; Bennett, J.; James, S.L. A double blind RCT of domperidone and metoclopramide as pro-lactational agents in mothers of preterm infants. In Proceedings of the Perinatal Society of Australia and New Zealand 5th Annual Conference, Canberra, Australia, 13–16 March 2001; p. 73.

71. Grzeskowiak, L.E.; Smithers, L.G.; Amir, L.H.; Grivell, R.M. Domperidone for increasing breast milk volume in mothers expressing breast milk for their preterm infants: A systematic review and meta-analysis. *BJOG* **2018**. [CrossRef] [PubMed]
72. Smolina, K.; Morgan, S.G.; Hanley, G.E.; Oberlander, T.F.; Mintzes, B. Postpartum domperidone use in British Columbia: A retrospective cohort study. *CMAJ Open* **2016**, *4*, E13–E19. [CrossRef] [PubMed]
73. Grzeskowiak, L.E.; Lim, S.W.; Thomas, A.E.; Ritchie, U.; Gordon, A.L. Audit of domperidone use as a galactogogue at an Australian tertiary teaching hospital. *J. Hum. Lact.* **2013**, *29*, 32–37. [CrossRef] [PubMed]
74. Grzeskowiak, L. Use of domperidone to increase breast milk supply: Are women really dying to breastfeed? *J. Hum. Lact.* **2014**, *30*, 498–499. [CrossRef] [PubMed]
75. Paul, C.; Zénut, M.; Dorut, A.; Coudoré, M.A.; Vein, J.; Cardot, J.M.; Balayssac, D. Use of domperidone as a galactagogue drug: A systematic review of the benefit-risk ratio. *J. Hum. Lact.* **2015**, *31*, 57–63. [CrossRef] [PubMed]
76. Sewell, C.A.; Chang, C.Y.; Chehab, M.M.; Nguyen, C.P. Domperidone for Lactation: What Health Care Providers Need to Know. *Obstet. Gynecol.* **2017**, *129*, 1054–1058. [CrossRef] [PubMed]
77. Hondeghem, L.M.; Logghe, N.H. Should Domperidone be Used as a Galactagogue? Possible Safety Implications for Mother and Child. *Drug Saf.* **2017**, *40*, 109–113. [CrossRef] [PubMed]
78. European Medicines Agency. *Domperidone-Containing Medicines*; European Medicines Agency: London, UK, 2014. Available online: http://www.ema.europa.eu/ema/index.jsp?curl=pages/medicines/human/referrals/Domperidone-containing_medicines/human_referral_prac_000021.jsp&mid=WC0b01ac05805c516f (accessed on 31 March 2018).
79. Health Canada. *Domperidone Maleate—Association with Serious Abnormal Heart Rhythms and Sudden Death (Cardiac Arrest)—For Health Care Professionals*; Health Canada: Ottawa, ON, Canada, 2015. Available online: http://hc-sc.gc.ca/dhp-mps/medeff/advisories-avis/prof/_2015/domperidone_hpc-cps-eng.php (accessed on 31 March 2018).
80. Smolina, K.; Mintzes, B.; Hanley, G.E.; Oberlander, T.F.; Morgan, S.G. The association between domperidone and ventricular arrhythmia in the postpartum period. *Pharmacoepidemiol. Drug. Saf.* **2016**, *25*, 1210–1214. [CrossRef] [PubMed]
81. Buffery, P.J.; Strother, R.M. Domperidone safety: A mini-review of the science of QT prolongation and clinical implications of recent global regulatory recommendations. *N. Z. Med. J.* **2015**, *128*, 66–74. [PubMed]
82. Hondeghem, L.M. Domperidone: Limited benefits with significant risk for cardiac death. *J. Cardiovasc. Pharmacol.* **2013**, *61*, 218–225. [CrossRef] [PubMed]
83. van Noord, C.; Dielman, J.P.; van Herpen, G.; Verhamme, K.; Sturkenboom, M.C. Domperidome and ventricular arrhythmia on sudden cardiac death: A population-based case-control study in the Netherlands. *Drug Saf.* **2010**, *17*, 1131–1136.
84. Parker, L.A.; Sullivan, S.; Krueger, C.; Kelechi, T.; Mueller, M. Effect of early breast milk expression on milk volume and timing of lactogenesis stage II among mothers of very low birth weight infants: A pilot study. *J. Perinatol.* **2012**, *32*, 205–209. [CrossRef] [PubMed]
85. Parker, L.A.; Sullivan, S.; Krueger, C.; Kelechi, T.; Mueller, M. Strategies to increase milk volume in mothers of VLBW infants. *MCN Am. J. Matern. Child. Nurs.* **2013**, *38*, 385–390. [CrossRef] [PubMed]

Human Milk Lipidomics: Current Techniques and Methodologies

Alexandra D. George [1], Melvin C. L. Gay [1], Robert D. Trengove [2] and Donna T. Geddes [1,*]

[1] School of Molecular Sciences, The University of Western Australia, Crawley, Perth, WA 6009, Australia; alexandra.george@research.uwa.edu.au (A.D.G.); melvin.gay@uwa.edu.au (M.C.L.G.)

[2] Separation Science and Metabolomics Laboratory, Murdoch University, Murdoch, Perth, WA 6150, Australia; R.Trengove@murdoch.edu.au

* Correspondence: donna.geddes@uwa.edu.au

Abstract: Human milk contains a complex combination of lipids, proteins, carbohydrates, and minerals, which are essential for infant growth and development. While the lipid portion constitutes only 5% of the total human milk composition, it accounts for over 50% of the infant's daily energy intake. Human milk lipids vary throughout a feed, day, and through different stages of lactation, resulting in difficulties in sampling standardization and, like blood, human milk is bioactive containing endogenous lipases, therefore appropriate storage is critical in order to prevent lipolysis. Suitable sample preparation, often not described in studies, must also be chosen to achieve the aims of the study. Gas chromatography methods have classically been carried out to investigate the fatty acid composition of human milk lipids, but with the advancement of other chromatographic techniques, such as liquid and supercritical fluid chromatography, as well as mass spectrometry, intact lipids can also be characterized. Despite the known importance, concise and comprehensive analysis of the human milk lipidome is limited, with gaps existing in all areas of human milk lipidomics, discussed in this review. With appropriate methodology and instrumentation, further understanding of the human milk lipidome and the influence it has on infant outcomes can be achieved.

Keywords: human milk; breastfeeding; lactation; lipids; lipidomics; mass spectrometry; chromatography; NMR spectroscopy

---

1. Introduction

Human milk (HM) is vital to the infant, providing both immune protection and energy required for optimal infant growth. Breastfeeding is associated with multiple benefits for both the infant and the mother, such as decreased risk of asthma, pneumonia, type 1 diabetes, and obesity and decreased incidence of breast and ovarian cancer, respectively [1–3]. Further, these breastfeeding benefits increase with the duration of breastfeeding [1,4].

The macronutrient composition of HM consists of approximately 7% carbohydrates, 5% lipids, 0.9% protein, and 0.2% minerals emulsified in an aqueous milk matrix [5]. While the lipid portion of HM makes up only 5% of mature milk, it contributes to over 50% of the infant's daily energy requirement [6]. These lipids are known to be involved in both neural and retinal tissue development as well as immune system development and defense in the infant [7–9]. Furthermore, the HM lipid profile impacts early growth in preterm infants [10].

Despite the importance of these lipids, the total lipid content in HM is highly variable, with large changes occurring throughout the day, between breasts, between women, and throughout the whole lactation period [11]. Interestingly, the total HM lipid content is not believed to be changed by maternal diet; however, diet influences the specific fatty acid (FA) composition. One example of this is docosahexaenoic acid (DHA)-containing triacylglycerides (TAGs) which have been found to be in higher concentrations in HM of women with high seafood intake [12,13]. The concentrations of DHA, docosapentaenoic acid (DPA), and arachidonic acid (AA) are also observed to decrease over the lactation period and these are the three FAs implicated in infant neural and retinal development [14].

Along with the variability of HM lipids, the complexity of the milk matrix and lipid hydrophobicity adds to the difficulty of a comprehensive lipidomic analysis. Further, over 40,000 biological lipid structures have been identified in various biological matrices such as human blood and plant material, leaving the possibility for thousands of lipids to be identified and deconvoluted in HM [15].

A number of basic analytical techniques have been employed over the years to investigate the lipid composition of HM; however, with the recent advancement of analytical techniques such as chromatography coupled with mass spectrometry and nuclear magnetic resonance spectroscopy, current analysis promises to be more comprehensive. Lipidomics is the research field in which complex lipidome analyses are carried out to produce a comprehensive and quantitative description of the lipid species present in a given matrix. While lipidomics is expanding exponentially in biological research, it is only recently being applied to HM. Lipids can be defined as FAs and their derivatives, or by their solubility in organic solvents and insolubility in inorganic solvents. Fat-soluble vitamins such as vitamin D are often included within this definition of lipids, but for the purpose of this review only standard lipid classes such as FAs, glycerolipids, glycerophospholipids, sphingolipids, sterols, prenols, which have been identified in HM will be discussed [16–20].

Additionally, this review will investigate the current status of HM lipidomic analysis and the new emerging techniques, methods, and instruments being used. It will focus on analysis of HM lipidome composition, rather than simply total lipids, which has commonly been estimated using creamatocrit or gravimetric methods [21]. With the present-day state of 'omics' techniques, the ability to comprehensively and quantitatively analyse the HM lipidome will allow a greater understanding of HM lipids. However, in order to make significant advances in HM analysis, quality control and standardised sampling must be routinely employed. Lipidomics platforms hold great promise to further elucidate HM lipid composition and the role of lipids with respect to infant health and disease.

2. Sampling

HM lipid content and composition, as mentioned above, is highly variable and constantly changing to meet the demands of the infant. The total lipid content of HM varies widely between women, throughout a feed, a day, and lactation, with reported values ranging widely from 11.4 g/L to 61.8 g/L [11,22,23]. While Jensen suggests that maternal age may influence HM lipid content, this has not been validated [11]. Similarly, diet has previously been suggested to influence lipid content, yet no studies exist to confirm this. In contrast, the FA composition of the lipids is influenced by maternal diet, where areas of China with high fish intake have significantly higher HM DHA than other provinces with lower fish intake, and DHA supplementation of breastfeeding women in Australia also led to an increase in HM DHA content [24,25]. While different ethnicity is thought to be another contributor to lipid composition variability, this too is most probably related to maternal diet. Other maternal health conditions, such as infections or metabolic diseases, have also been noted to reduce the total lipids in HM [6]. An obvious limitation to sampling protocols is that these studies are dealing with human participants, a mother feeding her infant, therefore sampling protocols should not negatively impact or interrupt infant feeding and sleeping patterns. Sampling protocols are non-invasive, involving expression of milk from the nipple either manually or using a breast pump. Differences between sampling methods and timing of collection of the sample may also contribute to complexity and variations within these results, therefore strict collection protocols should be implemented in order to obtain representative samples for HM studies. Details of the methods used in HM lipidomics studies, as well as the other methodology and identified lipids of existing studies, are summarised in Table 1.

2.1. Sampling with Respect to the Feed

Fat content increases as the breast is drained of milk, during a feed, therefore sampling pre-feed HM will give lower total fat content than mid- or post-feed samples [26]. Studies often do not take this into account and do not specify when samples are taken, often accepting random samples from nonspecified time points. Some studies will sample at a single time point with no further details, prescribed time points or will attempt to investigate feeds more thoroughly by collecting pre-, mid- and/or post-feed samples [27–31]. One frequently used sampling method to interrogate the entire feed is to drain the whole breast using a breast pump and then sample from the pumped milk [20,32,33]. However, as infants rarely drain the whole breast [34,35], this method will remove more milk from the end of the feed which is higher in fat content leading to an overestimation of the infant consumption [36].

2.2. Sampling over 24 h

As fat content increases with removal of milk from the breast subsequently the HM lipid content varies over a 24-h period, increasing from the first to the last feed of the day, higher in the evening than in the morning [37]. By sampling and test-weighing the infant before and after each feed in a 24-h period, milk production can be measured in addition to the actual amount of milk lipid ingested by the infant [38].

2.3. Sampling through Stages of Lactation

In general, the total HM lipid content increases throughout lactation, with Mitoulas et al. showing that lipids decrease from the first to second month but increase up to month 9 of lactation [26]. However, the mean amount of fat delivered to the infant remains constant as maternal milk production and infant intake changes across the months [26]. In order to account for the fat variations at different lactation stages, prescribed time points for sampling within a study, such as sampling on certain days (e.g., day 1, 14, and 42 post-partum) or sampling over a period of lactation (e.g., first 22–25 days of lactation) should be chosen, depending on the research question [13,29]. However, many studies either collect at different stages of lactation and pool their samples (such as [39]), or fail to mention when the samples are collected which makes comparison with other studies and understanding the lipidome difficult.

2.4. Ideal Sampling Routine

Due to these variations of both the total lipid content and lipid composition, lipidomic analysis at any given time has the potential to be very different. It is important that the aforementioned factors are all taken into account when sampling HM and that the study is defined in order to control these influences. This is rarely the case in HM studies, clearly outlined by the missing data in Table 2. We suggest defining the research question and then determining the appropriate samples in order to define and standardize sampling to minimize variables and confounding factors. Given that we know about the lipid variations at any given time, it is important that studies use sampling with 24-h test-weighing of the infant during breastfeeding (and expression) to provide more accurate interpretation of infant intake to determine the influence of these lipids on infant development [38]. This technique is not yet widely used but would greatly improve interpretation of research studies. Taking into account the published sampling methods, these are likely to contribute greatly to the large variation in reported lipids values [40].

Table 1. Summary of existing human milk (HM) lipidomics studies from 1959 to 2018, including HM sampling, storage, preparation, quality control (in- and out-of-sample) and instrumentation used (- indicates not reported).

Lipids Identified	Sampling	Storage	Sample Preparation	Quality Control	Instrumentation	Reference
Fatty acids ranging from 10:0 to 22:6, including some unknown at the time	6 hospital participants, mid-feed samples (for 24 h, pooled); 5 participants at home, random samples	4 °C (prior to pooling); −15 °C	1 or 2 mL human milk →LLE 95% ethanol-ethyl ether →Hydrolysis 5% methanolic-KOH →Derivatisation 5% methanolic-HCl	In: - Out: -	GC–FID Reoplex 400/Apiezon M column (Carrier gas: nitrogen)	Insull et al. (1959) [19]
Fatty acids ranging from 12:0 to 22:6	15 participant random samples (pooled)	-	4 mL human milk →TLC pre-separation →LLE chloroform:methanol (9:1) →Derivatisation BF_3	In: - Out: -	GC–FID, 50 m CP-Sil-88 column (Carrier gas: nitrogen)	Haug et al. (1983) [27]
Fatty acids ranging from 6:0 to 26:0	7 participants, sampled on day 20–22 (mid-feed)	On ice ≤2 h; 20 °C	-	In: C17:0 Out: -	GC–FID	van Beusekom et al. (1993) [28]
Polyunsaturated fatty acids ranging from 18:2 to 22:6; total saturated FAs; total monounsaturated FAs	23 participants 7-day samples from a single feed at weeks 6, 16, 30 (each time-point pooled)	−20 °C prior to delivery to laboratory	- mL human milk →Extracted - →Derivatisation 1% methanolic-H_2SO_4	In: - Out: -	GC 50 m BPX-70 column	Makrides et al. (1995) [14]
Fatty acids ranging from 10:0 to 22:6 including *cis* and *trans* isomers and some unknown at the time	198 samples, 3–4 weeks, mid-feed for a day (pooled)	-	5 g human milk →LLE chloroform:methanol (2:1) →0.02% BHT preservative →Derivatisation methanolic-BF_3	In: Triheptadecanoin (in extraction solvent) Out: -	GC–FID 100 m SP-2560 column (Carrier gas: hydrogen)	Chen et al. (1995) [41]
Fatty acids ranging from 10:0 to 22:6	Samples from 84 participants at day 3 and weeks 2, 4, and 6	−20 °C	2 g human milk →LLE chloroform:methanol (2:1) →Derivatisation methanolic-BF_3	In: Triheptadecanoin (in extraction solvent) Out: -	GC–FID 100 m SP-2560 column (Carrier gas: hydrogen)	Chen et al. (1997) [12]
31 Triglycerides	Pre- and post-feed samples from 11 participants between days 1–3, days 7–10, days 25–60 (47 samples)	−80 °C	1.5 mL human milk →LLE dicholoromethane-methanol (2:1)	In: C33:0 (after extraction) Out: -	LC–LSD, 250 mm Spherisorb ODS-2 column (Solvents: acetonitrile, dichloromethane, acetone)	Pons et al. (2000) [42]
Fatty acids ranging from 14:0 to 22:6	34 participants, samples on days 1, 4, 7, 14, 21, 28, at any time of day	−20 °C	≤2 mL human milk →LLE chloroform:methanol (2:1) →BHT preservative →Derivatisation methanolic-BF3	In: - Out: -	GC	Scopesi et al. (2001) [43]
Fatty acids ranging from 14:0 to 22:6	18 participants, days 1, 2, 3, 4, 5, 6, 7, 14, 28 between 0800–1000	4–8 °C (for <4 h), deep freeze, 1 freeze-thaw cycle	100 µL human milk →LLE chloroform:methanol →Derivatisation –	In: Pentadecanoic acid Out: -	GC–FID 40 m Cyanopropyl DB-23 column	Minda et al. (2004) [44]
1. Fatty acids ranging from 4:0 to 22:6 2. 18:1 *t* isomers	81 samples, from complete breast expression, between 0600 and 0800 in the first month	Room temperature (4 h); Lipid layer frozen at −20 °C	2 g human milk lipid layer →LLE chloroform:methanol (2:1) →Derivatisation sodium methoxide	In: - Out: -	1. GC–FID 100 m CP-Sil-88 column 2. GC–MS DB225 MS column	Mosley et al. (2005) [45]
Groups of FAMES and approximately 36 × specific FAMEs	1 random sample	−20 °C	1 mg human milk fat →LLE cyclohexane/ethylacetate, →Hydrolysis methanolic-KOH →Derivatisation BF_3 →SPE fractionation Ag^+-SPE	In: 14:0 and 17:0 Out: -	GC–EI–MS, 60 m SP2331 cyanosiloxane column (Carrier gas: helium)	Dreiucker et al. (2011) [46]

Table 1. *Cont.*

Lipids Identified	Sampling	Storage	Sample Preparation	Quality Control	Instrumentation	Reference
DHA and AA and other fatty acids	52 participants	-	1 mL human milk →Hydrolysis methanolic-KOH →Derivatisation H_2SO_4 →LLE hexane	In: C19:0 Out: -	GC–FID 50 m fused-silica CPSIL88 column (Carrier gas: helium)	Kelishadi et al. (2012) [47]
Fatty acids from 12:0 to 18:2	101 participant random samples over 3 days	−80 °C	20 μL human milk fat →Transesterification methanolic-BF_3	In: Tridecanoic acid (in extraction solvent) Out: -	GC 100 m HP88 column (Carrier gas: helium)	Akmar et al. (2013) [48]
Total saturated and unsaturated fatty acids, 18:2 *n*6, 18:3 *n*3, 20:4 *n*6, 22:6 *n*3	29 mid-feed samples (8–12 weeks post-partum) between 1200 and 1500	−80 °C	100 μL human milk. →Hydrolysis methanolic-NaOCH3 →Derivatisation methanolic-BF_3	In: - Out: -	GC–FID 40 m RTX-2330 (Carrier gas: helium)	Saphier et al. (2013) [49]
Free fatty acids between C10 and C24	23 term and 15 preterm participants/38 post-feed samples during days 0–7 day, 8–21, >21	Frozen	500 μL human milk →LLE chloroform methanol →transesterification methanolic-HCl	In: C17:0 Out: -	GC–MS 30 m Ultra Alloy-5 column (Carrier gas: helium)	Chuang et al. (2013) [50]
Fatty acids between 4:0 and 22:6	50 participants 4 weeks post-partum, provided one full breast expression	−80 °C	250 μL human milk →Transesterification methanolic-HCl	In: 11:0 FAME, 13:0 TAG Out: -	GC–FID 100m CP-Sil 88 column (Carrier gas: hydrogen)	Cruz-Hernandez et al. (2013) [32]
Phospholipid classes	50 participants, pre-, mid-, post-feed samples at 4 weeks	−80 °C	250 mg human milk →LLE chloroform:methanol (2:1) →Filtration PTFE filter	In: Phosphatidylglyceol Out: -	NP HPLC (ELSD) 2 × 250 mm Nucleosil 50-5 columns (Solvents: acetonitrile/methanol) NMR	Giuffrida et al. (2013) [20]
Polar and lipidic metabolites Tentative 287 lipids (positive mode), 126 lipids (negative mode)	52 samples between days 1 and 76, pooled. 10 participant samples at week 1, 9 participant samples at week 4	−80 °C (long term) −20 °C (short term)	50 μL human milk →LLE MTBE →Transesterification methanolic-HCl, BSTFA	In: C18:0 after extraction Out: Pooled HM	GC–Q–MS 30 m 122-5332G DVB5-MS column (Carrier gas: helium) LC–QTOF–MS (ESI) 15 cm EC-C8 column (Solvents: methanol water)	Villasenor et al. (2014) [51]
1. Fatty acids between 10:0 and 20:4 2. Triglycerides between 32:0 and 54:5	2 samples 4 random weeks post-partum	-	200 μL human milk →LLE (1) chloroform:methanol (2:1) →Transesterification with acid →LLE (2) chloroform: methanol: isopropanol (1:2:4)	In: 17:1–17:1–17:1 TAG, 17:0–14:1 PE, 17:0–14:1 PS, 17:0–14:1 PI, 18:1;2/17:0 SM (after extraction, for MS/MS) Out: -	1. GC–FID 60 m TRFRAME column (Carrier gas: helium) 2. MS/MS Triple TOF (positive and negative mode)	Sokol et al. (2015) [52]
Over 40 triglycerides	15 between-feed samples over days 1–5, 6–15 and >16		150 uL human milk →dichloromethane:methanol (2:1) →BHT preservative	In: - Out: -	HPLC–APCI–MS 150 mm Kinetex C18 column (Solvents: acetonitrile/n-pentanol)	Ten-Domenech et al. (2015) [53]
Fatty acids ranging from 10:0 to 22:6	477 participants gave pre-feed samples on days 1, 14, 42 between 1000 and 1100	−20 °C; −80 °C	200 μL human milk →LLE chloroform: methanol (1:1) →BHT preservative →Hydrolysis methanolic-KOH →Derivatisation methanolic-BF_3 →SPE Sep-pak silica column	In: - Out: -	GC–FID 60 m DB-23 Fused silica column (Carrier gas: nitrogen)	Jiang et al. (2016) [13]

Table 1. *Cont.*

Lipids Identified	Sampling	Storage	Sample Preparation	Quality Control	Instrumentation	Reference
8 long-chain polyunsaturated fatty acids	514 participants, between 0900 and 1100 for first 22–25 days	−80 °C	0.2 mL human milk fat →Transesterification methanolic-CH_3COCl	In: C17:0 Daturic acid Out: -	GC–FID 100 mm SP2560 column (Carrier gas: nitrogen)	Liu et al. (2016) [54]
1. Identified putative DHA-TAGs 2. Verified 56 DHA-TAGs ranging from $C_{45}H_{74}O_6$ to $C_{67}H_{116}O_6$	1 sample	-	0.2 mL human milk →LLE chloroform:methanol (2:1)	In: - Out: -	1. LC–ESI–triple quadrupole MS 250 mm synergi polar RP column 2. LC–ESI–LTQ–ORBI MS 2x 150 mm Poroshell 120 EC-C18 (Solvents: acetonitrile/water)	Liu et al. (2016) [29]
Polyunsaturated fatty acids	225 participants, provided pre- and/or post-feed milk at their own discretion, at 2 months	4 °C (≤24 h); −80 °C	200 uL human milk →Transesterification -	In: - Out: -	GC–FID	Rosenlund et al. (2016) [30]
Groups of fatty acids, Glycerophospholipids, Prenol lipids, Glycerolipids, Sphingolipids, Sterol lipids	1 participant provided samples, at 1 year	−80 °C	1 mL human milk →SPME C18, isopropanol elution	In: - Out: -	LC–ESI–QTOF–MS 50 mm SB-C18 column (Solvents: methanol, water, hexane, isopropanol)	Garwolinska et al. (2017) [55]
sn-glycero-3-phosphocholine (and other lipid derivatives)	37 mothers provided 15 (morning and evening) samples on days 9, 12, 24, 31, 60, 85, 86, 87	−20 °C (2–8 days); −80 °C	- mL human milk →LLE methanol:water	In: - Out: -	NMR	Wu et al. (2016) [56]
64 Triglycerides ranging from $C_{33}H_{62}O_6$ to $C_{65}H_{120}O_6$	27 participants provided a day 7 and day 42 sample	−20 °C	0.1 mL human milk →LLE hexane →Filtration 0.22 µm nylon filter	In: - Out: 4 commercial QC 18:2/18:2/18:2; 18:1/18:1/18:1; 16:0/16:0/16:0; 18:1/16:0/18:1 for calibration curves	SFC ESI–QTOF 100 mm BEH-2-Ethylpyridine column (Solvents: supercritical CO_2, methanol, acetonitrile)	Tu et al. (2017) [57]
Fatty acids ranging from 8:0 to 20:3	26 participants, left and a right sample at the same time on 3 consecutive days	−20 °C (≤1 week); −80 °C	- mL human milk →LLE chloroform:methanol (2:1) →Transesterification methanolic-H_2SO_4	In: - Out: -	GC–FID 50 mm BPX-70 column (Carrier gas: helium)	Gardner et al. (2017) [31]
1. Fatty acids ranging from 8:0 to 22:6 2. 2 × Ceramides; 7 × GlucosylCeramide; 22 × Phosphatidylcholine; 25 × Phosphatidylethanolamine; 5 × Phosphatidylglycerol; 2 × Phosphatidylinositol; 2 × Phosphatidylserine; Retinol; 9 × Diglycerides; 49×Triglycerideas; 11 × Sphingomyeline; 10 × Eicosanoids; 2×Cardiolipines; 10 × LysoPhosphatidylcholine/ Phosphatidylethanolamine	118 participants gave samples over 24 h (each participant pooled).	−80 °C	- mL human milk →LLE chloroform:methanol (1:1) →Transesterification -	In: - Out: pooled QC (10 participants pooled samples)	1. GC–FID 30 m fused silica column 2. LC-ESI-HRMS in positive and negative mode 100 mm CSH C18 column (Solvents: acetonitrile, water, isopropanol)	Alexandre-Gouabau et al. (2018) [10]

Abbreviations: LLE liquid-liquid extraction, GC gas chromatography, FID flame ionization detector, TLC thin-layer chromatography, BHT butyrated hydroxytoluene, LC liquid chromatography, LSD light scattering detector, MS mass spectrometry, EI electron ionization, FAME fatty acid methyl ester, SPE solid phase extraction, DHA docosahexaenoic acid, AA arachidonic acid, TAG triacylglyceride, NP normal phase, HPLC high pressure liquid chromatography, ELSD evaporative light scattering detector, NMR nuclear magnetic resonance spectroscopy, MTBE methyl-tert-butyl ether, Q quadrupole, ESI electrospray ionization, APCI atmospheric-pressure chemical ionization, TOF time of flight, LTQ linear trap quadrupole, ORBI orbitrap, SPME solid-phase microextraction, SFC supercritical fluid chromatography, HRMS high resolution mass spectrometry

Table 2. Summary of study sampling methods and corresponding total fat content in lactating women. All studies collected pre- and post-feed samples during a 24-h period. Studies that drained entire breast for samples were excluded. Total fat reported as a range, Mean, (SD or SE) where provided (- indicates not reported or taken into account).

	Sampling	During Feed		Time of Day				Lactation Stage							
Study	**i) Participant n ii) Sample n**	**Pre-Feed (g/L)**	**Post-Feed (g/L)**	**Morning (g/L)**	**Noon (g/L)**	**Afternoon (g/L)**	**Evening (g/L)**	**1 (g/L)**	**2 (g/L)**	**3 (g/L)**	**4 (g/L)**	**5 (g/L)**	**6 (g/L)**	**9 (g/L)**	**12 (g/L)**
Mitoulas et al., 2002 [26]	i) 17 initially ii) 76	-	-	-	-	-	-	39.9 (SE 1.4)	35.2 (SE 1.4)	-	35.4 (SE 1.4)	-	37.3 (SE 1.4)	40.7 (SE 1.4)	40.9 (SE 3.3)
Saarela et al., 2005 [22]	i) 20 ii) 483	21.0 (SD 8.4)	57.1 (SD 4.5)	-	-	-	-	19.7 (SD 8.2)	23.5 (SD 8.8)	21.0 (SD 8.4)	16.2 (SD 9.4)	11.4 (SD 6.2)	18.8 (SD 4.2)	-	-
Jackson et al., 1988 [39]	i) 25 ii) -	0.35–21.85 (SD 1.92)	-	17.9–50.6 31.4 (SD 6.6)	-	-	20.7–45.7 31.4 (SD 6.6)	-	-	-	-	-	-	-	-
Khan et al., 2013 [23]	i) 15 ii) -	32 (SD 12)	56 (SD 17)	18.4–69.2 29.3 (SD 10.9)	22.1–80.6 35 (SD 12.9)	21.2–72 31.6 (SD 10.4)	15.9–63.3 28.1 (SD 12.2)	-	-	-	-	-	-	-	-

3. Storage

As with lipidomic analysis of all biological samples, care must be taken to minimise lipolysis and lipogenesis during storage due to enzymes, such as lipase (bile salt-stimulated lipase and lipoprotein lipase), which are present endogenously in HM [58,59]. While immediate analysis of the lipidome is ideal to minimize any compositional changes by lipase activity, in reality this is not practical, therefore correct storage and sample preservation is imperative. Poor consideration of adequate storage affects the reproducibility and interpretation of HM study results and, as shown in Table 1, is something rarely considered in HM lipidomics.

3.1. Freezing

Maintaining the integrity of a HM sample is carried out by freezing samples at temperatures such as −20 °C, −70 °C or −80 °C. If the sample is not frozen adequately, endogenous lipases have the opportunity to cause lipid hydrolysis resulting in inaccurate and misrepresentative HM lipid content for measurement. Studies have shown that while freezing HM at −20 °C for 3 months resulted in a significant loss of lipids (up to 20%), storage at −70 °C or −80 °C stops enzyme activity within the samples and HM lipid integrity is best preserved [60–62]. Although one study showed major lipid loss in HM samples stored at −80 °C, Fusch et al. reported that this is likely an effect of poor experimental controls [63,64]. The duration of storage is not routinely reported in published studies but is obviously another factor affecting results. Another key factor is the number of freeze-thaw cycles that the sample underwent prior to analysis. In a study by Bitman et al., up to 20% fat loss was observed when HM underwent two freeze-thaw cycles, due to the resulting increase in lipolytic activity in HM during each of these cycles [65]. Therefore, steps during sample handling should be carefully planned such that all samples undergo the same number of freeze-thaw cycles.

3.2. Preservatives

HM has inherent antioxidant capacity to reduce and prevent oxidative degradation [66]. This degradation most commonly occurs in unsaturated fats, where the double bonds undergo cleavage by free radicals. In addition to freezing HM samples, antioxidant preservation of HM samples has also been used to maintain sample integrity. Phenol derivatives such as butyrated hydroxytoluene (BHT) have been used in previous studies to prevent lipid peroxidation [13,67]. BHT works by preferentially reacting with any oxygen present so that there is no opportunity for the lipids to be oxidatively degraded. There are currently no HM studies examining BHT efficacy for lipid preservation; however, studies of other biological samples such as red blood cells have used BHT with success, resulting in increased red blood cell FA preservation from 4 weeks to at least 17 weeks [68].

4. Lipid Extraction

Following appropriate HM sampling and storage for lipid analysis, sample preparation is essential to ensure accuracy and reproducibility of the results. For lipidomics analysis, mass spectrometry techniques, which will be discussed in Section 7.2, are commonly used. Therefore, clean-up steps such as liquid–liquid extraction and/or solid-phase extraction are essential to remove interferences such as proteins and sugars, as well as concentrate the lipids of interest. Sample preparation methods used in HM lipidomics studies are described in Table 1. Prior to lipid extraction, the sample must be homogenised, to ensure a uniform distribution of milk fat globules throughout the sample.

4.1. Liquid-Liquid Extraction

Liquid-liquid extraction (LLE) techniques are used to separate analyses by their relative solubility in different immiscible liquids. LLE is the classical choice of lipid extraction method used in HM analysis, with variations of the 1950s methods such as Folch [14,69] and Bligh–Dyer [70], using chloroform, methanol, and water in ratios 8:4:3 and 1:2:0.8 respectively, being most commonly used.

Other than the solvent ratio, the difference in these methods is that Bligh–Dyer uses smaller volumes of solvent and is a less time-consuming protocol [70]. While the Bligh–Dyer extraction was first developed on fish muscle, Folch extraction was developed on brain tissue, however both quoted as being easily adapted to other tissue types. When these solvents are added to HM, the lipids are dissolved into the organic phase (chloroform) and are separated from the aqueous phase (methanol and water, containing carbohydrates and salts) by a layer of cell debris and protein (Figure 1i).

While the use of these methods is well established, the drawbacks include the use of hazardous solvent, such as chloroform, and also the risk of contaminating or losing the lipid-containing lower phase when sampling through the aqueous phase or separating layers. These methods have been directly translated into HM studies or modified to either replace the use of hazardous solvent, such as chloroform with dichloromethane; or increase extraction efficiency with the introduction of centrifugation to enhance phase separation and the omission of water [27,29]. Recently a methyl-tert-butyl ether (MTBE) extraction method, initially developed for plasma lipid extraction, has been employed for HM lipid extraction for the analysis of both lipids and other HM metabolites [51]. This extraction, similar to the Folch and Bligh and Dyer method, separates lipids using phase separation. However, using the MTBE method, the organic phase containing lipids instead forms the upper layer, and the aqueous phase (containing the matrix pallet) forms the lower layer (Figure 1ii). This method has made extraction of lipids simpler and minimizes the potential of cross contamination.

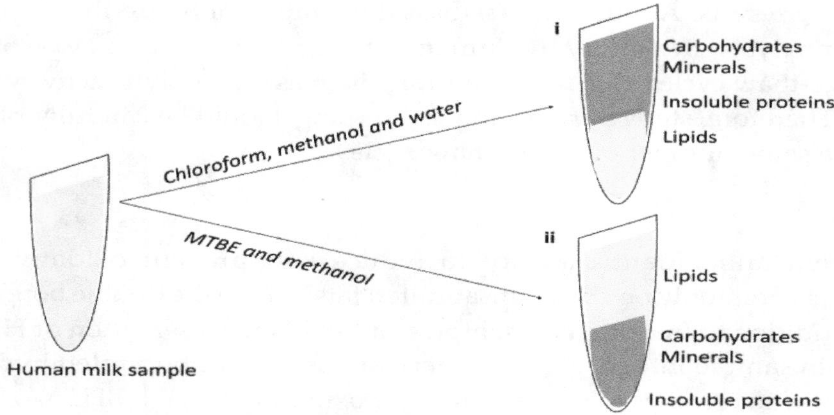

Figure 1. Liquid–liquid extraction of human milk lipids using (**i**) Folch extraction or (**ii**) Methyl-tert-butyl ether (MTBE) extraction.

4.2. Solid-Phase Extraction

The use of solid-phase extraction (SPE), a type of column chromatography, is gaining popularity for its rapid and efficient lipid extraction from biological fluids. In this process, HM is loaded into the cartridge with lipid analyses retained on the solid-phase sorbent, such as C18, packed in a cartridge, meanwhile the interfering milk matrix components are washed out. Lipids can then be eluted from the bonded phase using organic solvents (Figure 2) [71]. Only two published milk lipidome studies have successfully used SPE for lipid extraction from HM, extracting fatty acyls, glycolipids, sphingolipids, prenol lipids and sterol lipids for analysis [46,55]. The first study by Dreiucker and Vetter uses a silver-ion SPE to extract FAs separating them by their degree of saturation and isomeric configuration [46]. The FAs were then eluted with acetone-based solvents, which then allowed better measurement of preseparated FA isomers by GC–MS than in standard LLE extraction. While this silver-ion SPE method is more quantitative, it has limitations with reproducibility and standardization to ensure complete lipid extraction. In another study, a solid-phase micro extraction (SPME) technique was used. This SPME involves the immersion of a solid-phase sorbent-coated fiber into HM and then use of organic solvent (such as isopropanol) to desorb the lipids [55]. This technique has poor reproducibility for the amount and type of lipids absorbed by the fiber, even when other parameters such as time and elution solvent are standardized, thus rendering this method suitable for qualitative analyses only. These factors limit the current use of SPE in HM lipidomics; however, further optimisation could offer the possibility of SPE automation in a plate format, which would make this technique ideal for routine, high-throughput extraction of HM for lipidomics.

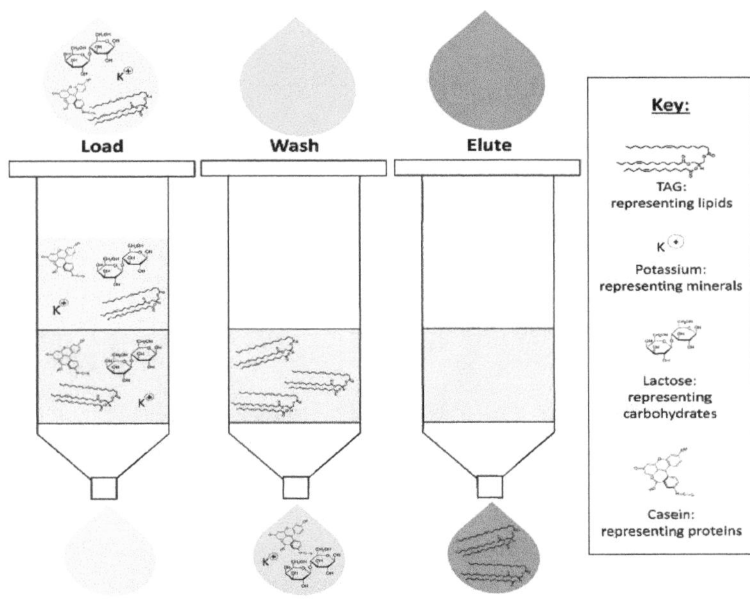

Figure 2. Solid-phase extraction of human milk lipids.

5. Lipid Transesterification

Following lipid extraction from HM samples, lipid transformation may be required for the analysis of non-volatile free or lipid-bound FAs. It is generally accepted that free FA in HM are artefacts of lipolysis, although only one study has investigated the FA from lipase hydrolysis of TAGs and other lipids (such as phospholipids and sphingolipids) [72]. This section will discuss only the analysis of FA that make up lipids, more specifically the FA composition of TAGs, which make up 98% of the lipids in HM, despite the methodology being poorly described (Table 1) [73]. Prior to the analysis of these FA, a two-part chemical transesterification is carried out, first hydrolysing the TAG, releasing three FA (Figure 3i), followed by derivatisation of the resulting FA to methyl esters (FAMEs) for GC analysis (Figure 3ii). This reaction can be either acid or base catalyzed. Derivatisation of FA is necessary for GC analysis as the high polarity of nonderivatised FA can result in hydrogen bond formation and therefore adsorption issues on a GC column, leading to band broadening and retention time shifting [74]. The resulting FAMEs have reduced polarity, able to be separated by a polar GC column.

The transesterification method is well-established and has been widely applied in FA analysis, where acidic transesterification using boron trifluoride (BF_3) is most commonly used, as first described in 1964 [75]. The early HM FA transesterification methods frequently use this BF_3 and methanol approach [10,12,13,43,48]. In other HM studies, transesterifications have used acid catalysis (methanolic-hydrogen chloride) or base catalysis (using methanolic-potassium hydroxide or sodium-methoxide) [19,32,45,72]. Although BF_3 is a hazardous chemical and could also interact with BHT preservatives in a sample, it is still widely used in HM preparation [32,76]. The primary drawbacks of transesterification for FAME analysis are the laborious and time-consuming steps involved, supporting the movement towards methods not involving such preparations (such as liquid chromatography–mass spectrometry).

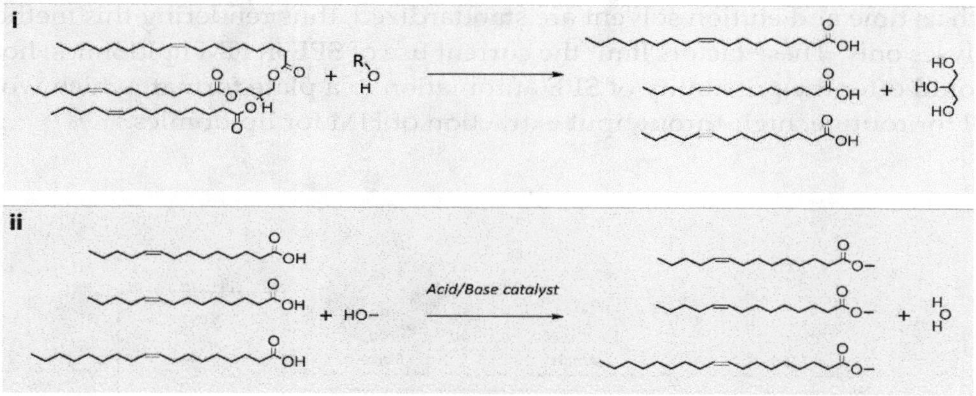

Figure 3. Transesterification reactions of triglyceride 14:1/14:1/18:1, one triglyceride commonly found in human milk. (**i**) Triglyceride hydrolysis, carried out with a base (such as KOH), resulting in glycerol and three free fatty acids; (**ii**) Resulting free fatty acid reaction with methanol and an acid/base catalyst producing three fatty acid methyl esters and water.

6. Quality Control

The use of quality control (QC) is essential to minimize influences, such as sample matrix effects and instrument variations that could cause issues with method accuracy and reproducibility. Despite the importance of QC in lipidomics, it is often overlooked in almost all, not just in HM, studies (as can be seen in Table 1). The QC measures are generally determined by several factors including the target lipid class of the study, the availability and cost of the standards and researcher preference. Several types of QC, which we have categorized as 'in-sample' and 'out-of-sample' QCs, should also be in place when lipidomic analyses are carried out and these are described below.

6.1. In Sample

This QC is added in known concentrations to HM during sample preparation and is also referred to as the internal standard (IS). For optimal lipidomics, more than one compound should be used as an IS. If these IS are added to HM prior to extraction, they can be used to assess variability that may occur in sample storage and extraction recovery. If the IS is added after sample extraction, it is used to monitor instrument performance and variability. The compound selected as an IS should be a labelled compound that is, or behaves as, the compound/s of interest. Due to limited availability of expensive commercial labelled lipid standards, to date no HM lipidomics studies have used labelled lipid standards. HM studies have, however, used a variety of unlabelled commercial lipids which are presumed not to be present in HM as an IS, for example heptadecanoic acid (C17:0) [28].

6.2. Out of Sample

QC samples should also be analyzed periodically within an experiment to monitor for any instrument abnormalities, such as sample degradation or loss of response. QCs are typically a pooled QC or commercial QC. A pooled QC is prepared by pooling aliquots of HM samples from the laboratory and analyzing these alongside a batch of samples. These QCs need to be rigorously prepared and stored in order to achieve reproducibility and for accurate monitoring of intra- and inter-batch variations. The pooled QC is the simplest and cheapest to prepare. Commercial QCs are known lipid analytes purchased to be run within a batch, like other out-of-sample QCs, confirming and identifying the retention time, m/z values and identity of these analyses. Additionally, these are often used to test an instrument for suitability. Out-of-sample QC should always be matrix matched to account for biological matrix effects, a condition that no HM lipidomic studies have yet met [77].

While there is currently no general consensus on the type of QC that should be used and the limits of variability within a lipidomics experiment, many studies will predefine the limits based on experience and the instruments used. Because of the vast number of lipids, untargeted HM lipidomics can only ever be semiquantitative [77].

7. Analytical Instrumentation for Lipidomic Analysis

Due to the complexity of lipids, complete lipidomic analysis requires more than one instrument platform. The choice of instrumentation for HM lipidomics therefore depends upon the study aims and the lipids of interest. Simple separation techniques have previously been used for qualitative analysis of lipids, such as thin-layer chromatography and gas chromatography (GC). Although GC is thought of as the gold standard for HM FA lipidomics, the availability and increasing prevalence of other separation techniques such as liquid chromatography (LC) and high-resolution mass analyzers, such as time-of-flight and Fourier Transform, means that the HM lipidome can be more comprehensively characterized [78]. The advantages and disadvantages of the instrumentation used in HM lipidomic analysis are summarized in Table 3. Consistent GC use in HM lipidomics can be seen in Table 1, with the slow emergence of mass spectrometry in recent years.

Table 3. Advantages and disadvantages of analytical instrumentation used in human milk lipidomics.

Separation/Detection Method	Advantages	Disadvantages
Gas chromatography	1. Fatty acid methyl ester analysis is well characterized 2. Flame ionisation detector is robust and easy to maintain	1. Sample derivatisation is required 2. Destructive 3. Isomers separation requires longer column and run time 4. Flame ionisation detector lacks mass selectivity
Liquid chromatography	1. No sample derivatisation required 2. Large selection of column chemistry available	1. Solvent system must be compatible with detector type
Supercritical fluid chromatography	1. No derivatisation required 2. Compatible with almost any detector type 3. Relatively inexpensive 4. Low waste output 5. Faster separation than in GC/LC 6. Higher resolution than in GC/LC	1. Polar lipid separation requires organic modifier
Thin-layer chromatography	1. Inexpensive	1. Qualitative lipid class separation only 2. Low separating resolution compared to GC and LC.
Mass spectrometry	1. High sensitivity and specificity 2. Qualitative and quantitative (with standards)	1. Expensive 2. Destructive
NMR spectroscopy	1. Non-destructive 2. Highly reproducible	1. Expensive 2. Signal overlapping in complex samples 3. Lower sensitivity than MS 4. Requires larger samples volume

7.1. Separation Methods

7.1.1. Gas Chromatography

GC coupled with a flame ionization detector (GC–FID) is the most routinely used separation method for FA analysis since the 1950s and is widely accepted for quantification of FA in many sample types, including HM [19]. Cyanopropyl-based columns ranging from 30 to 60 m in length are typically employed for FAME analysis. However, longer columns (up to 100 m) are used if separation of dietary FAME isomers such as *cis* C18:1 and *trans* C18:1 is desired. Therefore, the requirement for a longer GC column can extend both the method preparation and run time. The FID is generally used in FAME analysis as it is considerably cheaper to purchase and maintain compared to mass spectrometry (MS) detectors. Furthermore, the robustness of the FID allows the analysis of large numbers of samples before the need for any maintenance and does not have the same requirements and issues as MS (such as ionization source cleaning and ionization issues, as seen in mass spectrometry), discussed in Section 7.2. Mass Spectrometry [79]. Additionally, HM FAME analysis using GC is well characterized based on elution order and retention time, either requiring a limited number of standards or using Kovats retention index, as described in a HM study by Villasenor et al., for identification by comparing experimental and established retention indices [51]. Further, retention time locking can add to method reproducibility. However, GC–FID lacks mass selectivity, unlike MS, so it has been known to misidentify FAMEs in the presence of co-eluting compounds or contaminants that may be present in the sample, although this has not been investigated in HM studies [80,81].

7.1.2. Liquid Chromatography

While GC is widely used for FA analysis, LC, with an evaporative light-scattering detector (ELSD), charged aerosol detector (CAD), electrochemical detector, or coupled to mass spectrometry (MS), has been used in the analysis of intact lipids, such as TAGs and phospholipids [79]. Currently only one study has used LC–ELSD in HM lipidomics, to quantify phospholipids, while other LC methodology is most commonly carried out using mass spectrometry [20,53]. Due to the wide variety of lipids in HM, various stationary phases and solvent combinations are employed depending on the type of lipids and separation required. Lipid separation in biofluids, including HM, is most often carried out using a C18 stationary phase column but other silica-based stationary phases, such as C8, have also been used in HM analysis for separation of all lipid classes and phospholipids, respectively [20,51]. Reversed-phase LC separates intact lipids and free FA based on their specific FA polarity, degree of saturation and chain length, while normal-phase LC will separate lipids, such as glycerophospholipids, by their class [82]. In LC analyses, the solvent and stationary phase must be compatible with the detection method, for example MS, where ratios of organic and inorganic solvents such as acetonitrile, alcohol, and water are most commonly used. When MS is the chosen detector ammonium salts (formate or acetate) and formic acid will be added (discussed in Section 7.2. Mass Spectrometry). The main advantage of LC over GC is that transformation is not required and intact lipids such as triglycerides can be analyzed [83].

7.1.3. Supercritical Fluid Chromatography

Supercritical fluid chromatography (SFC) is another separation technique similar to LC, which, instead of using a liquid mobile phase, uses a supercritical fluid, such as carbon dioxide (CO_2), as the mobile phase. Supercritical fluids are formed when dense compressed gas is subjected to a specific pressure and temperature. CO_2 is the most commonly used supercritical solvent and its non-polar properties make it ideal for separating non-polar lipids like TAGs, shown by Laakso and Manninen in cow's milk, to separate TAGs by their molecular size [84]. Although SFC has been widely used in dairy milk fat research and oil separation, its use in HM is limited to one study where SFC was coupled to mass spectrometry [57]. Advantages of SFC include no requirement for derivatisation, and the ability for SFC to be coupled with all detector types, such as FID or MS, as well as its low cost and waste output relative to LC, using less organic solvents than LC, and allowing faster separation and higher resolution than LC and GC in metabolomics analyses [85]. These features all make SFC well suited to the analysis of multiple lipid classes in one sample that have a range of polarities [79].

7.1.4. Thin-Layer Chromatography

Like LC, thin-layer chromatography (TLC) may be qualitatively analytical but is more commonly used as a preparative step in human studies. HM studies often use TLC for separation of lipids into their individual classes, for example separation of short- and long-chain FAs prior to analysis [72]. This inexpensive technique is classically carried out using a silica plate and non-polar solvent for lipid class separation, and the classes can then be collected and analyzed using platforms such as GC or LC. As TLC does not have the separating resolution of GC or LC, its ability to perform identification is limited and thus may be the reason why TLC is not frequently used in HM lipidomics.

7.2. Mass Spectrometry

Mass spectrometry (MS) is the detection technique that identifies ionized compounds based on their mass-to-charge ratio (m/z). This is a destructive technique in which the sample is destroyed and cannot be used for future analysis. In HM lipidomics analysis, various types of mass analyzers, such as quadrupole, triple-quadrupole and time-of-flight, have been employed to identify and quantitate different lipids [79]. Given the increased sensitivity and specificity of MS in contrast to other detector types, such as FID and ELSD, it is possible to confirm the identity of known lipids, identify unknown lipids and to elucidate structural information of lipids using MS.

In order for lipids to be detected by MS, the compound needs to be ionized first using one of a variety of ionization techniques such as EI (electron ionization), ESI (electrospray ionization), CI (chemical ionization) or MALDI (matrix assisted laser desorption/ionization), which have been extensively reviewed [78,82]. These ionization methods can be carried out in either positive (EI, CI, or ESI) or negative (CI or ESI) mode, producing cations or anions respectively. In HM lipidomics, EI and ESI methods are commonly used. The EI technique is commonly used in conjunction with GC separation for FA analysis, where lipids are bombarded with a high-energy electron beam causing them to be ionized and fragmented in characteristic patterns. This is a hard ionization technique and generally only the fragment ions are observed [82]. Three HM studies have employed GC–MS since 2011, identifying and quantifying a large number of FAs as derivatised FAMEs, with MS having the added advantage of identifying many glycerolipids, glycerophospholipids, sphingolipids, prenol lipids, and sterol lipids not previously identified using GC–FID [46,50,51]. In contrast to EI–MS, ESI–MS is widely used in LC for HM lipidomics analysis [10,29,51,55]. This soft ionization technique involves pushing samples through a capillary with a voltage applied to it, creating a fine aerosol where ions are formed by desolvation. As ESI is a soft ionization technique, it is able to provide information on both the molecular ion (intact lipid, such as a triglyceride) as well as additional structural information by fragmenting the molecular ion, such as the FA composition of a specific triglyceride [82].

Additionally, LC–MS often uses additives such as ammonium formate and formic acid in the mobile phase as modifiers to promote ammonium adduct formation, these adducts being more stable than hydrogen adducts and easier to fragment than metal ions, and prevent retention time shifting [83]. The use of both positive and negative ionization mode in ESI–MS covers even more lipids, for example, identifying FAs using negative mode and phospholipids using positive mode [10].

Shotgun MS, which involves introducing a sample directly into the ion source and carrying out both positive and negative ionization mode MS, is a common technique for untargeted identification and structural characterization of lipids having been recently used for HM [52]. While this method is fast, sensitive and only requires a small amount of sample to be injected, the lack of chromatographic separation and ion suppression makes interpretation difficult. Ion suppression is a common effect where the response of a species of interest is suppressed due to endogenous matrix species such as proteins, or exogenous species such as plasticizers from plastic tubes/tube caps, in the sample compete for ionization [77]. This can be minimized with efficient lipid extraction during sample preparation, resulting in a cleaner and purer lipid extract. As lipid mixtures are challenging to interpret, chromatographic preseparation (GC or LC) is usually employed to further assist in separating lipids/isomers, providing additional orthogonal data for easier identification and more accurate quantification compared to the shotgun approach [79]. Additionally, untargeted analysis results in a large number of compounds to interrogate and often requires very specialized and expensive software.

7.3. Nuclear Magnetic Resonance Spectroscopy

Since the introduction of nuclear magnetic resonance spectroscopy (NMR) to the world of metabolomics, it has been used frequently in analyses of various biofluids and tissues, including muscle tissue and milk (such as in cows and camels) [86]. NMR is widely used in HM metabolomics to measure sugars, amino acids, and nucleotides; however, only one lipid (sn-glycero-3-phosphocholine), 12 phospholipid classes and a small number of lipid derivatives have been identified in HM by NMR [86,87]. NMR uses atomic magnetic properties, detecting every hydrogen/carbon/phosphorus-containing molecule and has the ability to provide valuable structural information for the intact lipid, such as structural differences between intact phospholipids [62,79]. In contrast to MS, NMR is a non-destructive technique, samples can be re-analyzed with NMR or other techniques [88]. However the drawbacks of NMR include signal overlapping, which can make discrimination of resonances from complex samples difficult, as well as larger sample volume requirements. While the use of NMR may be limited by its lower sensitivity than MS, NMR is highly reproducible and simple for a trained user to run [56]. Sample preparation may involve lipid extraction, such as with Folch extraction method, or simply whole milk may be analyzed. While preparation is simple, it can be difficult to run large numbers of samples with the same high-throughput capability of MS methods, unless an autosampler is available. The detected analyses can then be quantitated using the direct relationship between intensity of resonance and concentration [89].

8. Limitations and Future Perspectives

In addition to lipids being the most variable portion of HM, lipidomic analyses are limited by the number of samples analyzed, limiting the conclusions and relationships that can be identified in studies. Further, HM lipidomics would greatly benefit from standardized workflows for sample collection and preparation, analytical methodology on a wide number of platforms, data acquisition and data processing. The future of HM lipidomics needs higher lipid coverage on multiple platforms, allowing development of a HM metabolome/lipidome database similar to that of the Human Metabolome Database [90].

9. Conclusions

HM lipids are an essential macronutrient for the growth, development, and health of the infant; therefore, HM lipidomics are essential to provide a deeper understanding of short- and long-term infant health. The recent advances in instrumentation and methods in lipidomics will result in more comprehensive HM lipidomic investigations. Chromatography, MS, and NMR methods also offer potential for further lipid identification, structural elucidation, and investigation in HM. To develop better knowledge of the lipid changes in HM throughout lactation, more rigorous studies need to be carried out, employing stringent sampling and storage routines and advanced methodology with strict quality control. Rigorous protocols in HM investigations will allow more accurate assessment and investigation of the HM lipidome and the impact these lipids have on the infant.

Author Contributions: A.D.G. wrote the manuscript. M.C.L.G., R.D.T. and D.T.G. all critically reviewed the manuscript. All authors have read and approved the final manuscript.

References

1. Eidelman, A.I. Breastfeeding and the use of human milk: An analysis of the American academy of pediatrics 2012 breastfeeding policy statement. *Breastfeed. Med.* **2012**, *7*, 323–324. [CrossRef] [PubMed]
2. Layde, P.M.; Webster, L.A.; Baughman, A.L.; Wingo, P.A.; Rubin, G.L.; Ory, H.W. The independent associations of parity, age at first full term pregnancy, and duration of breastfeeding with the risk of breast cancer. Cancer and steroid hormone study group. *J. Clin. Epidemiol.* **1989**, *42*, 963–973. [CrossRef]
3. Collaborative Group on Hormonal Factors in Breast Cancer. Breast cancer and breastfeeding: Collaborative reanalysis of individual data from 47 epidemiological studies in 30 countries, including 50302 women with breast cancer and 96973 women without the disease. *Lancet* **2002**, *360*, 187–195. [CrossRef]

4. Victora, C.G.; Bahl, R.; Barros, A.J.; Franca, A.V.; Horton, S.; Krasevec, J.; Murch, S.; Sankar, M.J.; Walker, N.; Rollins, N.C. Breastfeeding in the 21st century: Epidemiology, mechanisms, and lifelong effect. *Lancet* **2016**, *387*, 475–490. [CrossRef]
5. Jenness, R. The composition of human milk. *Semin. Perinatol.* **1979**, *3*, 225–339. [PubMed]
6. Jensen, R.G. Lipids in human milk. *Lipids* **1999**, *34*, 1243–1271. [CrossRef] [PubMed]
7. Koletzko, B.; Agostoni, C.; Bergmann, R.; Ritzenthaler, K.; Shamir, R. Physiological aspects of human milk lipids and implications for infant feeding: A workshop report. *Acta Paediatr.* **2011**, *100*, 1405–1415. [CrossRef] [PubMed]
8. Innis, S.M. Dietary triacylglycerol structure and its role in infant nutrition. *Adv. Nutr.* **2011**, *2*, 275–283. [CrossRef] [PubMed]
9. Lauritzen, L.; Fewtrell, M.; Agostoni, C. Dietary arachidonic acid in perinatal nutrition: A commentary. *Pediatr. Res.* **2015**, *77*, 263–269. [CrossRef] [PubMed]
10. Alexandre-Gouabau, M.-C.; Moyon, T.; Cariou, V.; Antignac, J.-P.; Qannari, E.M.; Croyal, M.; Soumah, M.; Guitton, Y.; David-Sochard, A.; Billard, H.; et al. Breast milk lipidome is associated with early growth trajectory in preterm infants. *Nutrients* **2018**, *10*, 164. [CrossRef] [PubMed]
11. Jensen, R.G. The lipids in human milk. *Prog. Lipid Res.* **1996**, *35*, 53–92. [CrossRef]
12. Chen, Z.Y.; Kwan, K.Y.; Tong, K.K.; Ratnayake, W.M.N.; Li, H.Q.; Leung, S.S.F. Breast milk fatty acid composition: A comparative study between Hong Kong and Chongqing Chinese. *Lipids* **1997**, *32*, 1061–1067. [CrossRef] [PubMed]
13. Jiang, J.; Wu, K.; Yu, Z.; Ren, Y.; Zhao, Y.; Jiang, Y.; Xu, X.; Li, W.; Jin, Y.; Yuan, J.; et al. Changes in fatty acid composition of human milk over lactation stages and relationship with dietary intake in Chinese women. *Food Funct.* **2016**, *7*, 3154–3162. [CrossRef] [PubMed]
14. Makrides, M.; Simmer, K.; Neumann, M.; Gibson, R. Changes in the polyunsaturated fatty acids of breast milk from mothers of full-term infants over 30 wk of lactation. *Am. J. Clin. Nutr.* **1995**, *61*, 1231–1233. [CrossRef] [PubMed]
15. Sud, M.; Fahy, E.; Cotter, D.; Brown, A.; Dennis, E.A.; Glass, C.K.; Merrill, A.H., Jr.; Murphy, R.C.; Raetz, C.R.H.; Russell, D.W.; et al. LMSD: Lipid Maps structure database. *Nucleic Acids Res.* **2007**, *35*, D527–D532. [CrossRef] [PubMed]
16. Dotson, K.D.; Jerrell, J.P.; Picciano, M.F.; Perkins, E.G. High-performance liquid chromatography of human milk triacylglycerols and gas chromatography of component fatty acids. *Lipids* **1992**, *27*, 933–939. [CrossRef] [PubMed]
17. Kallio, M.J.; Siimes, M.A.; Perheentupa, J.; Salmenperä, L.; Miettinen, T.A. Cholesterol and its precursors in human milk during prolonged exclusive breast-feeding. *Am. J. Clin. Nutr.* **1989**, *50*, 782–785. [CrossRef] [PubMed]
18. Andreas, N.J.; Hyde, M.J.; Gomez-Romero, M.; Lopez-Gonzalvez, M.A.; Villaseñor, A.; Wijeyesekera, A.; Barbas, C.; Modi, N.; Holmes, E.; Garcia-Perez, I. Multiplatform characterization of dynamic changes in breast milk during lactation. *Electrophoresis* **2015**, *36*, 2269–2285. [CrossRef] [PubMed]
19. Insull, W. The fatty acids of human milk from mothers on diets taken ad libitum. *Biochem. J.* **1959**, *72*, 27–33. [CrossRef] [PubMed]
20. Giuffrida, F.; Cruz-Hernandez, C.; Flück, B.; Tavazzi, I.; Thakkar, S.K.; Destaillats, F.; Braun, M. Quantification of phospholipids classes in human milk. *Lipids* **2013**, *48*, 1051–1058. [CrossRef] [PubMed]
21. Du, J.; Gay, M.C.L.; Lai, C.T.; Trengove, R.D.; Hartmann, P.E.; Geddes, D.T. Comparison of gravimetric, creamatocrit and esterified fatty acid methods for determination of total fat content in human milk. *Food Chem.* **2017**, *217*, 505–510. [CrossRef] [PubMed]
22. Saarela, T.; Kokkonen, J.; Koivisto, M. Macronutrient and energy contents of human milk fractions during the first six months of lactation. *Acta Paediatr.* **2007**, *94*, 1176–1181. [CrossRef]
23. Khan, S.; Hepworth, A.R.; Prime, D.K.; Lai, C.T.; Trengove, N.J.; Hartmann, P.E. Variation in fat, lactose, and protein composition in breast milk over 24 hours: Associations with infant feeding patterns. *J. Hum. Lact.* **2013**, *29*, 81–89. [CrossRef] [PubMed]
24. Makrides, M.; Neumann, M.A.; Gibson, R.A. Effect of maternal docosahexaenoic acid (DHA) supplementation on breast milk composition. *Eur. J. Clin. Nutr.* **1996**, *50*, 352–357. [PubMed]

25. Ruan, C.; Liu, X.; Man, H.; Ma, X.; Lu, G.; Duan, G.; DeFrancesco, C.A.; Connor, W.E. Milk composition in women from five different regions of China: The great diversity of milk fatty acids. *J. Nutr.* **1995**, *125*, 2993–2998. [PubMed]
26. Mitoulas, L.R.; Kent, J.C.; Cox, D.B.; Owens, R.A.; Sherriff, J.L.; Hartmann, P.E. Variation in fat, lactose and protein in human milk over 24 h and throughout the first year of lactation. *Br. J. Nutr.* **2002**, *88*, 29–37. [CrossRef] [PubMed]
27. Haug, M.; Dieterich, I.; Laubach, C.; Reinhardt, D.; Harzer, G. Capillary Gas Chromatography of Fatty Acid Methyl Esters from Human Milk Lipid Subclasses. *J. Chromatogr. A* **1983**, *279*, 549–553. [CrossRef]
28. van Beusekom, C.M.; Nijeboer, H.J.; van der Veere, C.N.; Luteyn, A.J.; Offringa, P.J.; Muskiet, F.A.J.; Boersma, E.R. Indicators of long chain polyunsaturated fatty acid status of exclusively breastfed infants at delivery and after 20–22 days. *Early Hum. Dev.* **1993**, *32*, 207–218. [CrossRef]
29. Liu, Z.; Cocks, B.G.; Rochfort, S. Comparison of molecular species distribution of DHA-containing triacylglycerols in milk and different infant formulas by liquid Chromatography-Mass spectrometry. *J. Agric. Food Chem.* **2016**, *64*, 2134–2144. [CrossRef] [PubMed]
30. Rosenlund, H.; Fagerstedt, S.; Alm, J.; Mie, A. Breastmilk fatty acids in relation to sensitization-the ALADDIN birth cohort. *Allergy* **2016**, *71*, 1444–1452. [CrossRef] [PubMed]
31. Gardner, A.S.; Rahman, I.A.; Lai, C.T.; Hepworth, A.; Trengove, N.; Hartmann, P.E.; Geddes, D.T. Changes in fatty acid composition of human milk in response to cold-like symptoms in the lactating mother and infant. *Nutrients* **2017**, *9*, 1034. [CrossRef] [PubMed]
32. Cruz-Hernandez, C.; Goeuriot, S.; Giuffrida, F.; Thakkar, S.K.; Destaillats, F. Direct quantification of fatty acids in human milk by Gas Chromatography. *J. Chromatogr. A* **2013**, *1284*, 174–179. [CrossRef] [PubMed]
33. Daly, S.E.; Di Rosso, A.; Owens, R.A.; Hartmann, P.E. Degree of breast emptying explains changes in the fat content, but not fatty acid composition, of human milk. *Exp. Physiol.* **1993**, *78*, 741–755. [CrossRef]
34. Prime, D.K.; Kent, J.C.; Hepworth, A.R.; Trengove, N.J.; Hartmann, P.E. Dynamics of milk removal during simultaneous breast expression in women. *Breastfeed. Med.* **2012**, *7*, 100–106. [CrossRef] [PubMed]
35. Kent, J.C.; Ramsay, D.T.; Doherty, D.; Larsson, M.; Hartmann, P.E. Response of breasts to different stimulation patterns of an electric breast pump. *J. Hum. Lact.* **2003**, *19*, 179–186. [CrossRef] [PubMed]
36. Jensen, R.G.; Lammi-Keefe, C.J.; Koletzko, B. Representative sampling of human milk and the extraction of fat for analysis of environmental lipophilic contaminants. *Toxicol. Environ. Chem.* **1997**, *62*, 229–247. [CrossRef]
37. Lubetzky, R.; Littner, Y.; Mimouni, F.B.; Dollberg, S.; Mandel, D. Circadian variations in fat content of expressed breast milk from mothers of preterm infants. *J. Am. Coll. Nutr.* **2006**, *25*, 151–154. [CrossRef] [PubMed]
38. Kent, J.C.; Mitoulas, L.R.; Cregan, M.D.; Ramsay, D.T.; Doherty, D.A.; Hartmann, P.E. Volume and frequency of breastfeedings and fat content of breast milk throughout the day. *Pediatrics* **2006**, *117*, E387–e395. [CrossRef] [PubMed]
39. Jackson, D.A.; Imong, S.M.; Silprasert, A.; Ruckphaopunt, S.; Woolridge, M.W.; Baum, J.D.; Amatayakul, K. Circadian variation in fat concentration of breast-milk in a rural northern Thai population. *Br. J. Nutr.* **1988**, *59*, 349–363. [CrossRef] [PubMed]
40. Hassiotou, F.; Hepworth, A.R.; Williams, T.M.; Twigger, A.J.; Perrella, S.; Lai, C.T.; Filgueira, L.; Geddes, D.T.; Hartmann, P.E. Breastmilk cell and fat contents respond similarly to removal of breastmilk by the infant. *PLoS ONE* **2013**, *8*, E78232. [CrossRef] [PubMed]
41. Chen, Z.-Y.; Pelletier, G.; Hollywood, R.; Ratnayake, W.M. Trans fatty acid isomers in Canadian human milk. *Lipids* **1995**, *30*, 15–21. [CrossRef] [PubMed]
42. Pons, S.M.; Bargallo, A.C.; Folgoso, C.C.; Lopez Sabater, M.C. Triacylglycerol composition in colostrum, transitional and mature human milk. *Eur. J. Clin. Nutr.* **2000**, *54*, 878–882. [CrossRef] [PubMed]
43. Scopesi, F.; Ciangherotti, S.; Lantieri, P.B.; Risso, D.; Bertini, I.; Campone, F.; Pedrotti, A.; Bonacci, W.; Serra, G. Maternal dietary pufas intake and human milk content relationships during the first month of lactation. *Clin. Nutr.* **2001**, *20*, 393–397. [CrossRef] [PubMed]
44. Minda, H.; Kovacs, A.; Funke, S.; Szasz, M.; Burus, I.; Molnar, S.; Marosvolgyi, T.; Decsi, T. Changes of fatty acid composition of human milk during the first month of lactation: A day-to-day approach in the first week. *Ann. Nutr. Metab.* **2004**, *48*, 202–209. [CrossRef] [PubMed]

45. Mosley, E.E.; Wright, A.L.; McGuire, M.K.; McGuire, M.A. Trans fatty acids in milk produced by women in the United States. *Am. J. Clin. Nutr.* **2005**, *82*, 1292–1297. [CrossRef] [PubMed]
46. Dreiucker, J.; Vetter, W. Fatty acids patterns in camel, moose, cow and human milk as determined with GC/MS after silver ion solid phase extraction. *Food Chem.* **2011**, *126*, 762–771. [CrossRef]
47. Kelishadi, R.; Hadi, B.; Iranpour, R.; Khosravi-Darani, K.; Mirmoghtadaee, P.; Farajian, S.; Poursafa, P. A study on lipid content and fatty acid of breast milk and its association with mother's diet composition. *J. Res. Med. Sci.* **2012**, *17*, 824–827. [PubMed]
48. Daud, A.Z.; Mohd-Esa, N.; Azlan, A.; Chan, Y.M. The 'trans' fatty acid content in human milk and its association with maternal diet among lactating mothers in Malaysia. *Asia Pac. J. Clin. Nutr.* **2013**, *22*, 431–442. [PubMed]
49. Saphier, O.; Blumenfeld, J.; Silberstein, T.; Tzor, T.; Burg, A. Fatty acid composition of breastmilk of Israeli mothers. *Indian Pediatr.* **2013**, *50*, 1044–1046. [CrossRef] [PubMed]
50. Chuang, C.-K.; Yeung, C.-Y.; Jim, W.-T.; Lin, S.-P.; Wang, T.J.; Huang, S.-F.; Liu, H.-L. Comparison of free fatty acid content of human milk from Taiwanese mothers and infant formula. *Taiwan. J. Obstet. Gynecol.* **2013**, *52*, 527–533. [CrossRef] [PubMed]
51. Villasenor, A.; Garcia-Perez, I.; Garcia, A.; Posma, J.M.; Fernandez-Lopez, M.; Nicholas, A.J.; Modi, N.; Holmes, E.; Barbas, C. Breast Milk metabolome characterization in a single-phase extraction, multiplatform analytical approach. *Anal. Chem.* **2014**, *86*, 8245–8252. [CrossRef] [PubMed]
52. Sokol, E.; Ulven, T.; Færgeman, N.J.; Ejsing, C.S. Comprehensive and quantitative profiling of lipid species in human milk, cow milk and a phospholipid-enriched milk formula by GC and MS/MS(All). *Eur. J. Lipid Sci. Technol.* **2015**, *117*, 751–759. [CrossRef] [PubMed]
53. Ten-Doménech, I.; Beltrán-Iturat, E.; Herrero-Martínez, J.M.; Sancho-Llopis, J.V.; Simó-Alfonso, E.F. Triacylglycerol analysis in human milk and other mammalian species: Small-scale sample preparation, characterization, and statistical classification using HPLC-ELSD profiles. *J. Agric. Food Chem.* **2015**, *63*, 5761–5770.
54. Liu, G.; Ding, Z.; Li, X.; Chen, X.; Wu, Y.; Xie, L. Relationship between polyunsaturated fatty acid levels in maternal diets and human milk in the first month post-partum. *J. Hum. Nutr. Diet.* **2016**, *29*, 405–410. [CrossRef] [PubMed]
55. Garwolińska, D.; Hewelt-Belka, W.; Namieśnik, J.; Kot-Wasik, A. Rapid characterization of the human breast milk lipidome using a Solid-Phase Microextraction and liquid Chromatography-Mass Spectrometry-based approach. *J. Proteom. Res.* **2017**, *16*, 3200–3208. [CrossRef] [PubMed]
56. Wu, J.; Domellöf, M.; Zivkovic, A.M.; Larsson, G.; Öhman, A.; Nording, M.L. NMR-based metabolite profiling of human milk: A pilot study of methods for investigating compositional changes during lactation. *Biochem. Biophys. Res. Commun.* **2016**, *469*, 626–632. [CrossRef] [PubMed]
57. Tu, A.; Ma, Q.; Bai, H.; Du, Z. A comparative study of triacylglycerol composition in Chinese human milk within different lactation stages and imported infant formula by SFC Coupled with Q-TOF-MS. *Food Chem.* **2017**, *221*, 555–567. [CrossRef] [PubMed]
58. Zechner, R. Rapid and simple isolation procedure for lipoprotein lipase from human milk. *Biochim. Biophys. Acta (BBA) Lipids Lipid MeTable* **1990**, *1044*, 20–25. [CrossRef]
59. Freudenberg, E. Lipase of human milk; Studies on its enzymological and nutritional significance. *Bibl. Paediatr.* **1953**, *54*, 1–68.
60. Berkow, S.E.; Freed, L.M.; Hamosh, M.; Bitman, J.; Wood, D.L.; Happ, B.; Hamosh, P. Lipases and lipids in human milk: Effect of freeze-thawing and storage. *Pediatr. Res.* **1984**, *18*, 1257–1262. [CrossRef] [PubMed]
61. Chang, Y.-C.; Chen, C.-H.; Lin, M.-C. The macronutrients in human milk change after storage in various containers. *Pediatr. Neonatol.* **2012**, *53*, 205–209. [CrossRef] [PubMed]
62. Garcia-Lara, N.R.; Escuder-Vieco, D.; Garcia-Algar, O.; De la Cruz, J.; Lora, D.; Pallas-Alonso, C. Effect of freezing time on macronutrients and energy content of breastmilk. *Breastfeed. Med.* **2012**, *7*, 295–301. [CrossRef] [PubMed]
63. Lev, H.M.; Ovental, A.; Mandel, D.; Mimouni, F.B.; Marom, R.; Lubetzky, R. Major losses of fat, carbohydrates and energy content of preterm human milk frozen at −80 °C. *J. Perinatol.* **2014**, *34*, 396–398. [CrossRef] [PubMed]

64. Fusch, G.; Rochow, N.; Choi, A.; Fusch, S.; Poeschl, S.; Ubah, A.O.; Lee, S.-Y.; Raja, P.; Fusch, C. Rapid measurement of macronutrients in breast milk: How reliable are infrared milk analyzers? *Clin. Nutr.* **2015**, *34*, 465–476. [CrossRef] [PubMed]
65. Bitman, J.; Wood, D.L.; Mehta, N.R.; Hamosh, P.; Hamosh, M. Lipolysis of triglycerides of human milk during storage at low temperatures: A note of caution. *J. Pediatr. Gastroenterol. Nutr.* **1983**, *2*, 521–524. [CrossRef] [PubMed]
66. Tijerina-Saenz, A.; Innis, S.M.; Kitts, D.D. Antioxidant capacity of human milk and its association with vitamins A and E and fatty acid composition. *Acta Paediatr.* **2009**, *98*, 1793–1798. [CrossRef] [PubMed]
67. Boris, J.; Jensen, B.; Dalby Salvig, J.; Secher, N.J.; Olsen, S.F. A randomized controlled trial of the effect of fish oil supplementation in late pregnancy and early lactation on the n-3 fatty acid content in human breast milk. *Lipids* **2004**, *39*, 1191–1196. [CrossRef] [PubMed]
68. Magnusardottir, A.R.; Skuladottir, G.V. Effects of storage time and added antioxidant on fatty acid composition of red blood cells at −20 °C. *Lipids* **2006**, *41*, 401–404. [CrossRef] [PubMed]
69. Folch, J.; Lees, M.; Sloane Stanley, G.H. A simple method for the isolation and purification of total lipides from animal tissues. *J. Bio.l Chem.* **1957**, *226*, 497–509.
70. Bligh, E.G.; Dyer, W.J. A rapid method of total lipid extraction and purification. *Can. J. Biochem. Physiol.* **1959**, *37*, 911–917. [CrossRef] [PubMed]
71. Ruiz-Gutierrez, V.; Perez-Camino, M.C. Update on solid-phase extraction for the analysis of lipid classes and related compounds. *J. Chromatogr. A* **2000**, *885*, 321–341. [CrossRef]
72. Chappell, J.E.; Clandinin, M.T.; McVey, M.A.; Chance, G.W. Free fatty acid content of human milk: Physiologic significance and artifactual determinants. *Lipids* **1985**, *20*, 216–221. [CrossRef] [PubMed]
73. Meurant, G. *Handbook of Milk Composition*, 1st ed.; Jensen, R.G., Ed.; Academic Press: San Diego, CA, USA, 1995.
74. Orata, F. Derivatization reactions and reagents for Gas Chromatography analysis. *Adv. Gas Chromatogr.* **2012**, *5*, 83–108.
75. Morrison, W.R.; Smith, L.M. Preparation of fatty acid methyl esters and dimethylacetals from lipids with boron fluoride—Methanol. *J. Lipid Res.* **1964**, *5*, 600–608. [PubMed]
76. Christie, W.W. Preparation of ester derivatives of fatty acids for chromatographic analysis. *Adv. Lipid Method.* **1993**, *2*, 69–111.
77. Broadhurst, D.; Goodacre, R.; Reinke, S.N.; Kuligowski, J.; Wilson, I.D.; Lewis, M.R.; Dunn, W.B. Guidelines and considerations for the use of system suitability and quality control samples in mass spectrometry assays applied in untargeted clinical metabolomic studies. *Metabolomics* **2018**, *14*, 72. [CrossRef] [PubMed]
78. Yang, K.; Han, X. Lipidomics: Techniques, applications, and outcomes related to biomedical sciences. *Trends Biochem. Sci.* **2016**, *41*, 954–969. [CrossRef] [PubMed]
79. Jurowski, K.; Kochan, K.; Walczak, J.; Baranska, M.; Piekoszewski, W.; Buszewski, B. Analytical techniques in lipidomics: State of the art. *Crit. Rev. Anal. Chem.* **2017**, *47*, 418–437. [CrossRef] [PubMed]
80. Ackman, R.G. Misidentification of fatty acid methyl ester peaks in liquid canola shortening. *J. Am. Oil Chem. Soc.* **1990**, *67*, 1028. [CrossRef]
81. Hawrysh, Z.J.; Shand, P.J.; Lin, C.; Tokarska, B.; Hardin, R.T. Efficacy of tertiary butylhydroquinone on the storage and heat stability of liquid canola shortening. *J. Am. Oil Chem. Soc.* **1990**, *67*, 585–590. [CrossRef]
82. Waston, A.D. Thematic review series: Systems biology approaches to metabolic and cardiovascular disorders. Lipidomics: A global approach to lipid analysis in biological systems. *J. Lipid Res.* **2006**, *47*, 2101–2111.
83. Sommer, U.; Herscovitz, H.; Welty, F.K.; Costello, C.E. LC-MS-based method for the qualitative and quantitative analysis of complex lipid mixtures. *J. Lipid Res.* **2006**, *47*, 804–814. [CrossRef] [PubMed]
84. Laakso, P.; Manninen, P. Identification of milk fat triacylglycerols by capillary supercritical fluid chromatography-atmospheric pressure chemical ionization mass spectrometry. *Lipids* **1997**, *32*, 1285–1295. [CrossRef] [PubMed]
85. Taylor, L.T. Supercritical fluid chromatography. *Anal. Chem.* **2010**, *82*, 4925–4935. [CrossRef] [PubMed]
86. Garcia, C.; Lutz, N.W.; Confort-Gouny, S.; Cozzone, P.J.; Armand, M.; Bernard, M. Phospholipid fingerprints of milk from different mammalians determined by ^{31}p NMR: Towards specific interest in human health. *Food Chem.* **2012**, *135*, 1777–1783. [CrossRef] [PubMed]
87. Sundekilde, U.K.; Larsen, L.B.; Bertram, H.C. NMR-based milk metabolomics. *Metabolites* **2013**, *3*, 204–222. [CrossRef] [PubMed]

88. Guillén, M.D.; Ruiz, A. ^{1}H nuclear magnetic resonance as a fast tool for determining the composition of acyl chains in acylglycerol mixtures. *Eur. J. Lipid Sci. Technol.* **2003**, *105*, 502–507.
89. Wishart, D.S. Metabolomics: Applications to food science and nutrition research. *Trends Food Sci. Technol.* **2008**, *19*, 482–493. [CrossRef]
90. Wishart, D.S.; Feunang, Y.D.; Marcu, A.; Guo, A.C.; Liang, K.; Vazquez-Fresno, R.; Sajed, T.; Johnson, D.; Li, C.; Karu, N.; et al. HMDB 4.0: The human metabolome database for 2018. *Nucleic Acids Res.* **2018**, *46*, D608–D617. [CrossRef] [PubMed]

16

Human Milk Composition and Dietary Intakes of Breastfeeding Women of Different Ethnicity from the Manawatu-Wanganui Region of New Zealand

Christine A. Butts [1,*], Duncan I. Hedderley [1], Thanuja D. Herath [1], Gunaranjan Paturi [2], Sarah Glyn-Jones [3], Frank Wiens [4], Bernd Stahl [4] and Pramod Gopal [1,5]

1. The New Zealand Institute for Plant and Food Research Limited, Private Bag 11600, Palmerston North 4442, New Zealand; duncan.hedderley@plantandfood.co.nz (D.I.H.); hmth4@hotmail.com (T.D.H.); pramod.gopal@plantandfood.co.nz (P.G.)
2. The New Zealand Institute for Plant and Food Research Limited, Private Bag 92169, Auckland 1142, New Zealand; gunaranjan.paturi@plantandfood.co.nz
3. Danone Nutricia NZ Limited, 56-58 Aintree Avenue, Mangere, Auckland 2022, New Zealand; sarah.glyn-jones@danone.com
4. Danone Nutricia Research, Upsalalaan 12, 3584 CT Utrecht, The Netherlands; frank.wiens@danone.com (F.W.); bernd.stahl@danone.com (B.S.)
5. Riddet Institute, Massey University, Palmerston North 4442, New Zealand

* Correspondence: chrissie.butts@plantandfood.co.nz

Abstract: Human milk is nutrient rich, complex in its composition, and is key to a baby's health through its role in nutrition, gastrointestinal tract and immune development. Seventy-eight mothers (19–42 years of age) of Asian, Māori, Pacific Island, or of European ethnicity living in Manawatu-Wanganui, New Zealand (NZ) completed the study. The women provided three breast milk samples over a one-week period (6–8 weeks postpartum), completed a three-day food diary and provided information regarding their pregnancy and lactation experiences. The breast milk samples were analyzed for protein, fat, fatty acid profile, ash, selected minerals (calcium, magnesium, selenium, zinc), and carbohydrates. Breast milk nutrient profiles showed no significant differences between the mothers of different ethnicities in their macronutrient (protein, fat, carbohydrate, and moisture) content. The breast milk of Asian mothers contained significantly higher levels of polyunsaturated fatty acids (PUFAs), omega-3 (*n*-3) and omega-6 (*n*-6) fatty acids, docosahexaenoic acid (DHA), and linoleic acids. Arachidonic acid was significantly lower in the breast milk of Māori and Pacific Island women. Dietary intakes of protein, total energy, saturated and polyunsaturated fat, calcium, phosphorus, zinc, iodine, vitamin A equivalents, and folate differed between the ethnic groups, as well as the number of serves of dairy foods, chicken, and legumes. No strong correlations between dietary nutrients and breast milk components were found.

Keywords: human milk; breastfeeding; ethnicity; composition; diet

---

1. Introduction

Human milk usually provides all the nutrients a human infant requires for the first 6 months of life. As well as the essential macro and micro-nutrients, breast milk contains many distinctive bioactive molecules that protect the new-born against pathogens and inflammation, and contribute to immune system maturation, organ development, and healthy microbial colonization [1,2]. The benefits of breastfeeding on the health and wellbeing of the infant are well recognized and include the prevention of infections, optimal neurodevelopment, and may limit the development of allergy, obesity and diabetes later in life [3–5]. The World Health Organization (WHO) [6] and the national advisory bodies of many countries, including New Zealand (NZ) [7], actively support and promote breastfeeding by their strong recommendations that all infants should be exclusively breastfed for the first 6 months of life and that breastfeeding be continued with appropriate complementary foods for 2 years and beyond postpartum. For infants who are not breastfed, human milk composition is used as an important reference in decisions on the adequacy of surrogate infant nutrition products.

Human milk composition varies considerably within and between mothers and even within a single milk expression. This multidimensional variation in composition is believed to be an adaptation to the infants' changing needs [8–10], and geographical region and food supply [11,12]. The variations in human milk composition between individual women and populations have been reported to be in response to cultural differences such as diet and other lifestyle factors [13,14], environmental factors, such as mineral content of the soil that is then reflected in the mineral density of the foods grown there [15], and human genetic differences [16]. However, human milk composition data has not been collected from all world regions and populations. Therefore, studies of human milk composition in other regions and populations are important, particularly with regard to micronutrient concentrations and the proportions of specific lipids where a large variability has been noted from existing studies [14,17–19].

There is limited information available on the nutrient composition of breast milk from NZ mothers. Early research on breast milk from NZ women, by Deem [20,21], investigated diurnal variation in fat content and the influence of dietary macronutrient content on breast milk composition. Recent published information on breast milk composition in NZ women has focused on the levels of environmental contaminants in breast milk [22], the micronutrient iodine [23–26] and the macronutrient and amino acid compositions [27]. In the present study, we investigated the composition of breast milk of an ethnically mixed population of NZ women as a first representation of the New Zealand national population. The main ethnic groups in NZ are the indigenous Māori (14.9%) and three major immigrant populations from the Pacific Islands (7.4%), Asia (11.8%) and Europe (74.0%) [28]. We note here that some NZ citizens identify with more than one ethnic group resulting in the total being greater than 100%. The secondary aims of this study were to determine the dietary nutrient intakes of breastfeeding women, compare these to recommended intakes, to assess if the diets were different between different ethnic groups, and if this had any impact on breastmilk composition.

2. Materials and Methods

2.1. Study Design

This was an observational study with participating women providing samples of their breast milk as well as stool samples from themselves and their babies at 6–8 weeks postpartum. All participants gave their informed consent for inclusion before taking part in the study. The study was conducted in accordance with the Declaration of Helsinki and the protocol was approved by the New Zealand Human Disability and Ethics Committee (Application number 13/CEN/79/AM01).

One hundred and forty-six participants living in the Manawatū-Wanganui region of the North Island of New Zealand were screened for this study; 66 participants did not meet the recruitment criteria. A total of 80 women who fulfilled the inclusion and exclusion criteria were recruited into the study (Figure 1). The study was advertised through newspaper and radio, flyers displayed on community noticeboards, in midwifery and in childcare centers in and around the Palmerston North area. Interested participants were first contacted by phone and then visited in their homes to obtain informed consent and complete their enrolment into the study. Participant information regarding their ethnicity (self-identified), anthropometry, parity, recent pregnancy and childbirth experiences, general medical history, and recent breast-feeding practices, as well as previous pregnancies and birth history, were collected through questionnaires. Only breastfeeding women aged 18–55 years of Māori, Pacific Island, European, or Asian ethnicity permanently living in New Zealand were included.

Recruitment focused initially on women who were breast-feeding exclusively, however, if recruitment was slow we accepted women who were primarily breast-feeding and included no more than two formula feeds a day or water or medication. The mothers were asked to record exactly what method of feeding they used. Women with a pre-term childbirth or with infants who had required neonatal care were excluded from the study. Other exclusion criteria were active dieting, clinically significant renal, hepatic, endocrine, cardiac, pulmonary, pancreatic, neurological, hematologic, biliary, and mental health disorders as identified through their medical history.

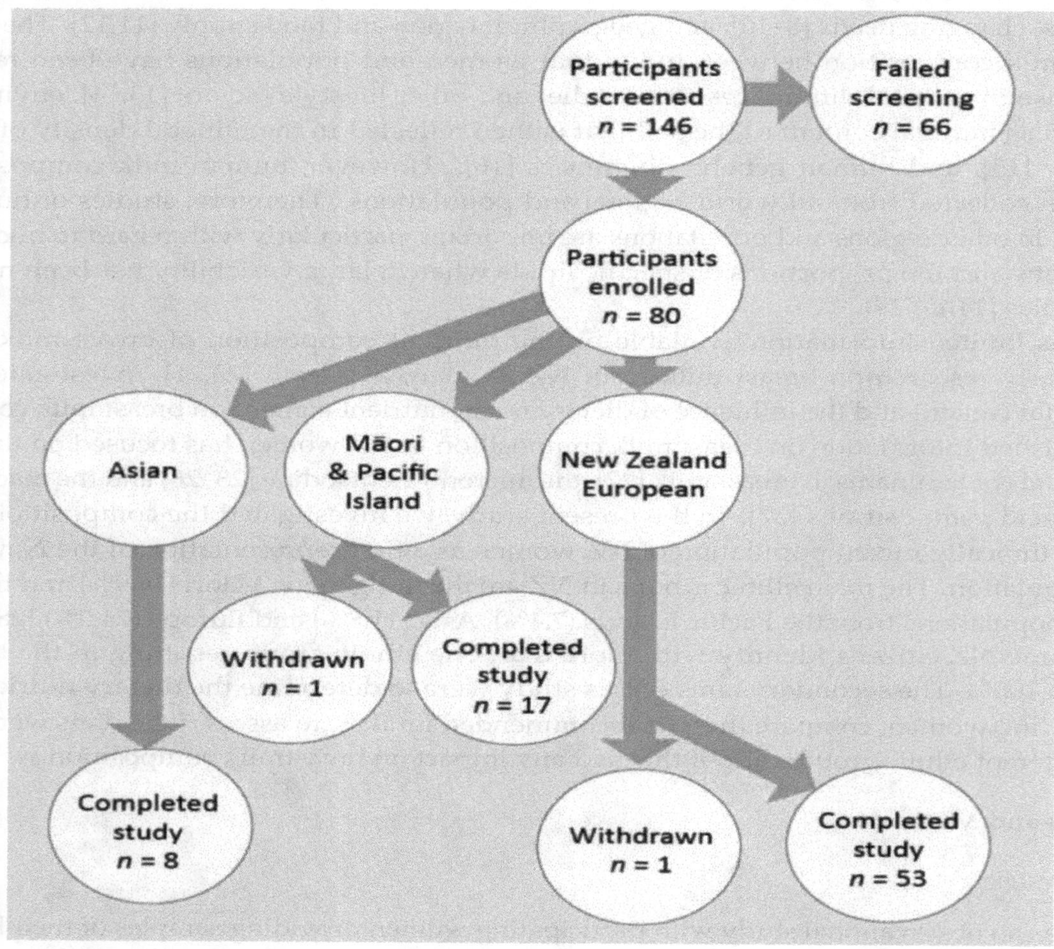

Figure 1. Study participant recruitment flow chart.

Following enrolment, each woman was asked to express three breast milk samples over a one-week period between six and eight weeks post-partum. Each sample of approximately 50 mL was collected from the first feed of the day (first feed after sunrise) into sterile containers and immediately frozen in household freezers at −18 °C. In order to guarantee enough milk supply to the infant, mothers fed their baby immediately before the collection of the expressed breast milk. Breast milk was collected by hand or breast pump, and the mode of expression was recorded. Subsequently, the three samples from each mother were thawed, pooled, aliquoted into smaller containers, and refrozen at −80 °C until analysis. In addition to breast milk, a fecal sample from both mother and infant was collected and frozen during the same week (rationale, methods and analyses will be reported elsewhere).

Each participating mother provided a diet record of every item she ate or drank and the quantities consumed over three consecutive days (two working days one non-working day) during the one week period of breast milk collection. Participants were reimbursed with grocery or fuel vouchers to compensate for their time commitment to this study.

2.2. Analysis of Breast Milk

Breast milk samples were analyzed for selected macronutrients (protein, carbohydrates, fat, polyunsaturated fatty acids; PUFAs) and micronutrients (calcium, magnesium, selenium, zinc). These analyses were carried out by the Nutrition Laboratory, Massey University, Palmerston North, NZ. Total protein was determined by the combustion method using a LECO analyzer (AOAC 968.06) [29] and the factor 6.38 to convert nitrogen content to protein. Total fat was measured using the Mojonnier method (AOAC 954.02) [29], and fatty acids were measured as their methyl esters by gas chromatography (Sukhija and Palmquist 1988). Ash was measured following incineration in a furnace at 550 °C (AOAC 942.05) [29]. Inductively coupled plasma mass spectroscopy (ICP-MS) was used to measure the individual minerals in breast milk. Following acid digestion, the samples were analyzed on a PerkinElmer Sciex Elan 6000 ICP-MS (PerkinElmer, Waltham, MA, USA). The system comprised a variable speed peristaltic pump, nebulizer, argon gas plasma (1500 W), vacuum chambers, quadrapole, and a combined pulse counting/analog detector. Each element was monitored at an isotope(s) chosen for its abundance/sensitivity and freedom from known interferences. The total carbohydrate content was estimated by the difference using the determined values for protein, fat, water, and ash [30].

2.3. Dietary Intake Analysis

The dietary intakes of the macro and micronutrients were calculated from the three-day food diaries completed by all participants. The data were entered into FoodWorks (Professional version 7.0 Xyris Software package, Brisbane, Australia) using the New Zealand Food Composition Database (2014).

2.4. Statistical Analysis

All data were transferred into an Excel database and summary statistics (means and standard deviations or standard errors) were calculated. The participants were grouped by ethnicity into three groups: Asians, Māori and Pacific Island, and NZ European. In NZ, population and government statistics distinguishes between indigenous Māori and immigrants from the Pacific Islands, however, for this study, we combined these two groups as both share a Polynesian background and the numbers of participants of Pacific Island ethnicity were small ($n = 2$). Demographic data, breast milk nutrients, dietary nutrient intakes, food serves, and the dietary supplements taken were compared between ethnic groups using an analysis of variance (ANOVA); where there was a significant ($p < 0.05$) difference between groups and multiple comparisons were made using the least significant difference. Where data were skewed, Kruskal-Wallis non-parametric ANOVA was also carried out. Nutrient data from the breast milk samples were analyzed in the same way. Analyses were carried out using Genstat (version 17, 2014, VSNi Ltd., Hemel Hempstead, UK) and the *R* package *gplots* (R Foundation for Statistical Computing, Vienna, Austria).

3. Results

3.1. Study Population

The demographic and baseline characteristics of all participants in this study are summarized in Tables 1 and 2. Of the 80 participants enrolled in the study, 78 completed the study; 68% of these were NZ Europeans, 22% Māori and Pacific Island and 10% Asian. One participant each of Māori and NZ European ethnicities withdrew from the study before completion as they were no longer able to provide the samples requested.

The mean age of the participants was 31 years, their mean body mass index (BMI) was 27, and the mean infant birth weight was 3.6 kg (Table 1). When analyzed based on ethnicity, there were no statistically significant differences in the age and heights of the women (Table 2), whereas there were significant differences in body weight ($p < 0.001$) and BMI ($p = 0.003$) of the mothers from the different ethnic groups. Asian women had the lowest mean body weight and BMI, and the Māori and Pacific Island mothers had the highest mean body weight and BMI (Table 2). It is important to note that the NZ Ministry of Health guidelines use different BMI [31] values to classify women of different ethnicities into normal, overweight and obese categories to those recommended by the WHO [32] (Table 3). Demographic distribution and baseline characteristics of the study population based on BMI classifications recommended by the NZ Ministry of Health are summarized in Table 4. Based on these criteria, the proportions of all participants in the normal, overweight and obese categories were 35%, 40%, and 25%, respectively. The Asian mothers had the highest proportion of women with normal BMI while the Māori and Pacific Island mothers had the lowest proportion in the normal BMI range.

Table 1. Demographics and baseline characteristics of the study participants.

Baseline Characteristics	Mean	Range
Mothers (n = 78)		
Age (years)	31 ± 5	19–42
Weight (kg)	74 ± 14	48–109
Height (m)	1.65 ± 0.06	1.52–1.87
Body mass index (kg/m^2)	27 ± 5	20–39
Babies (n = 79)		
Birth weight (kg)	3.6 ± 0.5	2.4–4.6
Weight at sample collection (kg)	4.8 ± 0.6	3.3–6.2

Data expressed as mean ± standard deviation.

Table 2. Demographics and baseline characteristics of the study participants according to ethnicity.

	Asian	Māori & Pacific Island	New Zealand European	p Value
Participants in group (n)	8	17	53	
Age (years)	30.4 ± 1.2	31.2 ± 1.5	30.7 ± 0.7	0.917
Weight (kg)	58.4 ± 3.1 ^{a}	80.8 ± 4.2 ^{b}	74.5 ± 1.6 ^{b}	<0.001
Height (m)	1.61 ± 0.02	1.65 ± 0.01	1.66 ± 0.01	0.162
Body mass index (kg/m^2)	22.5 ± 1.1 ^{a}	29.6 ± 1.5 ^{b}	27.2 ± 0.6 ^{b}	0.003
Birth weight (kg)	3.32 ± 0.13	3.63 ± 0.13	3.60 ± 0.06	0.255

Data expressed as mean ± standard error of the mean. Mean values with a different letter differ significantly, $p < 0.05$.

Table 3. World Health Organisation and New Zealand Ministry of Health classifications of body mass index (kg/m^2).

	World Health Organisation [1]	New Zealand Ministry of Health [2]		
	All Populations	Asian	Māori & Pacific	New Zealand European
Underweight	<18.50	<18.50	<18.50	<18.50
Normal	18.50–24.99	18.5–22.9	18.5–26	18.5–25
Overweight	≥25.00	23–27.4	26–32	25–30
Obese	≥30.00	>27.5	>32	>30

[1] Adapted from World Health Organisation 1995, 2000 and 2004 [32]. [2] Ministry of Health, New Zealand [31].

Table 4. Demographics and baseline characteristics of the study participants according to body mass index (BMI) classifications outlined by Ministry of Health, New Zealand.

	Normal	Overweight	Obese	p Value
Age (years)	30.3 ± 1.0	31.5 ± 0.8	30.2 ± 1.4	0.559
Weight (kg)	60.4 ± 1.2 ^{a}	74.7 ± 1.7 ^{b}	92.0 ± 2.0 ^{c}	<0.001
Height (cm)	165.0 ± 1.4	165.2 ± 1.0	164.6 ± 1.1	0.943
Baby's weight (kg)	3.52 ± 0.08	3.65 ± 0.09	3.54 ± 0.14	0.592
Participants in BMI category (%)	35	40	25	

Data expressed as mean ± standard error of the mean. Mean values with a different letter differ significantly, $p < 0.05$.

3.2. Nutrient Composition of Breast Milk

The nutrient profiles of the mothers' breast milk are presented in Table 5. The mean values for the three main macronutrients (protein, fat, carbohydrates) and water in the breast milk across all ethnicities were not significantly different between women of different ethnicities. There were no significant differences in the mean breast milk concentrations of the minerals calcium, selenium, and zinc, but there were significant differences in magnesium concentrations, where NZ European mothers had significantly higher concentrations than Māori and Pacific Island mothers ($p = 0.049$).

There were significant differences in the total PUFAs, n-3 and n-6 fatty acids present in the breast milk. Asian mothers had higher concentrations of these fatty acids than Māori and Pacific Island and NZ European mothers. The fatty acids contributing to these differences were docosahexaenoic acid (DHA) ($p < 0.001$), arachidonic acid ($p = 0.023$), and linoleic acid (*C18:2n6c*) ($p = 0.009$). DHA was significantly higher in Asian mothers' breast milk compared to Māori and Pacific Island and NZ European mothers, but there was no significant difference between the Māori and Pacific Island and NZ European mothers. For arachidonic acid, however, breast milk from Māori and Pacific Island mothers had significantly lower concentrations than Asian and NZ European mothers, and there was no significant difference between the breast milk concentrations from Asian and NZ European mothers.

The nutrient intakes of the study participants in this study determined from their 3-day diet records are summarized in Table 6. Protein intakes of Māori and Pacific Island mothers were significantly lower ($p = 0.023$) than the NZ European mothers. There were no significant differences in the intakes of energy, total fat, saturated, polyunsaturated or monounsaturated fats, carbohydrate, sugars, starch, or dietary fiber between the mothers from different ethnic groups. There were, however, some significant differences in the total energy and different types of fats consumed. The energy from saturated fat ($p = 0.019$) and the proportion of fat from saturated fat ($p = 0.010$) was significantly lower in the diets of Asian women compared to Māori and Pacific Island and NZ European women. Asian mothers consumed a significantly higher proportion of their total fat intake as monounsaturated fats ($p = 0.042$) than the other ethnic groups, and significantly more PUFAs ($p = 0.026$) than NZ European mothers.

Dietary intakes of calcium ($p = 0.007$), phosphorus ($p = 0.024$), and zinc ($p = 0.029$) were significantly higher in NZ European mothers than Asian and Māori and Pacific Island mothers. Iodine intakes were highest for the Asian mothers ($p = 0.027$). Dietary intakes of vitamins were similar except for folate (food; $p = 0.025$) and vitamin A equivalents ($p = 0.009$), where Asian mothers consumed significantly higher amounts than Māori and Pacific Island and NZ European mothers.

The association between specific dietary intakes of nutrients and breast milk composition was analyzed by Spearman rank-correlation (Figure 2). There were positive associations with breast milk concentrations of omega 6 (n-6) and PUFAs, and linoleic acid with polyunsaturated and monounsaturated fat consumption. Trans-fatty acid concentrations in breast milk were positively correlated with saturated fat intakes. Breast milk magnesium was positively associated with dietary magnesium intake as well as carbohydrate, energy, iodine, caffeine, iron, fiber, folate, and potassium dietary intake.

To further understand the dietary sources of nutrients eaten by the mothers, we examined the number of serves per day of the main food groups (Table 7) and found that these were similar across the ethnic groups—except for dairy products where NZ European mothers consumed significantly ($p = 0.009$) more serves. The numbers of serves of protein and fatty acid rich foods consumed by the mothers from the different ethnic groups were similar for lamb, beef, pork, fish, egg, and nuts (Table 8). Asian mothers, however, ate significantly ($p = 0.036$) more serves of chicken than Māori and Pacific Island mothers and more serves ($p = 0.027$) of legumes than NZ European mothers.

The percent recommended daily intake (RDI) of key nutrients are shown in Table 9. Recommended daily intake is the average amount of each nutrient that meets the daily needs of healthy people at a particular age, metabolic status (e.g., pregnant, lactating), and gender. For all the mothers in the study, the percent daily intakes for folate, selenium, iodine, and molybdenum were lower than the recommended levels for lactating mothers. Iodine intake for the Asian, Māori and Pacific Island, and NZ European mothers was particularly low at 53%, 23%, and 30%, respectively, of the recommended intake. In addition, Māori and Pacific Island mothers consumed less energy, protein, vitamin B_6, vitamin A, calcium, and zinc; Asian mothers consumed less calcium, and NZ European mothers consumed less energy, vitamin B_6, and vitamin A than recommended. There were significant differences in the percent RDI between mothers of different ethnicity for protein, vitamin C, vitamin A, calcium, phosphorus, and iodine. Asian mothers consumed a significantly higher percentage RDI's for vitamin C ($p = 0.016$), vitamin A ($p = 0.002$), and iodine ($p = 0.010$). Māori and Pacific Island mother's protein intake was the lowest ($p = 0.003$), and NZ European mothers consumed the highest RDI's for calcium ($p = 0.012$) and phosphorus ($p = 0.017$). Some mothers in the study consumed supplements (Table 10), which could have improved their %RDI's from those calculated from their diet records. Multivitamin, iodine and iron supplements were the most frequently taken dietary supplements. There were no significant differences ($p > 0.05$) in supplement consumption by the mothers of different ethnicity.

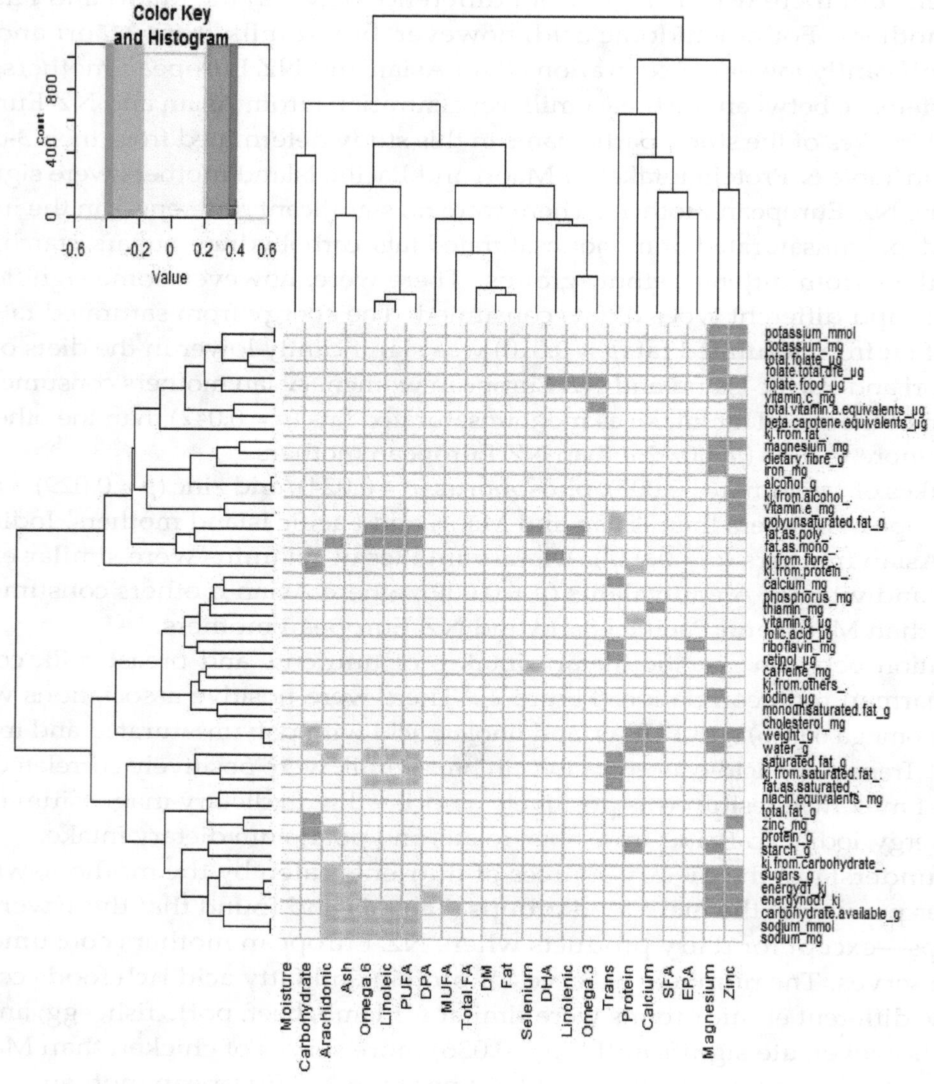

Figure 2. Spearman's rank-correlations between mother's dietary intake and breast milk nutrients. PUFAs, Polyunsaturated fatty acids; DPA, Docosapentaenoic acid; MUFA, Monounsaturated fatty acids; FA, fatty acid; DM, dry matter; DHA, Docosahexaenoic acid; SFA, Saturated fatty acids; and EPA, Eicosapentaenoic acid.

Table 5. Nutrient profiles of participant's breast milk.

Nutrient	Units	Asian	Māori & Pacific Island	New Zealand European	p Value
Moisture	%	86.6 ± 0.4	87.4 ± 0.4	87.4 ± 0.2	0.262
Ash	%	0.2 ± 0	0.2 ± 0	0.2 ± 0	0.927
Protein	%	1.13 ± 0.12	1.16 ± 0.07	1.20 ± 0.04	0.739
Fat	%	4.48 ± 0.45	3.72 ± 0.42	3.72 ± 0.16	0.296
Carbohydrate	%	7.61 ± 0.16	7.55 ± 0.06	7.53 ± 0.05	0.835
Calcium	mg/100 g	27.5 ± 1.3	29.1 ± 1.0	30.9 ± 0.7	0.086
Magnesium	mg/100 g	3.08 ± 0.08 [a,b]	3.01 ± 0.11 [a]	10.19 ± 6.20 [b]	0.049
Selenium	mg/100 g	0.016 ± 0.001	0.014 ± 0.001	0.013 ± 0.000	0.142
Zinc	mg/100 g	2.25 ± 0.29	2.27 ± 0.22	2.19 ± 0.12	0.953
Saturated fatty acids	g/100 g	1.81 ± 0.23	1.51 ± 0.16	1.50 ± 0.06	0.290
Trans-fatty acids	g/100 g	0.030 ± 0.009	0.031 ± 0.004	0.032 ± 0.002	0.948
Monounsaturated fatty acids	g/100 g	1.728 ± 0.145	1.396 ± 0.161	1.469 ± 0.063	0.302
Polyunsaturated fatty acids	g/100 g	0.658 ± 0.054 [a]	0.443 ± 0.048 [b]	0.466 ± 0.023 [b]	0.011
Omega-3 fatty acids	g/100 g	0.089 ± 0.012 [a]	0.057 ± 0.006 [b]	0.061 ± 0.003 [b]	0.012
Omega-6 fatty acids	g/100 g	0.562 ± 0.046 [a]	0.381 ± 0.042 [b]	0.401 ± 0.020 [b]	0.017
Eicosapentaenoic acid *C20:5n3*	g/100 g	0.005 ± 0.001	0.004 ± 0.000	0.004 ± 0.00	0.199
Docosahexaenoic acid *C22:6n3*	g/100 g	0.016 ± 0.004 [a]	0.006 ± 0.000 [b]	0.008 ± 0.001 [b]	<0.001
Linolenic acid *C18:3n3*	g/100 g	0.060 ± 0.009	0.045 ± 0.005	0.043 ± 0.002	0.055
Linoleic acid *C18:2n6c*	g/100 g	0.519 ± 0.045 [a]	0.349 ± 0.038 [b]	0.358 ± 0.018 [b]	0.009
Arachidonic acid *C20:4n6*	g/100 g	0.019 ± 0.002 [a]	0.012 ± 0.002 [b]	0.016 ± 0.001 [a]	0.023
Docosapentaenoic acid *C22:5n3*	g/100 g	0.006 ± 0.001	0.005 ± 0.000	0.005 ± 0.000	0.185
Capric acid *C10:0*	g/100 g	0.059 ± 0.019	0.047 ± 0.019	0.049 ± 0.019	0.309
Lauric acid *C12:0*	g/100 g	0.248 ± 0.109	0.196 ± 0.081	0.191 ± 0.070	0.177
Myristic acid *C14:0*	g/100 g	0.268 ± 0.159	0.216 ± 0.108	0.213 ± 0.074	0.320
Palmitic acid *C16:0*	g/100 g	0.929 ± 0.319	0.801 ± 0.339	0.780 ± 0.232	0.361
Palmitoleic acid *C16:1n7*	g/100 g	0.099 ± 0.027	0.098 ± 0.050	0.097 ± 0.038	0.991
Margaric acid *C17:0*	g/100 g	0.015 ± 0.006	0.014 ± 0.005	0.014 ± 0.006	0.959
Stearic acid *C18:0*	g/100 g	0.258 ± 0.094	0.243 ± 0.103	0.255 ± 0.082	0.872
Oleic acid *C18:1n9c*	g/100 g	1.507 ± 0.344	1.225 ± 0.557	1.294 ± 0.388	0.315
Vaccenic acid *C18:1n7t*	g/100 g	0.059 ± 0.020	0.048 ± 0.021	0.049 ± 0.016	0.314
Gondoic (11-Eicosenoic) acid *C20:1n9*	g/100 g	0.018 ± 0.004	0.014 ± 0.008	0.014 ± 0.005	0.148
Dihomo-γ-linolenic (*cis*-8,11,14-Eicosatrienoic acid) *C20:3n6*	g/100 g	0.013 ± 0.003	0.010 ± 0.006	0.015 ± 0.007	0.060
Total fatty acids (g/100 g)	g/100 g	4.20 ± 0.35	3.35 ± 0.36	3.44 ± 0.14	0.170

Data expressed as mean ± standard error of the mean. Mean values with a different letter differ significantly, $p < 0.05$.

Table 6. Nutrient intakes of the participants.

	Asian	Māori & Pacific Island	New Zealand European	*p* Value
Food weight (g)	3615 ± 369	2771 ± 254	3656 ± 263	0.175
Energy (no dietary fibre) (kJ)	9732 ± 1159	8762 ± 574	9940 ± 282	0.178
Energy dietary fibre (kJ)	10,008 ± 1208	8979 ± 586	10,124 ± 285	0.207
Protein (g)	85.4 ± 6.3 [a,b]	82.5 ± 5.0 [a]	97.8 ± 3.0 [b]	0.023
Total fat (g)	100.3 ± 14.0	88.9 ± 6.0	99.2 ± 3.8	0.407
Saturated fat (g)	34.6 ± 9.2	37.3 ± 2.3	41.7 ± 1.7	0.231
Polyunsaturated fat (g)	16.4 ± 2.5	12.8 ± 1.3	12.7 ± 1.0	0.338
Monounsaturated fat (g)	38.9 ± 6.0	32.7 ± 2.8	35.7 ± 1.7	0.471
Cholesterol (mg)	313 ± 32	286 ± 31	301 ± 15	0.831
Carbohydrate available (g)	275 ± 36	244 ± 19	272 ± 10	0.412
Sugars (g)	111 ± 24	105 ± 9	128 ± 6	0.132
Starch (g)	164 ± 14	139 ± 11	144 ± 6	0.408
Water (g)	3069 ± 348	2300 ± 235	3116 ± 266	0.221
Alcohol (g)	0.13 ± 0.08	0.74 ± 0.51	2.19 ± 1.05	0.555
Dietary fibre (g)	33.58 ± 5.80	25.96 ± 2.01	27.13 ± 1.18	0.155
Thiamine (mg)	1.56 ± 0.25	1.92 ± 0.19	1.75 ± 0.10	0.507
Riboflavin (mg)	2.14 ± 0.32	1.95 ± 0.14	2.31 ± 0.11	0.227
Niacin equivalents (mg)	37.25 ± 3.54	35.44 ± 2.61	42.44 ± 2.05	0.150
Vitamin C (mg)	156.80 ± 25.01	87.90 ± 18.03	118.70 ± 9.10	0.060
Vitamin D (μg)	3.83 ± 1.07	3.50 ± 0.52	4.42 ± 0.49	0.576
Vitamin E (mg)	13.37 ± 2.31	9.97 ± 0.82	11.91 ± 1.06	0.451
Total folate (μg)	421.30 ± 68.69	359.10 ± 36.03	348.40 ± 16.17	0.357
Folic acid (μg)	28.14 ± 13.47	87.27 ± 23.03	65.97 ± 9.50	0.173
Folate food (μg)	395 ± 67 [a]	273 ± 25 [b]	285 ± 13 [b]	0.025
Folate, total dietary folate equivalents (μg)	440 ± 72	418 ± 49	393 ± 20	0.693
Total Vitamin A equivalents (μg)	1583 ± 370 [a]	937 ± 80 [b]	988 ± 63 [b]	0.009
Retinol (μg)	668 ± 309	339 ± 32	427 ± 28	0.066
Beta-carotene equivalents (μg)	5483 ± 1880	3584 ± 462	3389 ± 312	0.118
Sodium (mg)	3138 ± 483	2914 ± 235	2889 ± 130	0.804
Sodium (mmol)	137 ± 21	127 ± 10	126 ± 6	0.804
Potassium (mg)	3609 ± 574	2971 ± 203	3551 ± 174	0.218
Potassium (mmol)	92 ± 15	76 ± 5	91 ± 4	0.218
Magnesium (mg)	406 ± 68	318 ± 24	401 ± 22	0.128
Calcium (mg)	736 ± 162 [a]	758 ± 56 [a]	1041 ± 53 [b]	0.007
Phosphorus (mg)	1489 ± 170 [a,b]	1356 ± 84 [a]	1648 ± 53 [b]	0.024
Iron (mg)	16.1 ± 1.9	13.3 ± 1.0	14.8 ± 0.7	0.328
Zinc (mg)	11.0 ± 0.9 [a,b]	10.7 ± 0.7 [a]	13.1 ± 0.5 [b]	0.029
Iodine (μg)	133.1 ± 56.4 [a]	61.1 ± 5.7 [b]	80.0 ± 5.8 [b]	0.027
KJ from protein (%)	15.3 ± 1.1	15.8 ± 0.5	16.6 ± 0.4	0.346
KJ from fat (%)	36.4 ± 2.2	36.6 ± 1.1	36.1 ± 0.8	0.956
KJ from saturated fat (%)	11.9 ± 1.6 [a]	15.0 ± 0.4 [b]	15.2 ± 0.4 [b]	0.019
KJ from carbohydrate (%)	45.8 ± 2.4	44.9 ±1.3	44.2 ± 0.9	0.753
KJ from alcohol (%)	0.03 ± 0.02	0.21 ± 0.14	0.62 ± 0.30	0.561
KJ from fibre (%)	2.55 ± 0.24	2.32 ± 0.12	2.14 ± 0.07	0.104
KJ from others (%)	0.12 ± 0.11	0.19 ± 0.05	0.22 ± 0.03	0.531
Fat as monounsaturated (%)	44.2 ± 3.4 [a]	39.0 ± 1.2 [b]	39.5 ± 0.7 [b]	0.042
Fat as polyunsaturated (%)	18.6 ± 1.8 [a]	15.7 ± 1.6 [a,b]	13.9 ± 0.6 [b]	0.026
Fat as saturated (%)	37.2 ± 4.7 [a]	45.3 ± 1.6 [b]	46.7 ± 1.1 [b]	0.010
Caffeine (mg)	13.9 ± 5.8	41.0 ± 10.8	118.5 ± 28.8	0.122

Data expressed as mean ± standard error of the mean. Mean values with a different letter differ significantly, $p < 0.05$. kJ—kilojoules.

Table 7. Number of food serves per day consumed by the participants.

	Asian	Māori & Pacific Island	New Zealand European	*p* Value
Fruit	2.48 ± 0.68	1.56 ± 0.55	1.48 ± 0.15	0.226
Vegetables	1.72 ± 0.46	2.38 ± 0.29	2.28 ± 0.17	0.437
Whole grains	2.88 ± 1.27	1.98 ± 0.34	1.84 ± 0.20	0.300
Meat and fish	1.21 ± 0.22	1.54 ± 0.13	1.58 ± 0.08	0.258
Egg	0.38 ± 0.12	0.27 ± 0.08	0.33 ± 0.06	0.849
Dairy	0.85 ± 0.26 [a]	1.09 ± 0.17 [a]	1.66 ± 0.13 [b]	0.009
Nuts and legumes	0.88 ± 0.25	0.28 ± 0.11	0.38 ± 0.10	0.107

Data expressed as mean ± standard error of the mean. Mean values with a different letter differ significantly, $p < 0.05$.

Table 8. Number of serves per day of foods rich in protein and fats consumed by the participants.

	Asian	Māori & Pacific Island	New Zealand European	p Value
Lamb	0.11 ± 0.11	0.49 ± 0.19	0.24 ± 0.09	0.231
Beef	0.67 ± 0.36	1.27 ± 0.37	1.77 ± 0.20	0.070
Pork	0.44 ± 0.29	1.58 ± 0.39	1.01 ± 0.18	0.082
Chicken	1.64 ± 0.33 [a]	0.54 ± 0.23 [b]	1.19 ± 0.19 [a,b]	0.036
Fish	0.90 ± 0.30	0.40 ± 0.24	0.58 ± 0.12	0.112
Egg	1.38 ± 0.32	1.27 ± 0.38	0.95 ± 0.19	0.255
Legumes	1.75 ± 0.74 [a]	0.48 ± 0.18 [a,b]	0.29 ± 0.09 [b]	0.027
Nuts	0.55 ± 0.23	0.67 ± 0.29	0.72 ± 0.25	0.394

Data expressed as mean ± standard error of the mean. Mean values with a different letter differ significantly, $p < 0.05$.

Table 9. Recommended daily intake (%) of the participants.

	Asian	Māori & Pacific Island	New Zealand European	p Value
Energy	107 ± 15	85 ± 6	96 ± 3	0.093
Protein	145 ± 18 [a]	96 ± 8 [b]	122 ± 4 [a]	0.003
Thiamine	116 ± 18	137 ± 14	124 ± 7	0.570
Riboflavin	148 ± 32	122 ± 9	143 ± 7	0.292
Niacin	225 ± 21	208 ± 15	247 ± 12	0.208
Vitamin C	209 ± 41 [a]	104 ± 21 [b]	140 ± 11 [b]	0.016
Vitamin B6	111 ± 17	88 ± 8	92 ± 5	0.303
Vitamin B12	118 ± 30	202 ± 94	190 ± 38	0.786
Folate, total dietary folate equivalents	92 ± 17	83 ± 10	78 ± 4	0.496
Total Vitamin A equivalents	154 ± 35 [a]	84 ± 7 [b]	89 ± 6 [b]	0.002
Magnesium	129 ± 22	99 ± 7	126 ± 7	0.111
Calcium	74 ± 16 [a]	78 ± 6 [a]	104 ± 5 [b]	0.012
Phosphorus	149 ± 17 [a,b]	132 ± 9 [a]	164 ± 5 [b]	0.017
Iron	164 ± 21	147 ± 11	163 ± 7	0.523
Zinc	99 ± 12	94 ± 6	108 ± 4	0.228
Selenium	68 ± 12	62 ± 6	70 ± 4	0.662
Iodine	53 ± 21 [a]	23 ± 2 [b]	30 ± 2 [b]	0.010
Molybdenum	80 ± 12	90 ± 11	74 ± 4	0.219

Data expressed as mean ± standard error of the mean. Mean values with a different letter differ significantly, $p < 0.05$.

Table 10. Number of participants taken dietary supplements.

	Asian	Māori & Pacific Island	New Zealand European	p Value
Total supplements	7	7	36	0.065
Multivitamin	3	3	8	0.361
Iodine	2	4	22	0.351
Iron	4	4	13	0.342
Vitamin C	1	1	11	0.405
Fish oil	2	1	5	0.342
Probiotics	2	0	4	0.099
Other	2	2	12	0.684

4. Discussion

This study is the first to measure and compare breast milk composition and nutrient intakes from an ethnically representative proportion of NZ mothers. We found that the breast milk nutrient profiles of women from different ethnicities were similar in their macronutrient composition, but there were differences in the concentrations of some fatty acids and magnesium. Dietary intakes were different for protein, total energy, saturated and polyunsaturated fat, calcium, phosphorus, zinc, iodine, vitamin A equivalents, and folate. The serves of dairy products, chicken and legumes consumed by the mothers were different between the ethnic groups. There were weak positive associations with breast milk concentrations of some fatty acids and magnesium with dietary fatty acid and magnesium intakes.

Our study population was representative of the main ethnic groups present in NZ. Recent census figures [28], reported that 74.0% of the NZ population identifies themselves as Europeans, 11.8% as Asian and 22.3% as Māori and Pacific Island. This is very similar to the proportions in our study population: 68% NZ European, 10% Asian, and 22% Māori and Pacific Island. Other demographic characteristics of the participants were also similar across the different ethnicities. Categorization of the participants' BMI was also representative of the NZ population with 40% classified as overweight and 30% as obese—reflecting the results reported by the NZ Ministry of Health [33] of 35% overweight and 30% obese. While the Māori and Pacific Island participants had significantly higher body weights and BMI in the present study, the actual values were lower or similar to those reported (BMI 28.7 vs. 32.8) in a recent national health survey [33]; as were the BMI's for Asian (BMI 22.5 vs. 24.4) and NZ European (BMI 27.2 vs. 27.9) participants. Weight gain during pregnancy is normal due to the growth of the fetus, placenta, and amniotic fluid [34], and postpartum weight loss may be influenced by infant nursing mode [35]. In normal weight mothers, the gestational weight gain has been found to be approximately 13 kg [36], and weight loss has been reported to be variable with between 8 and 9 kg at 1 month postpartum and 4 and 11 kg at 3 months postpartum [35,37]. Gestational weight gain is associated with ethnicity, socio-demographic, lifestyle, and pregnancy characteristics within populations but which of these factors is predominant is unknown [38]. We weighed the mothers in the present study at six weeks postpartum when postpartum weight loss may not be completed.

The macronutrient composition of human milk is known to vary within mothers and during lactation, and yet it is conserved across populations despite variations in maternal nutritional status [39,40]. We found no statistically significant differences in the macronutrient concentrations in the breast milk of NZ women of different ethnicity. Breast milk samples collected in this study had similar protein (1.2%), carbohydrate (7.5%), and fat (3.8%) concentrations to those reported in the literature for mature hind milk [6,8,40–42]. Lipids can be the most variable macronutrient of human breast milk. For example, hind milk, defined as the last milk of a feed, may contain higher concentrations (4.79–6.07 g/100 mL) of milk fat than that found in foremilk (1.14–2.63 g/100 mL), defined as the initial milk of a feed [43]. Milk fat content has also been reported to be significantly lower in night (37.2 g/L; 10:01 pm to 4:00 am) and morning (37.1 g/L; 4:01 am to 10:00 am) feed samples than those from day (42.8 g/L; 10:01 am to 4:00 pm) and evening (43.2 g/L; 4:01 to 10:00 pm) feeds [21,44]. Total fat, dry matter, and energy contents of human milk are also known to increase markedly during the feed (water content decreases accordingly) as the breast is emptied [45]. The breast milk samples in the present study were collected from the first feed of the day (first feed after sunrise) and after the baby was fed and were, therefore, samples of hind milk. The mean fat content of 3.79% found in the present study is within the ranges for hind milk and milk collected in the morning when milk fat content is lower [44].

Calcium, phosphorous and magnesium concentrations in maternal serum are tightly regulated and it has been reported that there is little effect of maternal dietary intake of these minerals on their concentrations in human milk [46,47]. The mean concentrations of calcium and magnesium in mature milk reported in the literature are approximately 280 mg/L and 35 mg/L, respectively [46,48,49]. The observed concentrations of calcium and magnesium in breast milk reported here are in agreement with these values. However, we found that the mean magnesium concentration of breast milk from NZ European mothers was significantly higher than for the Asian and Māori and Pacific Island mothers, though there was not a statistically significant difference in dietary magnesium intake between ethnicities. We did observe a weak positive association with breast milk magnesium content and dietary intake which is in contrast to the literature [46,47] and may warrant further investigation.

The mean concentrations of zinc and selenium in the breast milk collected in the present study were 2.21 mg/kg and 0.014 mg/kg, respectively, and there were no significant differences between mothers of different ethnicity. Zinc concentrations in human milk decrease over lactation and steeply decline over the first month of lactation from that found in colostrum (>10 mg/L) and then gradually to 0.5 mg/L by the twelfth month of lactation (Casey 1989). The dietary intake of zinc has mostly been reported in the literature as having little impact on the concentrations found in breast milk [14,48,50]. Two studies, however, reported that zinc supplementation may influence zinc concentration in late lactation [51,52], which is in agreement for the positive association found here (Figure 2). The selenium concentrations in mature breast milk have been reported to be between 10–30 μg/L [53], with higher concentrations found at the initiation of lactation (41 μg/L) and decreasing as lactation progresses [54]. Worldwide, there are major differences in the selenium content of soils and therefore in the food supply [15], and NZ has one of the lowest estimated adult selenium intakes and blood serum concentrations in the world [55]. Rural African women's selenium breast milk concentrations were low when their dietary selenium intakes were low [56]. In contrast, Debski et al. [57] reported that the selenium breast milk concentrations of lacto-ovo-vegetarian women (22.2 ng/mL) were greater than that of non-vegetarian women (16.8 ng/mL), but there was no significant differences in selenium intake between the two groups. We found no significant differences in breast milk selenium concentrations between the mothers of different ethnicity in the present study. No selenium dietary intake data are reported here as this data was not available for dietary analysis.

The composition of human milk has been observed to be consistent across ethnicities and countries in many parameters [58], but it is also known to be influenced by diet and particularly by intakes of fatty acids [14]. In the present study, we found that levels of PUFAs, *n*-3 and *n*-6 fatty acids, docosahexaenoic acid, and linoleic acid in the breast milk of Asian women were significantly higher compared to the other two ethnicities. While the intakes of the different types of dietary fat (monounsaturated, polyunsaturated, saturated) were similar between the different ethnic groups, the Asian women consumed fewer saturated fat and the proportion of dietary monounsaturated and polyunsaturated fats of total fat consumed was higher. This is supported by the lower number of dairy serves (higher in saturated fats) and higher number of serves of chicken (higher in polyunsaturated *n*-6 fatty acids) observed here in the Asian mothers. A similar result was observed for *n*-6 fatty acid contents in the breast milk of rural African women who consumed little animal fat [59].

Studies linking diet and breast milk fatty acid contents have not shown consistent results. Su et al. [60] found differences in breast milk fatty acid content between ethnicities, but the dietary intakes of *n*-3 and *n*-6 PUFAs for the different ethnicities were similar. Glew et al. [61] found no correlation between dietary intakes of α-linoleic acid and DHA and the amounts of these fatty acids in the breast milk of women from New Mexico. In contrast, a study in South Korea found that the dietary intakes of eicosapentaenoic acid (EPA), docosahexaenoic acid (DHA), omega 3 (*n*-3) fatty acids, omega 6 (*n*-6) fatty acids, saturated fatty acids (SFAs), and polyunsaturated fatty acids (PUFAs) were highly positively correlated, with the corresponding fatty acids in the breast milk samples [62], while a study in China found that dietary intakes and breast milk content of long chain *n*-3 PUFAs and linolenic were positively correlated [63]. Furthermore, other studies have shown that women who consume fish and other foods containing high levels of PUFA have relatively higher breast milk *n*-3 fatty acids and DHA concentrations compared to milk from women who consume diets that are low in these components [59,64,65]. In our study, the consumption of monounsaturated and polyunsaturated fats and fish were similar between the three ethnic groups. There were, however, correlations between dietary kilojoules from saturated fat, and *n*-6, linoleic and PUFAs in the breast milk. *Trans*-fatty acids in the milk were positively correlated with dietary saturated fat intake, and negatively correlated with polyunsaturated fat intake. Fatty acids in human milk are sourced not only from dietary fat but are also mobilized from maternal body fat and synthesized in the milk glands and hepatic cells. Therefore, the fatty acids found in human milk are likely to be influenced by short term and long term fatty acid dietary intake. The lack of consistency on the effect of dietary fatty acid intake on breast milk fatty acid composition in the literature is likely due to the collection of only short term fatty acid intake data, and not long term intakes, and the complex metabolic interdependencies between dietary and milk fatty acids.

The main strength of our study is that the breast milk nutrient composition and dietary nutrient intakes has been measured in NZ mothers of different ethnicity for the first time.

A strength and a limitation of this study is that our participant population was in only one region (Manawatū-Whanganui) of New Zealand. While the ethnic composition of our study population was similar to that found in the overall population of NZ, the study region included urban and rural areas but no major cities where diet and lifestyle could be different. The second limitation is the collection of breast milk after the infant had fed, as the time of milk collection is known to affect the measurement of the breast milk fat content where the concentration differs between the beginning and end of feeding and over the day night cycle. The breast milk samples in the present study comprised 1.2% protein, 3.8% fat, and 7.5% total carbohydrate, which is very similar to the data from mature breast milk (g/dL; protein 0.9–1.2, fat 3.2–3.6, lactose 7.2–7.8) collected from a number of studies reviewed by Ballard and Morrow [40]. The third limitation is the quantity of milk collected at each sampling (30 mL), which limited the quantity and therefore the range of nutrients that could be analyzed. This timing and quantity of breast milk collection were selected to ensure the infant had been fed and the infant's and mother's welfare were not compromised by the breast milk sampling.

5. Conclusions

We found that the nutrient composition of breast milk differed between ethnic groups for PUFAs, *n*-3, *n*-6, DHA, linoleic and arachidonic fatty acids and the mineral magnesium. Dietary intakes of protein, total energy, saturated and polyunsaturated fat, calcium, phosphorus, zinc, iodine, vitamin A equivalents, and folate differed between the ethnic groups, as well as the number of serves of dairy foods, chicken, and legumes. There were positive associations between breast milk concentrations of *n*-6, polyunsaturated and linoleic acid with dietary polyunsaturated and monounsaturated fats. The percent daily dietary intakes of folate, selenium, iodine, and molybdenum for the mothers in this study were less than that recommended for lactating women, which may negatively affect the health of these mothers and their infants. Additional dietary advice from health professionals such as midwives, registered nutritionists, and dietitians for pregnant and lactating mothers may improve their nutrient intakes ensuring the on-going health and well-being of NZ mothers and their babies.

Author Contributions: Data curation, T.D.H. and G.P.; Formal analysis, C.A.B., D.I.H. and G.P.; Investigation, C.A.B. and T.D.H.; Methodology, C.A.B., T.D.H. and G.P.; Project administration, C.A.B., S.G.-J. and P.G.; Resources, C.A.B.; Visualization, G.P.; Writing-original draft, C.A.B., D.I.H., T.D.H., P.G., and G.P.; Writing-review & editing, C.A.B., D.I.H., G.P., S.G.-J., F.W., B.S. and P.G.

Acknowledgments: We thank Juliet Ansell, Greg Ward and Berneace Steffens for the initial study design and plan. Our thanks to Alison Wallace and Sarah Eady for their contributions to the project scope and study design. We are grateful to Sheridan Martell and Hannah Dinnan for recruiting the study participants and encouraging and supporting the mothers to complete the questionnaires and collect the samples. We are grateful to Shila Shafaeizadeh and Leilani L. Muhardi of Nutricia Research Singapore for their comments on early versions of this manuscript.

References

1. Lönnerdal, B. Breast milk: A truly functional food. *Nutrition* **2000**, *16*, 509–511. [CrossRef]
2. Field, C.J. The immunological components of human milk and their effect of immune development in infants. *J. Nutr.* **2005**, *135*, 1–4. [CrossRef] [PubMed]
3. Victora, C.G.; Bahl, R.; Barros, A.J.D.; França, G.V.A.; Horton, S.; Krasevec, J.; Murch, S.; Sankar, M.J.; Walker, N.; Rollins, N.C. Breastfeeding in the 21st century: Epidemiology, mechanisms, and lifelong effect. *Lancet* **2016**, *387*, 475–490. [CrossRef]
4. Marseglia, L.; Manti, S.; D'Angelo, G.; Cuppari, C.; Salpietro, V.; Filippelli, M.; Trovato, A.; Gitto, E.; Salpietro, C.; Arrigo, T. Obesity and breastfeeding: The strength of association. *Women Birth* **2015**, *28*, 81–86. [CrossRef] [PubMed]

5. Manti, S.; Lougaris, V.; Cuppari, C.; Tardino, L.; Dipasquale, V.; Arrigo, T.; Salpietro, C.; Leonardi, S. Breastfeeding and IL-10 levels in children affected by cow's milk protein allergy: A restrospective study. *Immunobiology* **2017**, *222*, 358–362. [CrossRef] [PubMed]
6. World Health Organization. 10 Facts on Breastfeeding. Available online: http://www.who.int/features/factfiles/breastfeeding/en/ (accessed on 22 February 2018).
7. National Breastfeeding Advisory Committee of New Zealand. *National Strategic Plan of Action for Breastfeeding 2008–2012: National Breastfeeding Advisory Committee of New Zealand's Advice to the Director-General of Health*; Ministry of Health: Wellington, The New Zealand, 2009. Available online: http://www.moh.govt.nz (accessed on 20 February 2018).
8. Michaelsen, K.F.; Skafte, L.; Badsberg, J.H.; Jorgensen, M. Variation in macronutrients in human bank milk: Influencing factors and implications for human-milk banking. *J. Pediatr. Gastroenterol. Nutr.* **1990**, *11*, 229–239. [CrossRef] [PubMed]
9. Sauer, C.W.; Boutin, M.A.; Kim, J.H. Wide Variability in Caloric Density of Expressed Human Milk Can Lead to Major Underestimation or Overestimation of Nutrient Content. *J. Hum. Lact.* **2017**, *33*, 341–350. [CrossRef] [PubMed]
10. Fujita, M.; Roth, E.; Lo, Y.-J.; Hurst, C.; Vollner, J.; Kendell, A. In poor families, mothers' milk is richer for daughters than sons: A test of Trivers–Willard hypothesis in agropastoral settlements in Northern Kenya. *Am. J. Phys. Anthropol.* **2012**, *149*, 52–59. [CrossRef] [PubMed]
11. Hinde, K.; German, J.B. Food in an evolutionary context: Insights from mother's milk. *J. Sci. Food Agric.* **2012**, *92*, 2219–2223. [CrossRef] [PubMed]
12. Morrow, A.L.; Ruiz-Palacios, G.M.; Altaye, M.; Jiang, X.; Lourdes Guerrero, M.; Meinzen-Derr, J.K.; Farkas, T.; Chaturvedi, P.; Pickering, L.K.; Newburg, D.S. Human milk oligosaccharides are associated with protection against diarrhea in breast-fed infants. *J. Pediatr.* **2004**, *145*, 297–303. [CrossRef] [PubMed]
13. Prentice, A.; Prentice, A.M.; Whitehead, R.G. Breast-milk fat concentrations of rural african women: 1. Short-term variations within individuals. *Br. J. Nutr.* **1981**, *45*, 483–494. [CrossRef] [PubMed]
14. Bravi, F.; Wiens, F.; Decarli, A.; Dal Pont, A.; Agostoni, C.; Ferraroni, M. Impact of maternal nutrition on breast-milk composition: A systematic review. *Am. J. Clin. Nutr.* **2016**, *104*, 646–662. [CrossRef] [PubMed]
15. Zachara, B.A.; Pilecki, A. Selenium concentration in the milk of breast-feeding mothers and its geographic distribution. *Environ. Health Perspect.* **2000**, *108*, 1043–1046. [CrossRef] [PubMed]
16. Ameur, A.; Enroth, S.; Johansson, Å.; Zaboli, G.; Igl, W.; Johansson, A.C.; Rivas, M.A.; Daly, M.J.; Schmitz, G.; Hicks, A.A.; et al. Genetic Adaptation of Fatty-Acid Metabolism: A Human-Specific Haplotype Increasing the Biosynthesis of Long-Chain Omega-3 and Omega-6 Fatty Acids. *Am. J. Hum. Genet.* **2012**, *90*, 809–820. [CrossRef] [PubMed]
17. Yang, T.; Zhang, L.S.; Bao, W.; Rong, S. Nutritional composition of breast milk in Chinese women: A systematic review. *Asia Pac. J. Clin. Nutr.* **2018**, *27*, 491–502. [PubMed]
18. Fu, Y.Q.; Liu, X.; Zhou, B.; Jiang, A.C.; Chai, L.Y. An updated review of worldwide levels of docosahexaenoic and arachidonic acid in human breast milk by region. *Public Health Nutr.* **2016**, *19*, 2675–2687. [CrossRef] [PubMed]
19. Su, M.Y.; Jia, H.X.; Chen, W.L.; Qi, X.Y.; Liu, C.P.; Liu, Z.M. Macronutrient and micronutrient composition of breast milk from women of different ages and dietary habits in Shanghai area. *Int. Dairy J.* **2018**, *85*, 27–34. [CrossRef]
20. Deem, H.E. Effect of diet on human milk secretion. *Br. Med. J.* **1935**, *1935*, 80–81. [CrossRef]
21. Deem, H.E. Observations on the milk of New Zealand Women. *Arch. Dis. Child.* **1931**, *6*, 53–70. [CrossRef] [PubMed]
22. Bates, M.N.; Hannah, D.J.; Buckland, S.J.; Taucher, J.A.; Vanmaanen, T. Chlorinated organic contaminants in breast-milk of new-zealand women. *Environ. Health Perspect.* **1994**, *102*, 211–217. [CrossRef] [PubMed]
23. Brough, L.; Jin, Y.; Shukri, N.H.; Wharemate, Z.R.; Weber, J.L.; Coad, J. Iodine intake and status during pregnancy and lactation before and after government initiatives to improve iodine status, in Palmerston North, New Zealand: A pilot study. *Matern. Child Nutr.* **2015**, *11*, 646–655. [CrossRef] [PubMed]
24. Skeaff, S.A.; Ferguson, E.L.; McKenzie, J.E.; Valeix, P.; Gibson, R.S.; Thomson, C.D. Are breast-fed infants and toddlers in New Zealand at risk of iodine deficiency? *Nutrition* **2005**, *21*, 325–331. [CrossRef] [PubMed]
25. Mulrine, H.M.; Skeaff, S.A.; Ferguson, E.L.; Gray, A.R.; Valeix, P. Breast-milk iodine concentration declines over the first 6 mo postpartum in iodine-deficient women. *Am. J. Clin. Nutr.* **2010**, *92*, 849–856. [CrossRef] [PubMed]

26. Johnson, L.A.; Ford, H.C.; Doran, J.; Richardson, V.F. A survey of the iodide concentration of human-milk. *N. Z. Med. J.* **1990**, *103*, 393–394. [PubMed]
27. Darragh, A.J.; Moughan, P.J. The amino acid composition of human milk corrected for amino acid digestibility. *Br. J. Nutr.* **1998**, *80*, 25–34. [CrossRef] [PubMed]
28. Statistics New Zealand. *2013 Census QuickStats about Culture and Identity*; Statistics New Zealand: Wellington, New Zealand, 2014.
29. AOAC International. *Official Methods of Analysis of AOAC International*; AOAC International: Gaithersburg, MD, USA, 2005.
30. Food and Agriculture Organization of the United Nations. Analytical Methods for Carbohydrates in Foods. In *Food Energy—Methods of Analysis and Conversion Factors*; Food and Agriculture Organization of the United Nations: Rome, Italy, 2003; Volume 77.
31. Ministry of Health. *Food and Nutrition Guidelines for Healthy Pregnant and Breastfeeding Women: A Background Paper*; Ministry of Health: Wellington, New Zealand, 2006.
32. WHO. Global Datebase on Body Mass Index. Available online: http://apps.who.int/bmi/index.jsp?introPage=intro_3.html (accessed on 8 October 2017).
33. Ministry of Health. *Annual Update of Key Results 2014/15: New Zealand Health Survey*; Ministry of Health: Wellington, New Zealand, 2015.
34. Ministry of Health. *Guidance for Healthy Weight Gain in Pregnancy*; Ministry of Health: Wellington, New Zealand, 2014.
35. Martin, J.E.; Hure, A.J.; Macdonald-Wicks, L.; Smith, R.; Collins, C.E. Predictors of post-partum weight retention in a prospective longitudinal study. *Matern. Child Nutr.* **2014**, *10*, 496–509. [CrossRef] [PubMed]
36. Nomura, K.; Kido, M.; Tanabe, A.; Nagashima, K.; Takenoshita, S.; Ando, K. Investigation of optimal weight gain during pregnancy for Japanese Women. *Sci Rep.* **2017**, *7*, 2569. [CrossRef] [PubMed]
37. Whitaker, K.M.; Marino, R.C.; Haapala, J.L.; Foster, L.; Smith, K.D.; Teague, A.M.; Jacobs, D.R.; Fontaine, P.L.; McGovern, P.M.; Schoenfuss, T.C.; et al. Associations of Maternal Weight Status Before, During, and After Pregnancy with Inflammatory Markers in Breast Milk. *Obesity* **2017**, *25*, 2092–2099. [CrossRef] [PubMed]
38. Bahadoer, S.; Gaillard, R.; Felix, J.F.; Raat, H.; Renders, C.M.; Hofman, A.; Steegers, E.A.P.; Jaddoe, V.W.V. Ethnic disparities in maternal obesity and weight gain during pregnancy. The Generation R Study. *Eur. J. Obstet. Gynecol. Reprod. Biol.* **2015**, *193*, 51–60. [CrossRef] [PubMed]
39. Prentice, A.N.N. D—Regional Variations in the Composition of Human Milk A2—Jensen, Robert G. In *Handbook of Milk Composition*; Academic Press: San Diego, CA, USA, 1995; pp. 115–221. Available online: https://doi.org/10.1016/B978-012384430-9/50012-3pp (accessed on 23 February 2018).
40. Ballard, O.; Morrow, A.L. Human Milk Composition Nutrients and Bioactive Factors. *Pediatr. Clin. N. Am.* **2013**, *60*, 49–74. [CrossRef] [PubMed]
41. Hester, S.N.; Hustead, D.S.; Mackey, A.D.; Singhal, A.; Marriage, B.J. Is the Macronutrient Intake of Formula-Fed Infants Greater Than Breast-Fed Infants in Early Infancy? *J. Nutr. Metab.* **2012**, *2012*, 13. [CrossRef] [PubMed]
42. Wojcik, K.Y.; Rechtman, D.J.; Lee, M.L.; Montoya, A.; Medo, E.T. Macronutrient Analysis of a Nationwide Sample of Donor Breast Milk. *J. Am. Diet. Assoc.* **2009**, *109*, 137–140. [CrossRef] [PubMed]
43. Saarela, T.; Kokkonen, J.; Koivisto, M. Macronutrient and energy contents of human milk fractions during the first six months of lactation. *Acta Paediatr.* **2005**, *94*, 1176–1181. [CrossRef] [PubMed]
44. Kent, J.C.; Mitoulas, L.R.; Cregan, M.D.; Ramsay, D.T.; Doherty, D.A.; Hartmann, P.E. Volume and frequency of breastfeedings and fat content of breast milk throughout the day. *Pediatrics* **2006**, *117*, E387–E395. [CrossRef] [PubMed]
45. Michaelsen, K.F.; Larsen, P.S.; Thomsen, B.L.; Samuelson, G. The Copenhagen cohort study on infant nutrition and growth: Breast-milk intake, human-milk macronutrient content, and influencing factors. *Am. J. Clin. Nutr.* **1994**, *59*, 600–611. [CrossRef] [PubMed]
46. Vitolo, M.R.; Soares, L.M.V.; Carvalho, E.B.; Cardoso, C.B. Calcium and magnesium concentrations in mature human milk: Influence of calcium intake, age and socioeconomic level. *Arch. Latinoam. Nutr.* **2004**, *54*, 118–122. [PubMed]
47. Dorea, J.G. Calcium and phosphorus in human milk. *Nutr. Res.* **1999**, *19*, 709–739. [CrossRef]
48. Feeley, R.M.; Eitenmiller, R.R.; Jones, J.B.; Barnhart, H. Copper, iron, and zinc contents of human-milk at early stages of lactation. *Am. J. Clin. Nutr.* **1983**, *37*, 443–448. [CrossRef] [PubMed]

49. Fransson, G.B.; Lonnerdal, B. Zinc, copper, calcium, and magnesium in human-milk. *J. Pediatr.* **1982**, *101*, 504–508. [CrossRef]
50. Moser, P.B.; Reynolds, R.D. Dietary zinc intake and zinc concentrations of plasma, erythrocytes, and breast-milk in antepartum and postpartum lactating and nonlactating women—A longitudinal-study. *Am. J. Clin. Nutr.* **1983**, *38*, 101–108. [CrossRef] [PubMed]
51. Krebs, N.F.; Hambidge, K.M.; Jacobs, M.A.; Rasbach, J.O. The effects of a dietary zinc supplement during lactation on longitudinal changes in maternal zinc status and milk zinc concentrations. *Am. J. Clin. Nutr.* **1985**, *41*, 560–570. [CrossRef] [PubMed]
52. Karra, M.V.; Kirksey, A.; Galal, O.; Bassily, N.S.; Harrison, G.G.; Jerome, N.W. Effect of short-term oral zinc supplementation on the concentration of zinc in milk from american and egyptian women. *Nutr. Res.* **1989**, *9*, 471–478. [CrossRef]
53. Kumpulainen, J. Selenium: Requirement and supplementation. *Acta Paediatr. Scand.* **1989**, 114–117. [CrossRef]
54. Smith, A.M.; Picciano, M.F.; Milner, J.A. Selenium intakes and status of human-milk and formula fed infants. *Am. J. Clin. Nutr.* **1982**, *35*, 521–526. [CrossRef] [PubMed]
55. Combs, G.F. Selenium in global food systems. *Br. J. Nutr.* **2001**, *85*, 517–547. [CrossRef] [PubMed]
56. Funk, M.A.; Hamlin, L.; Picciano, M.F.; Prentice, A.; Milner, J.A. Milk selenium of rural african women: Influence of maternal nutrition, parity, and length of lactation. *Am. J. Clin. Nutr.* **1990**, *51*, 220–224. [CrossRef] [PubMed]
57. Debski, B.; Finley, D.A.; Picciano, M.F.; Lonnerdal, B.; Milner, J. Selenium content and glutathione-peroxidase activity of milk from vegetarian and nonvegetarian women. *J. Nutr.* **1989**, *119*, 215–220. [CrossRef] [PubMed]
58. Jenness, R. Composition of human-milk. *Semin. Perinatol.* **1979**, *3*, 225–239. [PubMed]
59. Koletzko, B.; Thiel, I.; Abiodun, P.O. The fatty acid composition of human milk in Europe and Africa. *J. Pediatr.* **1992**, *120*, S62–S70. [CrossRef]
60. Su, L.L.; Sk, T.C.; Lim, S.L.; Chen, Y.; Tan, E.A.; Pai, N.N.; Gong, Y.H.; Foo, J.; Rauff, M.; Chong, Y.S. The influence of maternal ethnic group and diet on breast milk fatty acid composition. *Ann. Acad. Med. Singap.* **2010**, *39*, 675–679. [PubMed]
61. Glew, R.H.; Wold, R.S.; Herbein, J.H.; Wark, W.A.; Martinez, M.A.; VanderJagt, D.J. Low Docosahexaenoic Acid in the Diet and Milk of Women in New Mexico. *J. Am. Diet. Assoc.* **2008**, *108*, 1693–1699. [CrossRef] [PubMed]
62. Kim, H.; Kang, S.; Jung, B.-M.; Yi, H.; Jung, J.A.; Chang, N. Breast milk fatty acid composition and fatty acid intake of lactating mothers in South Korea. *Br. J. Nutr.* **2017**, *117*, 556–561. [CrossRef] [PubMed]
63. Urwin, H.J.; Zhang, J.; Gao, Y.; Wang, C.; Li, L.; Song, P.; Man, Q.; Meng, L.; Frøyland, L.; Miles, E.A.; et al. Immune factors and fatty acid composition in human milk from river/lake, coastal and inland regions of China. *Br. J. Nutr.* **2012**, *109*, 1949–1961. [CrossRef] [PubMed]
64. Wang, L.W.; Shimizu, Y.; Kaneko, S.; Hanaka, S.; Abe, T.; Shimasaki, H.; Hisaki, H.; Nakajima, H. Comparison of the fatty acid composition of total lipids and phospholipids in breast milk from Japanese women. *Pediatr. Int.* **2000**, *42*, 14–20. [CrossRef] [PubMed]
65. Innis, S.M.; Kuhnlein, H.V. Long-chain *n*-3 fatty acids in breast milk of Inuit women consuming traditional foods. *Early Hum. Dev.* **1988**, *18*, 185–189. [CrossRef]

Permissions

All chapters in this book were first published by MDPI; hereby published with permission under the Creative Commons Attribution License or equivalent. Every chapter published in this book has been scrutinized by our experts. Their significance has been extensively debated. The topics covered herein carry significant findings which will fuel the growth of the discipline. They may even be implemented as practical applications or may be referred to as a beginning point for another development.

The contributors of this book come from diverse backgrounds, making this book a truly international effort. This book will bring forth new frontiers with its revolutionizing research information and detailed analysis of the nascent developments around the world.

We would like to thank all the contributing authors for lending their expertise to make the book truly unique. They have played a crucial role in the development of this book. Without their invaluable contributions this book wouldn't have been possible. They have made vital efforts to compile up to date information on the varied aspects of this subject to make this book a valuable addition to the collection of many professionals and students.

This book was conceptualized with the vision of imparting up-to-date information and advanced data in this field. To ensure the same, a matchless editorial board was set up. Every individual on the board went through rigorous rounds of assessment to prove their worth. After which they invested a large part of their time researching and compiling the most relevant data for our readers.

The editorial board has been involved in producing this book since its inception. They have spent rigorous hours researching and exploring the diverse topics which have resulted in the successful publishing of this book. They have passed on their knowledge of decades through this book. To expedite this challenging task, the publisher supported the team at every step. A small team of assistant editors was also appointed to further simplify the editing procedure and attain best results for the readers.

Apart from the editorial board, the designing team has also invested a significant amount of their time in understanding the subject and creating the most relevant covers. They scrutinized every image to scout for the most suitable representation of the subject and create an appropriate cover for the book.

The publishing team has been an ardent support to the editorial, designing and production team. Their endless efforts to recruit the best for this project, has resulted in the accomplishment of this book. They are a veteran in the field of academics and their pool of knowledge is as vast as their experience in printing. Their expertise and guidance has proved useful at every step. Their uncompromising quality standards have made this book an exceptional effort. Their encouragement from time to time has been an inspiration for everyone.

The publisher and the editorial board hope that this book will prove to be a valuable piece of knowledge for researchers, students, practitioners and scholars across the globe.

List of Contributors

Marie-Cécile Alexandre-Gouabau, Thomas Moyon, Agnès David-Sochard and Hélène Billard
INRA, UMR1280, Physiopathologie des Adaptations Nutritionnelles, Institut des maladies de l'appareil digestif (IMAD), Centre de Recherche en Nutrition Humaine Ouest (CRNH), Nantes F-44093, France

François Fenaille and Sophie Cholet
Service de Pharmacologie et d'Immunoanalyse, Laboratoire d'Etude du Métabolisme des Médicaments, CEA, INRA, Université Paris Saclay, MetaboHUB, F-91191 Gif-sur-Yvette, France

Anne-Lise Royer and Yann Guitton
LUNAM Université, ON;IRIS, Laboratoire d'Etude des Résidus et Contaminants dans les Aliments (LABERCA), USC INRA 1329, Nantes F-44307, France

Dominique Darmaun and Jean-Christophe Rozé
INRA, UMR1280, Physiopathologie des Adaptations Nutritionnelles, Institut des maladies de l'appareil digestif (IMAD), Centre de Recherche en Nutrition Humaine Ouest (CRNH), Nantes F-44093, France
CHU, Centre Hospitalo-Universitaire Hôtel-Dieu, Nantes F-44093, France

Clair-Yves Boquien
INRA, UMR1280, Physiopathologie des Adaptations Nutritionnelles, Institut des maladies de l'appareil digestif (IMAD), Centre de Recherche en Nutrition Humaine Ouest (CRNH), Nantes F-44093, France
EMBA, European Milk Bank Association, Milano I-20126, Italy

Carlos Zozaya, Victoria Sánchez-González and María Teresa Montes
Neonatology Department, La Paz University Hospital, Autonomous University of Madrid, 28046 Madrid, Spain

Alba García-Serrano and Javier Fontecha
Bioactivity and Food Analysis Department, Institute of Food Science Research (CIAL, CSIC-UAM), Autonomous University of Madrid, 28049 Madrid, Spain

Lidia Redondo-Bravo
Preventive Medicine and Public Health Department, La Paz University Hospital, Autonomous University of Madrid, 28046 Madrid, Spain

Miguel Saenz de Pipaón
Neonatology Department, La Paz University Hospital, Autonomous University of Madrid, 28046 Madrid, Spain
Carlos III Health Institute, Maternal and Child Health and Development Research Network, 48903 Barakaldo, Bizkaia, Spain

Amanda de Sousa Rebouças and Roberto Dimenstein
Department of Biochemistry, Federal University of Rio Grande do Norte, 59078-970 Natal-RN, Brazil

Ana Gabriella Costa Lemos da Silva, Amanda Freitas de Oliveira, Lorena Thalia Pereira da Silva, Vanessa de Freitas Felgueiras and Karla Danielly da Silva Ribeiro
Department of Nutrition, Federal University of Rio Grande do Norte, 59078-970 Natal-RN, Brazil

Marina Sampaio Cruz and Vivian Nogueira Silbiger
Department of Pharmacy, Federal University of Rio Grande do Norte, 59012-570 Natal-RN, Brazil

Camille Davisse-Paturet, Juliette Pierson, Sandrine Lioret and Blandine de Lauzon-Guillain
Université de Paris, CRESS, INSERM, INRA F-75004 Paris, France

Karine Adel-Patient
UMR Service de Pharmacologie et Immunoanalyse, CEA, INRA, Université Paris-Saclay, 91191 Gif-sur-Yvette, France

Amandine Divaret-Chauveau
Unité d'allergologie pédiatrique, Hôpital d'enfants, CHRU de Nancy, 54500 Vandoeuvre-lès-Nancy, France
EA3450, DevAH-Department of Physiology, Faculty of Medicine, University of Lorraine, 54500 Vandoeuvre-lès-Nancy, France

Marie Cheminat and Marie-Noëlle Dufourg
Ined, Inserm, Joint Unit Elfe F-75020 Paris, France

Marie-Aline Charles
Université de Paris, CRESS, INSERM, INRA F-75004 Paris, France
Ined, Inserm, Joint Unit Elfe F-75020 Paris, France

Agnieszka Bzikowska-Jura, Aneta Czerwonogrodzka-Senczyna and Dorota Szostak-Węgierek
Department of Clinical Dietetics, Faculty of Health Sciences, Medical University of Warsaw, E Ciolka Str. 27, 01-445Warsaw, Poland

Edyta Jasińska-Melon and Hanna Mojska
Department of Metabolomics Food and Nutrition Institute, 61/63 Powsińska Str., 02-903Warsaw, Poland

Gabriela Olędzka
Department of Medical Biology, Faculty of Health Sciences, Medical University of Warsaw, Litewska Str. 14/16, 00-575 Warsaw, Poland

Aleksandra Wesołowska
Laboratory of Human Milk and Lactation Research at Regional Human Milk Bank in Holy Family Hospital, Faculty of Health Sciences, Department of Neonatology, Medical University of Warsaw, Zwirki I Wigury Str. 63A, 02-091Warsaw, Poland

Jonneke Hollanders, Lisette R. Dijkstra, Joost Rotteveel, Martijn J.J. Finken and Alyssa A. Toorop,
Emma Children's Hospital, Amsterdam UMC, Pediatric Endocrinology, Vrije Universiteit Amsterdam, 1000-1183 Amsterdam, The Netherlands

Bibian van der Voorn
Department of Paediatric Endocrinology, Obesity Center CGG, Sophia Children's Hospital, 3000-3099 Rotterdam, The Netherlands

Stefanie M.P. Kouwenhoven and Johannes B. van Goudoever
Emma Children's Hospital, Amsterdam UMC, Department of Pediatrics, Vrije Universiteit Amsterdam, 1000-1183 Amsterdam, The Netherlands

Maria Grunewald, Christian Hellmuth, Franca F. Kirchberg, Katharina Werkstetter, Berthold Koletzko and Hans Demmelmair
Ludwig-Maximilians-Universität, Division of Metabolic and Nutritional Medicine, Dr. von Hauner Children's Hospital, University of Munich Medical Center, 80337 Munich, Germany

Maria Luisa Mearin, Sabine L. Vriezinga
Department of Paediatrics, Leiden University Medical Center, 2300 Leiden, The Netherlands

Renata Auricchio
Department of Medical Translational Sciences and European Laboratory for the Investigation of Food-Induced Diseases, University Federico II, 80131 Naples, Italy

Gemma Castillejo
Department of Pediatric Gastroenterology Unit, Hospital Universitari Sant Joan de Reus, URV, IIPV, 43201 Reus, Spain

Ilma R. Korponay-Szabo
Celiac Disease Center, Heim Pál Children's Hospital, 1089 Budapest, Hungary

Isabel Polanco
Department of Pediatric Gastroenterology and Nutrition, La Paz University Hospital, 28033 Madrid, Spain

Maria Roca
U. Enfermedad Celiaca e Inmunopatología Digestiva, Instituto de Investigación Sanitaria La Fe, 46026 Valencia, Spain

Jennifer Hahn-Holbrook and Adi Fish
Department of Psychology, University of California, Merced, 5200 North Lake Rd, Merced, CA 95343, Canada

Laura M. Glynn
Department of Psychology, Chapman University, Orange, CA 92866, USA

Alecia-Jane Twigger
Institute for Stem Cell Research, Helmholtz Center Munich, 85764 Munich, Germany

Gwendoline K. Küffer and Luis Filgueria
Faculty of Science and Medicine, University of Fribourg, 1700 Fribourg, Switzerland

Donna T. Geddes
School of Molecular Sciences, Faculty of Science, The University of Western Australia, Perth 6009, Australia

Maria Lorella Gianni, Beatrice Letizia Crippa, Daniela Morniroli, Nadia Liotto and Paola Roggero and Fabio Mosca
Fondazione IRCCS Ca' Granda Ospedale Maggiore Policlinico, NICU, via Commenda 12, 20122 Milan, Italy
Department of Clinical Sciences and Community Health, University of Milan, Via San Barnaba 8, 20122 Milan, Italy

Maria Enrica Bettinelli
Department of Clinical Sciences and Community Health, University of Milan, Via San Barnaba 8, 20122 Milan, Italy

Priscilla Manfra, Gabriele Sorrentino, Elena Bezze, Laura Plevani, Giacomo Cavallaro, Genny Raffaeli and Lorenzo Colombo
Fondazione IRCCS Ca' Granda Ospedale Maggiore Policlinico, NICU, via Commenda 12, 20122 Milan, Italy

Eduardo Villamor
Department of Pediatrics, Maastricht University Medical Center (MUMC+), School for Oncology and Developmental Biology (GROW), 6202 AZ Maastricht, The Netherlands

Paola Marchisio
Fondazione IRCCS Ca' Granda Ospedale Maggiore Policlinico, 20122 Milan, Italy
Department of Pathophysiology and Transplantation, University of Milan, 20122 Milan, Italy

Adriana V. Gaitán and Fan Zhang
Louisiana State University and Louisiana State University Agricultural Center, Baton Rouge, LA 70803, USA

JodiAnne T. Wood and Alexandros Makriyannis
Center for Drug Discovery, Northeastern University, Boston, MA 02115, USA

Carol J. Lammi-Keefe
Louisiana State University and Louisiana State University Agricultural Center, Baton Rouge, LA 70803, USA
Pennington Biomedical Research Center, Baton Rouge, LA 70803, USA

Sucheta Telang
Division of Neonatology, Department of Pediatrics, University of Louisville, Louisville, KY 40202, USA
Division of Hematology/Oncology, Department of Medicine, James Graham Brown Cancer Center, University of Louisville, Louisville, KY 40202, USA

Elizabeth V. Asztalos
Department of Newborn and Developmental Paediatrics, Sunnybrook Health Sciences Centre, University of Toronto, M4N 3M5 Toronto, ON, Canada

Alexandra D. George, Melvin C. L. Gay and Donna T. Geddes
School of Molecular Sciences, The University of Western Australia, Crawley, Perth, WA 6009, Australia

Robert D. Trengove
Separation Science and Metabolomics Laboratory, Murdoch University, Murdoch, Perth, WA 6150, Australia

Christine A. Butts, Duncan I. Hedderley and Thanuja D. Herath
The New Zealand Institute for Plant and Food Research Limited, Private Bag 11600, Palmerston North 4442, New Zealand

Gunaranjan Paturi
The New Zealand Institute for Plant and Food Research Limited, Private Bag 92169, Auckland 1142, New Zealand

Sarah Glyn-Jones
Danone Nutricia NZ Limited, 56-58 Aintree Avenue, Mangere, Auckland 2022, New Zealand

Frank Wiens and Bernd Stahl
Danone Nutricia Research, Upsalalaan 12, 3584 CT Utrecht, The Netherlands

Pramod Gopal
The New Zealand Institute for Plant and Food Research Limited, Private Bag 11600, Palmerston North 4442, New Zealand
Riddet Institute, Massey University, Palmerston North 4442, New Zealand

Index

Printed in the USA
CPSIA information can be obtained
at www.ICGtesting.com
JSHW051358091023
49903JS00006B/191